Clinical Pediatric Neurosciences

for Primary Care

Agustín Legido, MD, PhD, MBA, and Joseph H. Piatt Jr, MD
Editors

D1523768

American Academy of Pediarics
141 Northwest Point Blvd
Elk Grove Village, IL 60007-1098

Library of Congress Control Number: 2009920367
ISBN: 978-1-58110-296-3
MA0440

The recommendations in this publication do not indicate an exclusive course of treatment or serve as a standard of medical care. Variations, taking into account individual circumstances, may be appropriate.

9-206/0509

Last digit is the print number: 9 8 7 6 5 4 3 2 1

Contributors

Chandra Matadeen-Ali, MD
Section of Neurology
St Christopher's Hospital for Children
Drexel University College of Medicine
Philadelphia, PA

Karen S. Carvalho, MD
Section of Neurology
St Christopher's Hospital for Children
Drexel University College of Medicine
Philadelphia, PA

Marcos Cruz, MD
Section of Neurology
St Christopher's Hospital for Children
Drexel University College of Medicine
Philadelphia, PA

Suzanne Debrosse, MD
Pediatric Neurology
Rainbow Babies & Children's Hospital
Case Western Reserve University School
 of Medicine
Cleveland, OH

Jatinder S. Goraya, MD
Section of Neurology
St Christopher's Hospital for Children
Philadelphia, PA

H. Huntley Hardison, MD
Section of Neurology
St Christopher's Hospital for Children
Drexel University College of Medicine
Philadelphia, PA

Navasuma Havaligi, MD, MPH
Section of Neurology
St Christopher's Hospital for Children
Drexel University College of Medicine
Philadelphia, PA

R. Guy Hudson, MD
Pediatric Urology
Swedish Medical Center
Seattle, WA

Andrew Jea, MD
Division of Neurosurgery
The Hospital for Sick Children
Toronto, ON
Canada

**Christos D. Katsetos, MD, PhD,
 FRCPath**
Section of Neurology and Department
 of Pathology
St Christopher's Hospital for Children
Drexel University College of Medicine
Philadelphia, PA

Divya S. Khurana, MD
Section of Neurology
St Christopher's Hospital for Children
Drexel University College of Medicine
Philadelphia, PA

Sanjeev V. Kothare, MD
Section of Neurology
St Christopher's Hospital for Children
Drexel University College of Medicine
Philadelphia, PA

Abhaya V. Kulkarni, MD, PhD
Division of Neurosurgery
The Hospital for Sick Children
Toronto, ON
Canada

Agustín Legido, MD, PhD, MBA
Section of Neurology
St Christopher's Hospital for Children
Drexel University College of Medicine
Philadelphia, PA

Joseph Madsen, MD
Department of Neurosurgery
Children's Hospital Boston
Boston, MA

Harold G. Marks, MD
Section of Neurology
St Christopher's Hospital for Children
Drexel University College of Medicine
Philadelphia, PA

Joseph J. Melvin, DO
Section of Neurology
St Christopher's Hospital for Children
Drexel University College of Medicine
Philadelphia, PA

Robert Owen, MD
Department of Neurosurgery
University of Kentucky Chandler
    Medical Center
Lexington, KY

Alexander Papanastassiou, MD
Department of Neurosurgery
Children's Hospital Boston
Boston, MA

Joseph H. Piatt Jr, MD
Section of Neurosurgery
St Christopher's Hospital for Children
Drexel University College of Medicine
Philadelphia, PA

Thomas Pittman, MD
Department of Neurosurgery
University of Kentucky Chandler
    Medical Center
Lexington, KY

Shenandoah Robinson, MD
Pediatric Neurosurgery
Rainbow Babies & Children's Hospital
Case Western Reserve University School
    of Medicine
Cleveland, OH

R. Michael Scott, MD
Department of Neurosurgery
Children's Hospital Boston
Boston, MA

Steven R. Skoog, MD
Department of Urology
Oregon Health & Sciences University
Portland, OR

Nathan R. Selden, MD, PhD
Department of Neurological Surgery
Oregon Health & Sciences University
Portland, OR

Edward R. Smith, MD
Department of Neurosurgery
Children's Hospital Boston
Boston, MA

Duncan Stearns, MD
Section of Oncology
St Christopher's Hospital for Children
Drexel University College of Medicine
Philadelphia, PA

Ignacio Valencia, MD
Section of Neurology
St Christopher's Hospital for Children
Drexel University College of Medicine
Philadelphia, PA

Sabrina W. Yum, MD
Section of Neurology
St Christopher's Hospital for Children
Drexel University College of Medicine
Philadelphia, PA

Table of Contents

Preface

This volume has been prepared for the general pediatrician.

Complaints and concerns related to the head and spine and the nervous system that they contain are very common in primary pediatric practice, but a trainee can complete a program accredited by the American Board of Pediatrics without a clinical rotation in pediatric neurology. A programmatic exposure to pediatric neurosurgery is truly exceptional. Yet a very large fraction of the practice of pediatric neurology and neurosurgery is office work: elective consultations about common problems at the request of a primary pediatrician or management of chronic disease in cooperation with the patient's primary medical home. Hospital work as well is largely derived from complications of common pediatric conditions. We feel that the pediatric neurosciences sit at the heart of pediatrics, and that our subspecialty practices are organic elaborations arising out of general pediatric practice. We hope that our book exemplifies this unity of knowledge and experience.

If this volume proves useful to general pediatricians who turn to it to fill in lacunae from their postgraduate training, it may be useful as well to pediatric residents. We have tried to be concise rather than encyclopedic, although references and suggestions for further reading have proliferated at the end of chapters rather beyond our original intention. The medical student who wishes to read everything that is known about a narrow topic will do better with one of the standard texts.

A unique feature of this volume is the collaboration of its medical and surgical authors. There are many handbooks and brief texts of pediatric neurology. Necessarily, these texts either avoid neurosurgical topics or handle them on the basis of hearsay. We hope readers find that the complementary perspectives presented here make this volume more comprehensive and authoritative than its predecessors.

If readers find this volume helpful, our contributing authors deserve the credit. We are deeply grateful for their labor and patience. If readers find portions of this volume to be confusing or wrong, we editors deserve the blame. Hoping that the reception of this volume justifies a second edition someday, we welcome critical comments.

Agustín Legido, MD, PhD, MBA
Joseph H. Piatt Jr, MD

St Christopher's Hospital for Children
Philadelphia, PA

Chapter 1

Neonatal Neurologic and Neurosurgical Disorders

Suzanne Debrosse, MD
Shenandoah Robinson, MD
Agustín Legido, MD, PhD, MBA

Introduction

Neonatal neurologic and neurosurgical disorders encompass a wide range of conditions, both of the premature and term infant, originating before, during, and in the days after birth. Many affected infants will receive care in the neonatal intensive care unit, while others might be encountered in the regular newborn nursery. Most neonatal neurologic and neurosurgical disorders are uncommon, and some are life threatening. Parents are often understandably anxious about any problems afflicting their infant, and conditions diagnosed in the newborn may have medicolegal implications. Because of these factors, and the need in some infants for medical or surgical intervention, early specialist consultation is encouraged. Even if no intervention is needed, consultation reassures parents and establishes parameters for follow-up with the specialist.

Perinatal Hypoxic-Ischemic Encephalopathy

Perinatal hypoxic ischemia is the most common cause of neurologic disease during the neonatal period (hypoxic-ischemic encephalopathy [HIE]), and it is associated with a high mortality and morbidity rate, including cerebral palsy, mental retardation, and seizures. Hypoxic-ischemic encephalopathy occurs in the setting of perinatal asphyxia, which is a multiorgan system disease. The incidence of perinatal asphyxia is about 1.0% to 1.5% in most hospitals and is usually related to gestational age and birth weight. It occurs in 9.0% of infants less than 36 weeks' gestation.

Hypoxemia indicates a low content of oxygen in the blood. *Ischemia* is a diminished amount of blood perfusing the brain. Both can occur as a result of *asphyxia,* which refers to respiratory dysfunction that causes hypoxemia, carbon dioxide retention, and acidosis.

Etiology

The etiology of perinatal HIE includes those circumstances that can affect the cerebral blood flow (CBF) in the fetus and newborn, compromising the supply of oxygen to the brain. They may develop antepartum (20%), intrapartum (30%), intrapartum and antepartum (35%), or postpartum (10%). Box 1-1 displays the most common causes of decreased availability of brain oxygen in the fetus and newborn.

It is likely that the contribution of prenatal causes to perinatal asphyxia has been underappreciated in the past. The Collaborative Perinatal Project of the National Institute of Neurologic Disorders showed that one-third of newborns with intrapartum asphyxia had some type of congenital malformation, suggesting that prenatal disorders can predispose to perinatal hypoxia-ischemia. As the methods for evaluating the neurologic status of the fetus have improved, prenatal causes of perinatal asphyxia are becoming more relevant.

Pathogenesis

The basic mechanism of HIE is cerebral oxygen deprivation. Lack of oxygen leads to an increase in anaerobic metabolism, a decrease in the production of high-energy compounds, and accumulation of toxic metabolites that contribute to neuronal damage.

Circulatory Factors

The impairment of CBF regulation plays a major role in the pathogenesis of neuronal injury in HIE. The ability of the brain to maintain an almost constant CBF, in spite of fluctuations in the cerebral perfusion pressure, which depends on the systemic blood pressure, is called *autoregulation.* This mechanism is maintained by change in the resistance of cerebral arterioles, the regulation of which depends on multiple factors: myogenic (constriction of smooth muscle of cerebral blood vessels), biochemical (oxygen, carbon dioxide, pH, potassium, calcium osmolarity, hemoglobin), and neuron-hormonal

---

Box 1-1. Etiology of Perinatal Hypoxic-Ischemic Encephalopathy

Prenatal
Maternal hypotension/hypertension
Preeclampsia/toxemia
Drugs (cocaine)
Uterine anomalies
Abruptio placentae
Cerebral thrombosis/embolus
Congenital encephalitis
Congenital malformations

Intrapartum
Placental anomalies/hemorrhage
Umbilical cord prolapse/compression
Umbilical artery thrombosis
Craniocerebral injury
Cerebral thrombosis/embolus

Postnatal
Congenital heart disease
Cardiac arrhythmia
Severe lung disease
Severe apnea
Cerebral thrombosis/embolus
Anemia/polycythemia
Sepsis/disseminated intravascular coagulation
Meningitis/encephalitis

(sympathetic and cholinergic nervous system, prostaglandins, arginine vasopressin, renin-angiotensin, vasointestinal polypeptide, substance P, opioids).

A persistent or severe asphyxia causes loss of cerebrovascular autoregulation, and the CBF becomes passively sensitive to changes in blood pressure. Passive elevations of CBF are produced by stimulating nursing maneuvers, such as tracheal suction, or by seizures. The persistence or severity of asphyxia may finally affect the heart and cause bradycardia and decreased cardiac output, with secondary hypotension and compromise of cerebrovascular autoregulation. The collapse of systemic blood pressure depresses CBF, which can cause ischemic neuronal damage.

Metabolic Factors

Hypoxemia and ischemia cause a decrease in brain glycogen and phospho-creatine and an increase in lactate, which is followed by decreased cerebral production of glucose and adenosine triphosphate (ATP). These changes are the consequence of dysfunction of high energy phosphate mitochondrial metabolism. As a compensatory mechanism, anaerobic glycolysis is accelerated, and glycogenolysis and glucose use are increased. Despite this acceleration, brain energy demands cannot be met, and brain glucose and ATP decrease. The deficit of high energy compounds triggers a series of mechanisms, the ultimate effect of which is cell death. Moreover, hypoglycemia, probably by stimulating the release of glutamate, and hyperlactacidemia may also cause neuronal damage.

Biochemical Factors

Excitatory Amino Acids

Following asphyxia there is an increase in the release of excitatory amino acids, aspartate and glutamate, in the cerebral extracellular space. Such an increase is related to the failure of the energy metabolism, which causes release of excitatory amino acids by neuronal depolarization and failure of postsynaptic uptake. As a consequence, there is a prolongation of the neuroexcitotoxic effects of glutamate on glutamatergic receptors, mainly the N-methyl-D-aspartate (NMDA) receptor, but also the quisqualate and kainate receptors. Hypoglycemia, which follows hypoxia-ischemia, can also cause neuronal injury by increasing the levels of excitatory amino acids. Excitatory amino acids are also toxic to the astroglia and oligodendroglia. Glia, particularly astrocytes, play a crucial role in uptake of glutamate from the synapses and prevention of excessive accumulation in the synaptic cleft. Therefore, destruction of glia can augment neuronal damage in those circumstances where there is an important elevation of neuroexcitatory amino acids.

The mechanisms of neuronal death mediated by glutamate are several. The activation of non-NMDA glutamatergic receptors causes cell depolarization, which facilitates the intracellular flux of Cl^-, Na^+, and water causing osmotic lysis of the cell. On the other hand, the activation of NMDA receptors facilitates the intracellular flux of calcium, which causes progressive neuronal necrosis.

Oxygen Free Radicals

A free radical is an atom or molecule with an uneven number of electrons in its outermost orbit. Examples of free radicals are hydrogen, glutathione, superoxide, hydroxide, lipid peroxide, and nitric oxide.

During the phase of hypoxia-ischemia, stores of ATP are progressively degraded into adenosine diphosphate, adenosine monophosphate, adenosine, inosine, and hypoxanthine. During the oxygenation-reperfusion phase, hypoxanthine is metabolized to xanthine by the enzyme xanthineoxidase, a reaction that generates the free radical superoxide. Calcium participates in this process by activating a protease that transforms the enzyme xanthinedehydrogenase into xanthineoxidase.

Oxygen free radicals produce peroxidation and fragmentation of cell membrane phospholipids through the activation of phospholipases; this produces the anatomical and functional impairment of cell membranes. Free radicals can also destroy DNA molecules. Additionally, phospholipase activation releases polyunsaturated free fatty acids from cell membranes. Oxidation of these fatty acids through the cyclooxygenase and lipooxygenase pathways produces thromboxanes, prostaglandins, and leukotrienes, which induce chemotaxis and inflammatory responses, and release of more free radicals.

Intracellular Calcium

The mechanism of cell death induced by calcium depends on the activation of lipases, proteases, and endonucleases, which cause irreversible damage of the structure of the cell and the mitochondria. Ionic calcium also activates phospholipases that produce the destruction of the structural components of the cell membrane. It has also been shown that the intracellular flux of calcium potentiates the activation of the NMDA glutamate receptors, which produce more ionic abnormalities and subsequent cell death. Moreover, ionic calcium contributes to the release of oxygen free radicals through the synthesis of xanthine and prostaglandins. Finally, intracytoplasmic calcium can transfer into the nucleus and activate the caspase-dependent system of apoptosis, causing DNA fragmentation and apoptotic cell death. Thus it is possible that impairment of calcium homeostasis may be the common final pathway for many mechanisms of neuronal damage in perinatal hypoxia-ischemia.

Clinical Manifestations

The American Academy of Pediatrics Committee on Fetus and Newborn and the American College of Obstetricians and Gynecologists have agreed on criteria for recognizing perinatal asphyxia of sufficient severity to have the potential to cause neurologic damage.

1) Profound metabolic acidosis (pH<7.0) on an umbilical cord arterial sample
2) Persistence of an Apgar score of 0 to 3 for 5 minutes
3) Clinical neurologic sequelae in the immediate neonatal period to include seizures, hypotonia, or coma
4) Evidence of multiorgan dysfunction in the immediate neonatal period
5) Exclusion of other identifiable etiologies such as trauma, coagulation disorders, infectious conditions, or genetic disorders

Many clinical symptoms that can be seen in perinatal asphyxia are nonspecific. The evaluation of the newborn with suspected asphyxia should begin with review of the obstetric data and the results of prenatal and intrapartum monitoring.

The clinical manifestations of perinatal HIE depend on its severity:

Mild HIE: There is transitory lethargy, followed by jitteriness. There is mild head lag on traction. Usually there are no seizures. Symptoms are maximal in the first 24 hours. The prognosis is good.

Moderate HIE: There is obtundation possibly progressing to coma. The infant has a hypotonic posture at rest. Seizures may or may not be present. Symptoms are maximal at 48 to 72 hours. The prognosis is guarded.

Severe HIE: The newborn is stuporous or comatose. There is severe hypotonia at rest and on traction. Seizures are usually a constant feature. Symptoms are maximal from birth to 72 hours. The prognosis is poor.

Diagnosis

Neurologic Examination

The neurologic examination should focus on

A) *Mental status:* Presence or absence of spontaneous eye opening, response to tactile or auditory stimuli, and quality of the response (absent, normal, or hyperactive).

B) *Respirations:* Need for assisted ventilation, episodes of apnea.

C) *Brain stem function:* Pupillary reactivity, ocular movements (spontaneous and provoked), corneal reflexes, symmetry of the face, sucking and swallowing reflex, lingual fasciculations.

D) *Motor system:* Quality and symmetry of spontaneous movements, passive muscle tone, intensity and symmetry of deep tendon reflexes, distribution of motor impairment.

E) *Primitive reflexes:* Presence and quality.

F) *Presence of seizures:* Seizures are associated with moderate and severe HIE. The diagnosis of seizures in the neonatal period may be difficult, because some epileptic motor activity can be mistaken for normal motor activity or jitteriness. In general, epileptic motor activity in newborns is not triggered by stimuli, is not suppressed by holding the affected area, and is frequently accompanied by signs of autonomic dysfunction (changes in heart rate, respiratory rate, or blood pressure). Also, most neonatal seizures are "occult," that is, they appear as epileptic activity on the electroencephalogram (EEG) without clinical correlation; vice versa, some clinical manifestations of seizures are not accompanied by epileptic activity on the EEG.

Biochemical Evaluation

The postnatal analysis of the acid-base status is useful to determine the persistence and severity of perinatal asphyxia. The cerebrospinal fluid (CSF) should be examined in newborns with HIE to rule out infection or hemorrhage.

Frequent biochemical abnormalities that are seen in patients with HIE—and that contribute to the neurologic symptoms—are hypoglycemia, hypocalcemia, hyponatremia, and hyperammonemia. Other substances that have been found elevated in blood of asphyxiated newborns are creatine phosphokinase (isoenzyne BB), hypoxanthine, vasopressin, erythropoietin, and triglycerides. In the CSF, there have been reported high levels of lactate, neuronal enolase, protein S-100, and myelin basic protein. In the urine, an excessive secretion of urine organic acids, protein S100B and β_2-microglobulin has been found. Creatine phosphokinase BB, erythropoietin, and β_2-microglobulin are prognostic indicators of long-term outcome.

Electroencephalogram

The EEG findings in perinatal HIE parallel the severity of the encephalopathy. In cases of mild to moderate hypoxia-ischemia, the voltage may be slightly decreased (10–15 μV/mm) and slightly discontinuous; sharp waves of multifocal distribution may be present. In newborns with a more severe HIE, the EEG voltage decreases below 5 μV/mm and the tracing becomes more discontinuous, acquiring the aspect of burst suppression, where periods of very low voltage (<5μV/mm), lasting several seconds, alternate with other shorter periods (1–10 seconds) of generalized bursts of high amplitude electrical activity. In the more severe cases, the interburst periods become more prolonged and progress to a flat EEG.

Paroxysmal EEG abnormalities superimposed on an otherwise stable background are most frequently seizures. Epileptic activity can be recognized as sudden, repetitive, evolving stereotyped waveforms of variable amplitude and frequency with a clear onset, middle, and end. Their minimal duration is 10 seconds (mean 2 minutes), and they are separated by interictal periods of variable duration (mean 8 minutes).

Because of the difficulty in diagnosing neonatal seizures, the gold standard for confirmation of the epileptic nature of seizures in the newborn is continuous video/EEG monitoring with conventional EEG. There is also intense current interest in continuous EEG monitoring with the amplitude-integrated EEG, a device that uses 2 channels (one per hemisphere) to monitor the EEG background and the presence of seizures.

Evoked Potentials

Evoked potentials represent electrical activity induced in the brain by sensory stimulation (auditory, visual, or somatosensory). They provide information about the function of these sensory pathways from the peripheral receptors to the brain.

Brain stem auditory evoked responses (BAERs) consists of a series of vertex-positive waves, designated I to VII, registered within the first 10 milliseconds after an acoustic stimulus. In newborns, waves I, III, and V are registered. Wave I originates in the auditory nerve and wave V most likely in the inferior colliculi. The I to V interpeak latency indicates brain stem conduction time. Waves I and V latencies, interpeak latencies I to V, and ratio of wave V to I are used to assess hearing and neurologic impairment. Because many newborns are intubated and get middle ear effusions, in many cases BAERs are not reliable.

Visual evoked responses (VERs) can be elicited by a flashing light (stroboscopic lamp) or light-emitting diode (goggles) or by pattern stimuli (reversing onset/offset, checks, bars, pinwheels). In preterm infants, the initial wave emerging at 24 weeks is largely negative at 300 milliseconds, N300 or N2. After about 27 weeks of gestation, a positive wave emerges, the P450 or P3, and after 32 to 35 weeks an earlier positivity, the P200 or P2, appears. In asphyxiated newborns, VER abnormalities include abnormal wave morphology, prolongation of latencies, absence of some components, or total lack of response. Visual evoked responses are difficult to perform in newborns and require technical and professional expertise.

Somatosensory evoked responses are a series of positive and negative potentials that can be detected following stimulation of the median or popliteal nerves. The path for sensory information from periphery to cortex includes peripheral nerve; plexus; dorsal roots; posterior columns; the cuneate and gracilis nuclei; and, after decussation, the medical lemniscus, thalamus, and parietal cortex. In asphyxiated newborns, there can be found an increase in the latency of the components N19 (thalamus) and P22 (cerebral cortex), prolonged interval N13–N19 (cervical spinal cord-thalamus), and N19–N22 (thalamus-cerebral cortex), as well as a flat response. Somatosensory evoked responses are probably the easiest evoked potentials to record in newborns, the most reliable, and the ones that have the best correlation with neurologic outcome.

Anatomical Neuroimaging Studies

The improvement of anatomical neuroimaging techniques and the development of functional neuroimaging techniques have provided more accurate means of evaluating the neurologic consequences of perinatal hypoxia-ischemia.

Transfontanel Ultrasound

Head ultrasound examination is very useful and easy to perform at the crib side. It is the first choice for the evaluation of premature newborns to diagnose intraventricular hemorrhage (IVH), periventricular leukomalacia (PVL), and posthemorrhagic hydrocephalus. In full-term newborns, transfontanel ultrasound can also be very useful to visualize cerebral edema, subcortical leukomalacia, focal or multifocal necrosis, and lesions of the basal ganglia and thalamus.

Computed Tomography

The optimum diagnostic value of the computed tomography (CT) scan is attained in asphyxiated newborns beyond term age. In preterm infants, the high water content of the brain tissue and the high protein content of the CSF are reflected as normal areas of hypodensity on the CT scan, particularly in the periventricular region; therefore, it is difficult to differentiate them from abnormal hypodensities. Diffuse cortical and subcortical necrosis is seen as generalized hypodensity during the first days, reflecting neuronal necrosis and edema (Figure 1-1).

Weeks later the lesion progresses to cortical atrophy and increased ventricular size secondary to loss of white matter. Focal and multifocal necrosis appears on CT scans as areas of hypodensity in the distribution of one or several vascular territories, most frequently the middle cerebral artery. Lesions of the basal ganglia are visualized as hypodensity in cases of ischemia and necrosis, and hyperdensity when there is increased vascularity or calcification. Computed tomography is also very useful to detect intracranial hemorrhagic complications, which are frequently associated with HIE.

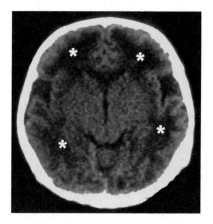

Figure 1-1.
Non-contrast head computed tomography in a full-term newborn with severe asphyxia performed at 48 hours of life. Diffuse cortical and subcortical hypodensities (white asterisks). (Courtesy of Eric N. Faerber, St Christopher's Hospital for Children, Philadelphia, PA.)

Magnetic Resonance Imaging

A discussion of the physics of magnetic resonance imaging (MRI) is beyond the scope of this chapter, but the distinctive feature of this technology is that images can be tuned to reflect various physical aspects of the environment of aqueous protons throughout the brain. T1-weighting causes CSF to appear darker ("low signal") and white matter to appear lighter ("high signal") relative to gray matter. T1-weighted images are optimal for demonstrating anatomical detail, and they are sensitive to the presence of fresh hemorrhage. T2-weighting causes CSF to appear bright and white matter to appear relatively dark. T2-weighted images display brain edema vividly, they are useful for assessment of myelination, and they are very sensitive in the demonstration of hemosiderin at sites of old hemorrhage. Fluid attenuated inversion recovery is a T2-weighted technique modified by suppression of signal in regions of free water, such as the ventricular cavities. Fluid attenuated inversion recovery facilitates clear definition of periventricular structures and is therefore very useful in demonstration of diseases of white matter. Diffusion-weighted imaging distinguishes cytotoxic edema from other states of brain water and is thus the standard for determination of infarction. Magnetic resonance imaging is generally more sensitive and specific than head ultrasound and CT scan in HIE. Magnetic resonance imaging allows the visualization of all neuropathologic lesions that are associated with HIE: ischemic necrosis, multi-cystic encephalomalacia, parasagittal "watershed" lesions, basal ganglia injury, and periventricular leukomalacia (Figure 1-2). The complementary information obtained from the many different techniques or "sequences" that can be employed in MRI make it the superior technology for demonstrating the lesions of HIE and their course. The burden of MRI is that image acquisition is slow, so neonates who are not comatose and flaccid require prolonged sedation. Furthermore, physiological monitoring and mechanical ventilation in the neighborhood of the device's powerful magnet require specialized, nonferromagnetic equipment.

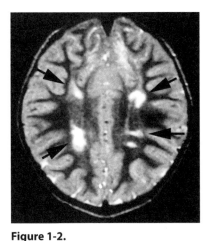

Figure 1-2.
Brain magnetic resonance imaging of a 2-year-old girl with history of perinatal asphyxia. A T2-weighted image shows periventricular high signal lesions (black arrows) compatible with residual leukomalacia. (Courtesy of Eric N. Faerber, St Christopher's Hospital for Children, Philadelphia, PA.)

Functional Neuroimaging Studies

Positron Emission Tomography

This technique uses radiopharmaceuticals labeled with positron-emitting isotopes generated by an on-site cyclotron. One commonly employed compound is ^{18}F-fluorodeoxyglucose, which is taken up by brain tissue in proportion to regional glucose metabolism. Regional glucose metabolism is in turn very closely linked under most circumstances to regional CBF. Overall, studies in children with perinatal asphyxia have shown that brain areas of metabolic dysfunction are more extensive than what might be predicted by the anatomical involvement on CT or MRI or on the basis of neurologic examination.

Single-Photon Emission Computed Tomography

Single-photon emission computed tomography (SPECT) examines cerebral function by imaging regional CBF. It is less expensive and more widely available than positron emission tomography (PET). Brain SPECT uses radiopharmaceuticals that emit a single photon with each nuclear decay. The best compounds for brain studies are ^{99m}Tc-hexamethylpropylene amine oxime and I[123]-iodoamphetamine. Studies in asphyxiated newborns have shown specific patterns of CBF distribution that correspond to the different patterns of neuropathology, including selective neuronal necrosis, parasagittal "watershed" ischemia, focal ischemia, PVL, and mixed lesions. Also, like PET, SPECT generally demonstrates more extensive involvement in cases of focal ischemic or hemorrhagic lesions than CT and MRI (Figure 1-3).

Magnetic Resonance Spectroscopy

Phosphorus (^{31}P) magnetic resonance spectroscopy (MRS) identifies 7 peaks corresponding to the major phosphorus metabolites important for cellular energy metabolism: phosphomonoesters; inorganic phosphate (Pi); phosphodiesters; phosphocreatine (PCr); and the gamma, alpha, and beta phosphorous nuclei of ATP. Newborns with perinatal asphyxia have abnormalities in the spectra, including decreased PCr/Pi and total ATP/total phosphorous, indicating impaired oxidative phosphorylation.

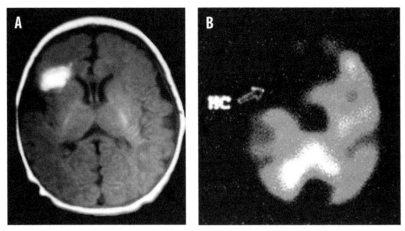

Figure 1-3.
Head magnetic resonance imaging (MRI) and single-photon emission computed tomo-graphy (SPECT) of a 4-day-old full-term newborn with meconium aspiration requiring extracorporeal membrane oxygenation. **A.** MRI shows a high signal lesion in the right frontal region on T1-weighted images compatible with acute intraparenchymal hemor-rhage. **B.** SPECT shows a more extensive area of decreased cerebral blood flow in the same region. (Courtesy of Drs Stephen Baumgart, Heman Desai, and Chan Park, Jefferson Medical College, Philadelphia, PA.)

Proton (^{1}H) MRS spectra of the neonatal brain show peaks correspond-ing to myoinositol, N-acetylaspartate (NAA, a neuronal marker), choline-containing compounds (Cho), and creatine plus phosphocreatine (Cr). Asphyxiated newborns show low NAA/Cho and NAA/Cr ratios.

Near Infrared Spectroscopy

This technique allows measurement of the cerebral content of oxyhemo-globin, deoxyhemoglobin, and oxidized cytochrome oxidase, which is the terminal compound of the mitochondrial respiratory chain. From changes in concentration of oxyhemoglobin and deoxyhemoglobin, cerebral blood vol-ume (CBV) can be calculated. Therefore, near infrared spectroscopy allows a continuous monitoring of brain function as reflected in CBV among new-borns with HIE.

Treatment

Supportive Treatment

Maintaining Effective Ventilation

Maintenance of normoxemia and normocapnia is an important goal of the treatment of HIE and requires adequate ventilation with minimal manipulation to avoid important fluctuations of blood gases.

Maintaining Adequate Cerebrovascular Perfusion

Maintenance of a stable cardiovascular status is important to maintain an effective CBF. In addition to hypoxemia, hyperviscosity, heart failure, persistence of ductus, and episodes of apnea-bradycardia can contribute to decreased CBF. Hypertension must be treated to avoid intracranial hemorrhage.

Maintaining Adequate Blood Glucose

Oral glucose is capable of sustaining energy metabolism in the brain under conditions of advanced cerebral edema because of its capacity for consumption by anaerobic glycolysis with the production of lactic acid and ATP. Maintenance of adequate levels of glucose is important to ensure a normal neuronal metabolism. The effects of hyperglycemia in the neonatal hypoxic-ischemic brain are controversial, but some studies have suggested that it can exacerbate brain damage.

Treatment of Complications

Cerebral edema: Although cerebral edema is seldom such a severe problem that it requires treatment for its own sake, it may occur in cases of severe ischemic necrosis. Hyperosmolar agents such as mannitol and hypertonic saline are the treatments of choice. Fluid restriction may be considered, but it must not be allowed to compromise cardiac output. Hyperventilation can lower intracranial pressure transiently, but only by lowering CBF and CBV. This intervention risks exacerbation of ongoing cerebral ischemia.

Seizures: The most frequent cause of neonatal seizures is HIE. There is some clinical and experimental evidence suggesting that seizures may increase the brain damage caused by hypoxia-ischemia. Therefore, neonatal seizures, clinical and subclinical, should be treated aggressively, ideally with simultaneous video/EEG monitoring. Phenobarbital, fosphenytoin, and lorazepam should be used to stop not only the clinical but also the subclinical epileptic activity.

Neuroprotection

Although many experimental studies have investigated multiple compounds that have shown neuroprotective effects in the laboratory, translation to the clinical arena has been disappointing.

To date only allopurinol has been subjected to clinical trials in humans—as prophylaxis against brain damage in newborns undergoing cardiac surgery for congenital heart disease: Allopurinol decreased the number of bad neurologic outcomes in a subgroup of patients with hypoplastic left heart syndrome.

Also, a small study comparing the neurologic and neuroimaging outcomes of asphyxiated newborns treated or not with opioids has suggested that they may have a neuroprotective effect.

There is a great interest in new antiepileptic drugs (eg, levetiracetam and topiramate) as possible neuroprotective agents for HIE, but clinical trials remain to be conducted.

From a practical clinical standpoint, the only real advance in neuroprotection for perinatal asphyxia has been hypothermia. Two large, multi-institutional investigations, using head cooling or systemic cooling, have demonstrated that hypothermia may be neuroprotective if initiated within 6 hours of birth for newborns without the most severe degrees of asphyxia. A head cooling system has been approved by the US Food and Drug Administration, and its use is expanding in neonatal intensive care units.

Prognosis

The outcome of term infants with perinatal HIE is directly related to the severity of the neonatal neurologic syndrome. Thus infants with mild, moderate, or severe encephalopathy have a 100%, 71%, and 0% of good outcome, respectively. Seizures increase the risk of neurologic sequelae by as much as 40-fold. The severity of EEG, evoked potential, and neuroimaging abnormalities also correlates well with long-term neurologic impairment, including cerebral palsy, mental retardation, and epilepsy.

Intraventricular Hemorrhage in the Preterm Infant

The IVH characteristic of the premature infant, germinal matrix-IVH (GM-IVH), is distinct from IVH of the term infant discussed later in this chapter. Germinal matrix IVH is defined as hemorrhage into the germinal matrix of the premature brain, an area of both fragile vessels and important precursor cells. About half of extremely low birth weight (<1,000 g) infants in the 1990s experienced IVH.

Most commonly—especially with smaller lesions—infants have asymptomatic GM-IVH, with very subtle or no signs, although a drop in hematocrit may be seen. Less common are changes in level of consciousness, changes in movement, low tone, and abnormal eye movements, which evolve over many hours and which may have a "stuttering" course. Rarely, infants become rapidly symptomatic, with progression over minutes to hours to stupor or coma, respiratory irregularities and apnea, seizures, posturing, and other signs of elevated intracranial pressure. Systemic disruptions of homeostasis and unstable vital signs may be seen. The differential diagnosis of GM-IVH includes other intracranial bleeding, including subdural hematoma (SDH), as well as conditions such as sepsis or meningitis.

Several schemes for grading GM-IVH have been published. Four grades are recognized. There are inconsistencies among the various schemes in the definition of the intermediate grades, but there is agreement about the mildest (germinal matrix hemorrhage) and the most severe (hemorrhagic destruction of periventricular brain parenchyma). Box 1-2 presents a modification of the popular system of Volpe. Note that posthemorrhagic ventricular dilatation does not feature in this classification. For reasons of safety, convenience, and diagnostic sensitivity, transfontanel ultrasound is the brain imaging modality of choice for the premature infant. Ultrasounds are typically performed sequentially to assess for expansion of the hemorrhage and development of hydrocephalus (Figure 1-4). Also well demonstrated

---

Box 1-2. Intraventricular Hemorrhage

Grade I: Hemorrhage limited to the germinal matrix
Grade II: Hemorrhage spilling into the ventricle
Grade III: Hemorrhage filling and distending the ventricle
Grade IV: Hemorrhage destroying periventricular brain parenchyma (hemorrhagic infarction)

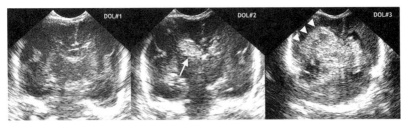

Figure 1-4.
Sequential, coronal, transfontanel ultrasound images of an individual premature infant on the first 3 days of life. The study on the first day of life (DOL#1) is normal. On the second day (DOL#2) there is intraventricular hemorrhage on both sides, larger on the right (white arrow), with distention of the frontal horn of the ventricle that justifies the designation grade III. On the third day (DOL#3) there is a massive, grade IV hemorrhage with extension into the basal ganglia and periventricular white matter on the right (white arrow heads).

by ultrasound is periventricular leukomalacia, a form of ischemic injury to white matter in the walls of the lateral ventricles distinctive to prematurity and a frequent fellow traveler with IVH.

For a minority of infants with progressive ventriculomegaly, the ventricles may stabilize spontaneously without intervention. The remainder will require intervention for symptomatic hydrocephalus. Symptomatic progression is assessed by sequential ultrasound scans, measurements of head circumference on a preterm infant chart, and palpation of fontanel fullness and cranial suture separation. Clinical signs of symptomatic hydrocephalus usually appear after ventricular expansion is noted by ultrasound. Consultation with a pediatric neurosurgeon is appropriate when IVH is associated with progressive ventriculomegaly on cranial ultrasounds, head circumference measurements that cross percentiles, and a full fontanel with split sutures.

Because permanent ventriculoperitoneal shunts are not usually placed in infants weighing less than 1,500 g due to high rates of failure and frequent wound complications, temporizing measures are often employed until the infant either no longer needs CSF diversion or grows large enough for a permanent shunt. The first choice as a temporizing option is sequential lumbar punctures. In many infants with progressive ventriculomegaly, sequential lumbar punctures will be sufficient to halt progression and allow normalization of CSF dynamics.

For infants in whom lumbar punctures fail to control ventriculomegaly or are contraindicated, options include a ventriculosubgaleal shunt, a ventricular reservoir with sequential percutaneous needle aspirations of

CSF, external ventricular drainage, and ventricular punctures. A dominant consideration in choosing among these options is to minimize the risk of bacterial ventriculitis, which is associated with additional risk of neurologic impairment. External ventricular drainage has a high rate of infection, and sequential ventricular taps can be associated with the later development of loculated hydrocephalus. Currently, both ventriculosubgaleal shunts (Figure 1-5) and ventricular reservoirs with sequential taps are popular measures for control of posthemorrhagic ventricular dilatation when lumbar punctures fail. Ventriculosubgaleal shunts and reservoirs have similar risks and complication rates.

These temporary shunts are typically converted to, or replaced by, a permanent ventriculoperitoneal shunt shortly before the newborn is discharged home, but if symptomatic hydrocephalus resolves spontaneously, a permanent shunt is not required. Roughly 1 out of every 3 premature babies who requires a subgaleal shunt or reservoir for posthemorrhagic ventricular dilation will stabilize by term and escape a permanent ventriculoperitoneal shunt. Subgaleal devices are not removed routinely, as removal is of

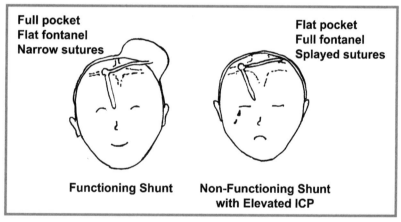

Figure 1-5.
A functioning ventriculosubgaleal shunt diverts cerebrospinal fluid (CSF) from the lateral ventricle to the subgaleal space in the scalp. The scalp pocket containing CSF is often full and can become quite large, while the fontanel remains slack, and the sutures apposed. If the shunt becomes obstructed or if the scalp scars down to the surface of the skull while hydrocephalus persists, then the scalp pocket disappears, the fontanel becomes full, and the sagittal and coronal sutures become separated. Ventriculosubgaleal shunts typically include a reservoir, so when the subgaleal pocket disappears, treatment can often be continued by sequential needle aspiration of CSF.

no real benefit to the patient. Premature babies with GM-IVH and some degree of posthemorrhagic ventricular dilatation who reach term without active hydrocephalus seldom require treatment at a later date, but clinical and imaging follow-up through the first year of life is prudent to detect the occasional infant with delayed, insidious progression.

Neurologic impairment in children who had GM-IVH is correlated with the severity of GM-IVH, but more powerfully with the degree of parenchymal injury due to hemorrhagic infarction or periventricular leukomalacia. Even though less damage appears to be present with low-grade IVH, children with grade I/II GM-IVH often have impaired development compared with children with normal ultrasounds. Children born prematurely with IVH need to be followed proactively for developmental delay, cognitive disability, cerebral palsy, and epilepsy.

Intraventricular Hemorrhage in the Term Infant

Intraventricular hemorrhage in the term infant has a pathogenesis and clinical course distinct from that of the premature infant. In term infants, IVH often stems from bleeding in the choroid plexus, and may be associated with thrombosis of the internal cerebral veins and their tributaries. There may be overlap with other types of brain hemorrhage in these infants, with blood originating from parenchymal bleeding or infarction. Trauma may be a contributing factor. A full hematologic evaluation may be indicated if the etiology is uncertain. In contrast to the minority of premature infants with GM-IVH requiring CSF diversion, 50% of term infants with IVH will require a shunt for symptomatic hydrocephalus. A large proportion will also have neurologic deficits and epilepsy.

Birth Trauma

For the purposes of the following discussion, the term birth *trauma* refers to injuries caused by mechanical factors during labor and delivery. Although some lesions may be more common with certain types of difficult delivery (eg, instrumental delivery), underlying factors that may have precipitated a difficult or traumatic delivery, such as preexisting antenatal neurologic abnormality, must be considered as well. Not every neurologic abnormality in the newborn has been caused necessarily by trauma during parturition.

Cephalic Trauma

Trauma to the scalp is a very common—perhaps even a normal—consequence of a cephalic presentation and a vaginal delivery. The most prevalent lesion is caput succedaneum, an edematous, ecchymotic swelling of the scalp over the presenting portion of the head caused by compression of the surrounding scalp by the edge of the dilated cervix during the latter stages of labor. It resolves without treatment.

Cephalohematoma is a clot under the periosteum of the skull, almost always over the parietal bone. It accompanies as many as 5% of all deliveries, and its distinctive anatomical feature is delimitation by the calvarial sutures, where the periosteum adheres tightly to the borders of the skull bones. Cephalohematomas may be associated with underlying skull fractures. They never require surgical treatment, even when infrequently the elevation of the periosteum leads to ossification: The osseous bump will gradually recede with growth and remodeling of the skull.

The most threatening scalp lesion associated with the birth process is subgaleal hematoma. The space between the galea and the periosteum of the skull is large, extending from ear to ear and from the nasion to the line of insertion of the cervical muscles on the occiput, and it is filled by very insubstantial areolar tissue and tiny bridging vessels. These vessels may be the origin of smaller hematomas, but larger hemorrhages are probably the consequence of laceration of a dural venous sinus. There is a statistical association between subgaleal hematoma and the use of vacuum extractors, particularly the older metal designs. That application of a vacuum might pull the scalp off the skull and cause hemorrhage is easy to imagine, but the use of a vacuum extractor may simply be a marker of difficulty in the delivery. The subgaleal space does not tamponade hemorrhage very effectively, and an expanding hematoma encounters little resistance as it dissects through it. A newborn can lose a substantial fraction of total blood volume into the subgaleal space in a short time. Coagulopathy accompanies hypotension and acidosis, and as the larger hemorrhages are associated with difficult deliveries, there may be superimposed hypoxic-ischemic encephalopathy. The principal issue in the management of subgaleal hematoma, therefore, is recognition of hypovolemic shock and resuscitation from it. Drainage of the hematoma is seldom undertaken, as it precipitates more hemorrhage.

Calvarial trauma in the neonate is common and typically results from compression of the skull against maternal structures or, more rarely, by instruments such as forceps. Skull fractures may be linear, depressed, or diastatic and may be visualized on plain radiographs or head CT. They may be an incidental finding, and uncomplicated linear skull fractures usually are asymptomatic.

Computed tomography is the preferred imaging modality for the evaluation of calvarial trauma. Magnetic resonance imaging does not display osseous structures, is not very sensitive to the presence of subarachnoid hemorrhage, and requires commitment of a long period in an environment where the ill neonate is difficult to monitor. A head CT should be obtained in infants with both a linear skull fracture and a large cephalohematoma, as blood may accumulate under the fracture to form an epidural hematoma that may require evacuation. A circular depressed skull fracture (the so-called ping-pong fracture) represents a buckling inward of the flexible neonatal bone. Neurosurgical consultation is recommended, and CT scan should be obtained to rule out any accompanying hemorrhage or bone fragments in the brain. Surgical elevation is seldom required, and few fractures result in sequelae. A traumatic pseudomeningoencephalocele, or *growing skull fracture,* is a rare complication and occurs after fewer than 1 in 500 fractures (Figure 1-6). The necessary pathological substrate for a growing skull fracture includes a contusion of the underlying brain and a laceration of the underlying dura. The radiologic hallmark of dural laceration is diastasis of the fracture, and the brain contusion itself is well demonstrated by CT scanning. The

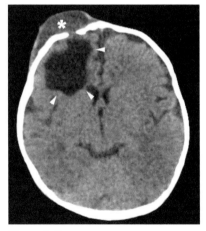

Figure 1-6.
A traumatic pseudomeningoencephalocele or *growing skull fracture.* Growing skull fractures typically appear as scalp swellings 1 to 3 months after injury. The necessary conditions are a diastatic fracture, laceration of the underlying dura, and a contusion of the subjacent brain. The swelling (white asterisk) represents cerebrospinal fluid and possibly gliotic brain tissue contained by a meningeal cicatrix. The low-density lesion of the right frontal lobe (white arrow heads) is the encephalomalacic residuum of the earlier contusion.

brain contusion evolves into an area of encephalomalacia, which becomes a focus of exaggerated brain pulsatility that is transmitted through the dural laceration to the edges of the fracture. The pulsatile cerebral cicatrix erodes the edges of the bone and herniates under the scalp. Growing skull fractures are often associated with neurologic deficits and seizures, and because the scarring of the brain and erosion of the skull evolve over a few months, recognition is usually delayed. Growing skull fractures can occur in infancy and early childhood as well, and in these age groups are commonly, but not exclusively, the consequence of battery.

Epidural hematoma is uncommon and is often associated with skull fracture or cephalohematoma as discussed previously. Affected infants may have signs of elevated intracranial pressure and show focal symptoms such as seizures, but most are asymptomatic. Computed tomography reveals the epidural hematoma. Some require surgical evacuation, but long-term problems are rare.

Subdural hematoma in the term neonate is most often asymptomatic. Prospective studies show otherwise unsuspected SDH is in up to a quarter of vaginally delivered newborns, and these hemorrhages seem to have no clinical consequences. Subdural hematoma is also the most common intracranial hemorrhage related to birth trauma. It can occur over the convexities of the hemispheres, as seen in traumatic brain injury among older patients, but in the neonate SDH more commonly appears layered over the tentorium or adjacent to the falx in the posterior interhemispheric fissure. This distinctive pattern of hemorrhage reflects the forces applied to the neonatal skull during passage through the birth canal in an ordinary vertex presentation. The skull is compressed from front and back. The frontal and occipital bones are forced toward each other, and the squeezed brain pushes the parietal bones away from the skull base, placing the tentorium and the falx under tension. If the compressive forces are not excessive, what results is normal birth molding of the skull, with the parietal bones overriding the frontal and occipital bones. Excessive compressive forces and excessive deformation of the junction of the tentorium and the falx, however, can cause laceration of these structures and rupture of the vein of Galen or its tributaries (Figure 1-7). Extreme compression of the occiput can dislocate the flat, supraoccipital portion of the occipital bone from the basal, exoccipital bone, an insult termed *occipital osteodiastasis* and often associated with posterior fossa SDH or even laceration of the cerebellum.

Infants with SDH usually become symptomatic within 24 hours of birth, but the presentation may be delayed. Symptoms may include ventilatory depression, seizures, and focal deficits. Subdural hematoma over the convexity of the hemisphere can cause a herniation syndrome, just as in older patients, with hemiparesis and ipsilateral papillary dilation. If it is massive enough to cause symptoms, SDH along the tentorium or in the posterior fossa may cause ventilatory depression or bradycardia. In many cases the clinical picture is overshadowed by global neurologic

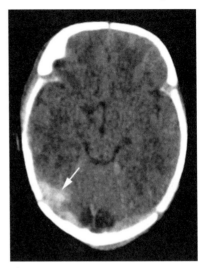

Figure 1-7.
This computed tomography scan of a term neonate shows subdural hemorrhage layered on the tentorium (white arrow).

depression from concomitant birth asphyxia. Computed tomography is the preferred imaging modality. Management of SDH includes prompt neurosurgical consultation, although surgery is rarely needed. Hydrocephalus may be a complication, particularly of posterior fossa SDH.

Spinal Trauma

Birth-related spinal cord injury is seldom associated with radiographically visible fracture or dislocation of the vertebrae. The elasticity of the ligaments of the neonatal cervical spine is greater than the elasticity of the spinal cord itself, and the ligaments can withstand deformations of the spinal column during the birth process that are sufficient to tear or rupture the spinal cord. The prevalence of spinal cord injury among newborns has been estimated at 1 per 70,000 live births. High cervical lesions are more common with vertex deliveries, and lower cervical or upper thoracic lesions are more common with breech deliveries. Symptoms vary with the level and completeness of the lesion, but affected infants may demonstrate flaccid extremities with loss of reflexes, atonic anal sphincter and distended bladder, and a sensory level.

Neurologic signs can be asymmetrical. With high cervical lesions, there may be ventilatory distress or failure from diaphragmatic paralysis. Thoracic lesions may be associated with Horner syndrome. A sensory level is a key factor in differentiating this injury from other causes of neonatal low tone, such as neonatal spinal muscular atrophy (Werdnig-Hoffman disease). The diagnosis is frequently delayed, especially in the setting of associated HIE. The development of complex-appearing reflex movements after resolution of initial flaccidity can be particularly confusing if the absence of behavioral arousal to painful stimulation of the active limb is overlooked.

Magnetic resonance imaging and neurosurgical consultation are important to exclude a surgically correctable problem such as a vertebral dislocation or an epidural hematoma, but treatable lesions are seldom identified. The effects of high-dose steroid treatment in neonatal spinal cord injury have not been studied. As the benefits of steroids for adult spinal cord injury are controversial, and as steroids can be detrimental to the developing brain, they should be withheld. Treatment of spinal cord trauma is supportive, especially ventilatory support for infants with diaphragmatic paralysis. As for spinal cord injury in older patients, immobilization of the spine is desirable. There are no neck braces for neonates, but custom-fitted thermoplastic infant carriers can be fabricated to maintain a neutral position for 6 to 12 weeks. Orthopedic consultation and physical and occupational therapy services are indicated to preserve range of motion and to minimize musculoskeletal deformity. Complete spinal cord injury in infancy is complicated almost invariably by scoliosis later in childhood. Prognosis depends on the degree of completeness of the injury, which can be very difficult to determine in the newborn. Uncertainty about prognosis creates painful ethical issues surrounding the ventilator-dependent neonate with high cervical spinal cord injury.

Brachial Plexus Injury

Injury to the brachial plexus is relatively common in term infants, with an incidence fairly constant over time, despite varying trends in obstetrical practice, at roughly 1 per 1,000 live term births. The cause is believed to be stretching of the brachial plexus by extreme lateral traction. Root involvement reflects a gradient of severity from superior to inferior. The more common and milder injuries involve the C5 and C6 roots and the upper trunk and cause the characteristic clinical picture of Erb palsy with the "waiter's tip" posture: adduction and internal rotation of the shoulder, extension of the elbow, pronation of the forearm, and flexion at the wrist. Severe injuries may affect the entire plexus and cause a flaccid extremity. Isolated injury of the C8 and T1 roots, so-called Klumpke palsy, is so rare that it is unknown in many large clinical experiences, despite the existence of a popular eponym. Diaphragmatic paralysis is a rare but potentially serious complication, and can often be identified with a chest radiograph. Injuries that affect the entire plexus can interrupt the sympathetic chain at the level of the T1 root to cause Horner syndrome with miosis of the ipsilateral pupil and ptosis of the eyelid.

In the first days of life, the limb should be handled gently but immobilization is not recommended. After 10 to 14 days, gentle passive range-of-motion exercises should begin to prevent contractures, and supportive wrist splints may be used. Physical or occupational therapists should see the infant before hospital discharge to provide instruction to the parents for daily exercises.

Most infants experience significant spontaneous recovery, and those who recover often begin to show improvement within a few weeks. Rate and degree of recovery depends largely on whether there is damage to nerve sheaths, axons (more serious), or both (most serious). If nerve roots are completely avulsed from the cord, there is essentially no chance of spontaneous recovery. Infants with total plexus involvement have a worse prognosis than infants with only partial involvement.

Sequential neurologic examinations are important. If monthly sequential examinations fail to show the start of improvement by 3 months, surgical referral is indicated. Plastic surgeons, pediatric orthopedists, and pediatric neurosurgeons may possess the necessary set of skills for microsurgical reconstruction of the infant brachial plexus; the referring physician must make inquiries regarding interest and experience. Magnetic resonance imaging and electromyography are important in perioperative planning for surgical repair, but because they often require sedation and special instructions, these studies are best ordered by the surgeon. Surgery is considered typically only for those infants who have had minimal progress toward recovery, and is usually performed between 6 and 12 months of age. Surgery can render a nonfunctional limb useful, but it cannot restore a normal limb. Infants who fail to make a complete early recovery typically experience some degree of long-term musculoskeletal limitation, even if plexus reconstruction has resulted in recovery of voluntary muscle control. Contracture and deformity of the glenohumeral joint are associated with limited external rotation and abduction, and limited supination of the forearm is common as well. Continuing follow-up by a pediatric orthopedist is essential for attainment of optimal function.

Bibliography

Andersen J, Watt J, Olson J, Van Aerde J. Perinatal brachial plexus palsy. *Paediatr Child Health.* 2006;11:93–100

Bassan H, Feldman HA, Limperopoulos C, et al. Periventricular hemorrhagic infarction: risk factors and neonatal outcome. *Pediatr Neurol.* 2006;35:85–92

Delivoria-Papadopoulos M, Mishra OP. Nuclear mechanisms of hypoxic cerebral injury in the newborn. *Clin Perinatol.* 2004;31:91–105

Dykes FD, Dunbar B, Lazarra A, Ahmann PA. Posthemorrhagic hydrocephalus in high-risk preterm infants: natural history, management, and long-term outcome. *J Pediatr.* 1989;114: 611–618

Fenger-Gron J, Kock K, Nielsen RG, Leth PM, Illum N. Spinal cord injury at birth: a hidden causative factor. *Acta Paediatr.* 2008;97:824–826

Fritz KI, Delivoria-Papadopoulos M. Mechanisms of injury to the newborn brain. *Clin Perinatol.* 2006;33:573–591

Hudgins RJ, Boydston WR, Gilreath CL. Treatment of posthemorrhagic hydrocephalus in the preterm infant with a ventricular access device. *Pediatr Neurosurg.* 1998;29:309–313

Inder TE, Volpe JJ. Mechanisms of perinatal injury. *Semin Neonatol.* 2000;5:3–16

Legido A. Perinatal hypoxic ischemic encephalopathy: recent advances in diagnosis and treatment. *Int Pediatr.* 1994;9:114–136

Levine MG, Holroyde J, Woods JR Jr, Siddiqi TA, Scott M, Miodovnik M. Birth trauma: incidence and predisposing factors. *Obstet Gynecol.* 1984;63:792–795

Looney CB, Smith JK, Merck LH, et al. Intracranial hemorrhage in asymptomatic neonates: prevalence on MR images and relationship to obstetric and neonatal risk factors. *Radiology.* 2007;242:535–541

MacKinnon JA, Perlman M, Kirpalani H, Rehan V, Sauve R, Kovacs L. Spinal cord injury at birth: diagnostic and prognostic data in twenty-two patients. *J Pediatr.* 1993;122:431–437

McComb JG, Ramos AD, Platzker AC, Henderson DJ, Segall HD. Management of hydrocephalus secondary to intraventricular hemorrhage in the preterm infant with a subcutaneous ventricular catheter reservoir. *Neurosurgery.* 1983;13:295–300

Ment LR, Bada HS, Barnes P, et al. Practice parameter: neuroimaging of the neonate: report of the Quality Standards Subcommittee of the American Academy of Neurology and the Practice Committee of the Child Neurology Society. *Neurology.* 2002;58:1726–1738

Menticoglou SM, Perlman M, Manning FA. High cervical spinal cord injury in neonates delivered with forceps: report of 15 cases. *Obstet Gynecol.* 1995;86:589–594

Perrin RG, Rutka JT, Drake JM, et al. Management and outcomes of posterior fossa subdural hematomas in neonates. *Neurosurgery.* 1997;40:1190–1199

Piatt JH Jr. Birth injuries of the brachial plexus. *Pediatr Clin North Am.* 2004;51:421–440

Pollina J, Dias MS, Li V, Kachurek D, Arbesman M. Cranial birth injuries in term newborn infants. *Pediatr Neurosurg.* 2001;35:113–119

Van Bel F, Groenendaal F. Long-term pharmacologic neuroprotection after birth asphyxia: where do we stand? *Neonatology.* 2008;94:203–210

Volpe J. *Neurology of the Newborn.* 5th ed. Philadelphia, PA: Saunders Elsevier; 2008

Volpe JJ. Perinatal brain injury: from pathogenesis to neuroprotection. *Ment Retard Dev Disabil Res Rev.* 2001;7:56–64

Zafeiriou DI, Psychogiou K. Obstetrical brachial plexus palsy. *Pediatr Neurol.* 2008;38:235–242

Chapter 2

Chronic Static Encephalopathies

Agustín Legido, MD, PhD, MBA

In contrast to chronic progressive encephalopathies, the static encephalopathies are characterized by signs of cerebral dysfunction that do not get worse with time. Any function of the brain that is affected in a static way might be classified under the term *chronic static encephalopathy,* but this chapter focuses on 4 patterns of static brain dysfunction that represent most patients seen in a pediatric neurology clinic with this type of problem: global developmental delay or intellectual disability, autism spectrum disorders, attention-deficit/hyperactivity disorder (ADHD), and cerebral palsy. What follows is a practical approach to the description of these disorders emphasizing, whenever appropriate, practice parameters and guidelines promulgated by relevant professional societies such as the American Academy of Neurology (AAN) and American Academy of Pediatrics (AAP).

Global Developmental Delay or Intellectual Disability

Definition

Global developmental disability is a subset of developmental disabilities defined as significant delay in 2 or more of the following developmental domains: gross/fine motor, speech/language, social/personal, and activities of daily living. Significant delay is defined as performance 2 standard deviations or more below the mean on age-adjusted scales. The term *global developmental delay* is usually reserved for younger children (typically <5 years), whereas the term *mental retardation* is usually applied to older children among whom IQ testing is more valid and reliable. Available valid instruments for assessing intelligence (such as the Stanford-Binet or Wechsler Preschool Primary Scale of Intelligence) are not generally applicable for children younger than 3 years. Although the use of the term *delay* within global developmental delay suggests the possibility of maturational catch-up, the reality as revealed by recent longitudinal studies suggests otherwise.

According to a recent consensus statement, *mental retardation* is defined as "a disability characterized by significant limitation both in intellectual functioning and in adaptive behavior as expressed in conceptual, social, and practical adaptive skills." More recently, the term *intellectual disability* has emerged to replace *mental retardation*.

Initial screening is important not only in identifying children with developmental delay, but also it is the first step in determining whether a child has global delay, a language disorder, or an autistic spectrum disorder. Accumulating evidence demonstrates the benefits of early intervention through a variety of programs (eg, Head Start) with respect to short-term outcomes and suggests that early diagnosis of a child with global delay may improve outcome.

Evaluation

History

Developmental surveillance is recognized as an integral component of pediatric care. The history is the most important element in the evaluation of a child with global developmental delay or intellectual disability. The first questions are whether there is true delay and whether it is global. Sometimes the child may be normal but may seem delayed in comparison to an older sibling, a cousin, or a neighbor. Sometimes the child may have a specific developmental deficit (eg, a language delay because of repeated ear infections), but such focal deficits must be distinguished from global developmental delay or chronic encephalopathy.

The next question is whether the symptoms have been progressive. If the answer is positive, it implies an underlying condition that continues actively to damage the brain, and the diagnostic investigation veers in the direction of chronic progressive encephalopathies. Chronic progressive encephalopathies are considered elsewhere in this volume but, briefly, 3 main processes need to be considered: metabolic disorders, heredodegenerative disorders, and postinfectious diseases. The family history is critical in relation to possible metabolic or heredodegenerative disorders, as metabolic conditions have a genetic basis. The presence of symptoms such as failure to thrive, vomiting, avoidance of certain foods, and the observation of distinctive body odors and typical hair abnormalities (notably, kinky hair) raise suspicions of inborn errors of metabolism. Chronic progressive encephalopathy as an infectious or postinfectious process is extremely rare but must be considered in the setting of a history of measles in early childhood (subacute sclerosing panencephalitis) or previous treatment with cadaver pituitary-derived growth hormone (Jakob-Creutzfeldt disease).

In the absence of progressive symptoms and in the absence of actual developmental or intellectual regression, diagnostic concern is channeled toward chronic static encephalopathy. Identification of a specific prenatal, perinatal, or early postnatal brain insult supports this concern. A detailed history of events during pregnancy must be elicited. Among the prenatal causes of brain damage, genetic conditions, intrauterine infections, fetal exposure to drugs or alcohol, and malformative processes such as fetal cerebral infarction and hemorrhage must be considered. Detailed information about labor and delivery must be sought. The 3 main causes of perinatal brain damage are cerebral hypoxia-ischemia, trauma, and infection, to which prematurity-related complications must be added. Postnatal events must be noted in detail, particularly in relation to these same 3 etiologies of brain damage: hypoxia-ischemia, trauma, and infection. The social history may be illuminating as well: Good parenting in a stimulating and loving environment is essential for a normal brain development and, conversely, extreme environmental deprivation can arrest development and can give the false impression of fixed encephalopathy.

Physical Examination

The focus of the general physical examination is on growth and dysmorphisms. The child should be examined naked. Length or height, weight, and head circumference should be obtained and plotted on normative percentile graphs. For example, microcephaly and computed tomography (CT) scan documentation of intracranial calcifications suggest congenital infection with toxoplasmosis or cytomegalovirus. The presence of facial dysmorphic features must be noted and described. Many syndromes are associated with typical dysmorphic facies, but in the context of static encephalopathy, interpupillary distance deserves particular attention. Diminished interpupillary distance may herald the presence of holoprosencephaly, while increased interpupillary distance is commonly seen in association with anterior basal encephaloceles. Normative percentile charts are available. Body asymmetries and anomalies and deformities of the extremities must be documented. Joint motion and extensibility must be noted. Skin must be examined for any type of vascular lesion, and hypermelanotic or hypomelanotic macules; ultraviolet illumination by Wood light accentuates such irregularities of pigmentation. Abnormal skin laxity must also be documented. Abnormalities of hair and dentition must be noted. The spine must be examined both for deformity and for cutaneous signs of dysraphism. Cardiac murmurs direct attention to the possibility of congenital heart disease, a frequent component of many developmental syndromes. Abdominal examination must pay particular attention to the presence of hepatomegaly or splenomegaly, which suggests the possibility of a metabolic storage disease.

Neurologic Examination

The level of alertness of the child and the interaction with the family and the examiner are very informative with respect to rate and course of development. Autistic behaviors are often apparent within moments of the first patient contact. Assessment of the cranial nerves must include documentation of ocular motility; esotropia and exotropia are seen frequently among children with developmental disabilities. Pupillary examination includes notation of the color of the irides and assessment of reactivity to light. Funduscopy can provide data critical to the recognition of a variety of genetic, developmental, and neurodegenerative syndromes, but a dilated examination by a pediatric ophthalmologist may be necessary to appreciate such findings as malformation or hypoplasia of the optic nerves, anomalies of the retinal vessels, pigmentary changes of the retina, and the so-called cherry red spot of Tay-Sachs disease. Normal vision and hearing must be documented, and clinical assessment must sometimes be supplemented by visual evoked responses or brain stem auditory evoked responses. The movement of the facial muscles needs to be evaluated, and the presence of any asymmetry noted. Normal oropharyngeal function must be investigated from history and through active examination. Motor examination includes assessment of abnormalities of muscle tone and their distribution. In general, patients with chronic encephalopathy often exhibit hypotonia of the neck and trunk and hypertonia of the extremities. Symmetry and complexity of movements must be noted. Muscle strength can be assessed by inspection and by active, confrontational examination of individual muscle groups. The intensity of deep tendon reflexes must be quantified, and the symmetry or asymmetry must be described. The presence of pyramidal signs must be noted, recalling that the Babinski sign is normal through the first year of age. Gait must be described. The presence of any involuntary movements must also be noted.

Neurodevelopmental Assessment

The Denver Developmental Screening Test (DDST) is an efficient and reliable method for assessing development in the physician's office. It rapidly assesses 4 different components of development: personal-social, fine motor adaptive, language, and gross motor. Additional psychometric tests can amplify the results, but the DDST, in combination with the neurologic assessment, provides sufficient information to initiate further diagnostic studies. A consultation with a developmental pediatrician or a developmental or school psychologist will provide important additional information, using the appropriate tests (Table 2-1).

Tests

A likely diagnosis is usually apparent after a detailed history and physical and neurologic examination, so in most instances additional laboratory and imaging investigations are confirmatory rather than exploratory. Studies have shown that roughly one-third of etiologic diagnoses are made on the basis of history and examination alone.

Neuroimaging Studies

Advances in magnetic resonance imaging (MRI) have shown that this neuroimaging technique is very useful in demonstrating brain dysgenesis with regular 1.5 Tesla machines, but it is even more sensitive with the newer 3.0 Tesla machines. Magnetic resonance imaging also provides information about certain metabolic disorders such as leukodystrophies and mitochondrial disorders. Magnetic resonance spectroscopy can add confirmatory biochemical information. Some studies suggest that MRI makes a critical contribution to diagnosis in up to 50% of children who have a neurodevelopmental disability.

Genetic Studies

In the case of the child with developmental delay or intellectual disability for whom no diagnosis can be made on the basis of history and examination, investigation with neuroimaging, high-resolution band karyotyping, and testing for FMR1 triplet repeat for fragile X syndrome will identify a specific

Table 2-1. Measures for Evaluation of Neurodevelopmental, Intellectual, and Behavioral Progress[a]

Type of Test	Age
Developmental Tests	
Bailey Scales of Infant Development, Second Edition (Bayley II)	16 days to 3 years 6 months 15 days
Bayley Infant Neurodevelopmental Screener (BINS)	3 months to 24 months
Denver Developmental Screening Test II (Denver II)	Birth to 6 years
Intelligence or Cognitive Tests	
Wechsler Intelligence Scale for Children Fourth Edition (WISC-IV)	6 years 0 months 0 days to 16 years 11 months 30 days
Wechsler Preschool and Primary Scale of Intelligence, Third Edition (WPPSI-III)	2 years 6 months 0 days to 16 years 11 months 30 days
Standford-Binet Intelligence Scales, Fifth Edition (SB5)	2 years 0 months to 85+ years
Differential Ability Scales (DAS)	2 years 6 months to 17 years 11 months
Leiter International Performance Scale, Revised (Leiter-R)	2 years 0 months to 20 years 11 months
Comprehensive Test of Nonverbal Intelligence (CTONI)	6 years to 90 years
Neuropsychological Tests	
NEPSY (NE for neuro and psychology)	3 years 0 months to 12 years 11 months
Delis-Kaplan Executive Function System (D-KFES)	8 years to 89 years
Indirect Functional Ratings by Parent or Caregiver	
Vineland Adaptive Behavior Scales,	0 to 89 years (parents/caregivers)
Second Edition (Vineland-II)	3 to 21 years 11 months (teachers)
Infant Development Inventory	Birth to 18 months
Child Development Inventory	15 months to 6 years

[a]Modified from Sherr EH, Shevell MI. Mental retardation and global developmental delay. In: Swaiman KF, Ashwal S, Ferriero DM, eds. *Pediatric Neurology. Principles and Practice.* Philadelphia, PA: Mosby and Elsevier; 2006:802–804, with permission from Elsevier.

etiology in 17%. Overall, 10% of children who have a global developmental delay or intellectual disability have an underlying associated cytogenetic abnormality. Among children with negative routine cytogenetic testing, comprehensive FISH (fluorescent in situ hybridization) techniques to detect microscopic subtelomeric rearrangements can produce an etiologic diagnosis in approximately 7.5%. The diagnosis of Rett syndrome must be considered in females with unexplained moderate to severe mental retardation, and suspicious patients can be tested for the *MECP2* gene deletion. The role of routine use of gene microarray to evaluate patients with global developmental delay or intellectual disability is being studied, and maybe in the near future specific indications for its use will maximize its diagnostic potential.

Metabolic Studies

At present, unselected metabolic screening cannot be justified in the context of global developmental delay or intellectual disability. It can be considered when there is suspicion of chronic progressive encephalopathy, either from the family history or from the clinical course of the patient. Neonatal screening programs for metabolic disorders, particularly since the advent of tandem mass spectrometry, have eroded the indications for unselected metabolic testing in older children. Routine screening for inborn errors of metabolism in children with global developmental delay has a yield of about 1%. In the presence of specific clinical indicators or in the context of homogenous or isolated populations, the yield may be as high as 5%. When stepwise screening is performed, the yield may increase to about 14%.

Other Tests

Lead screening. Current consensus guidelines with respect to lead testing in children recommend a strategy of targeted screening of all children with identifiable risk factors. These risk factors emphasize potential sources of environmental exposure and socioeconomic disadvantage. Developmental delay alone is not presently recognized as a risk factor within these guidelines.

Thyroid screening. Implementation of newborn screening programs has been extremely successful in eliminating hypothyroidism-related cognitive sequelae, with very few cases reported in which the diagnosis was not established in the newborn period. In the absence of systematic newborn screening, congenital hypothyroidism may be responsible for approximately 4% of cases of cognitive delay. Unless there are systemic features suggestive of thyroid dysfunction, there is no need for routine screening of children with developmental delay.

Electroencephalogram (EEG). An EEG can be obtained when a child with global developmental delay has a history or physical examination suggesting the presence of epilepsy or a specific epileptic syndrome. There is no evidence to recommend performing an EEG in a patient with global developmental delay but without suspicion of epilepsy.

Figure 2-1 summarizes a diagnostic algorithm from the AAN practice parameter "Evaluation of the Child With Global Developmental Delay."

Autism

Definition

Autism is a behaviorally distinct syndrome with many known and unknown causes. The severity of involvement in individual cases is extremely variable. Therefore, the term *autism spectrum disorders (ASDs),* or *autisms,* is appropriate. The *Diagnostic and Statistical Manual of Mental Disorders, 4th Edition Text Revision (DSM-IV-TR)* and the 10th edition of the *International Classification of Diseases of the World Health Organization* refer to the autism spectrum as *pervasive developmental disorders* (PDDs) and refer to *autistic disorder* (AD) or *autism,* as the term is used commonly in the literature, as the classic, more severe end of the spectrum.

Autism symptoms may be noted from infancy or become evident after a period of normal or nearly normal development. The clinical constellation affects 3 key areas, as described by Rapin and Tuchman: (1) impaired sociability, empathy, and ability to read other people's moods and intentions, with resulting inadequate or inappropriate social interactions; (2) rigidity and perseveration, including stereotypies (purposeless repetitive movements and activities), the need for sameness, and resistance to change; (3) impaired language, communication, and imaginative play.

Most individuals with autism also manifest mental retardation, typically moderate mental retardation with IQs between 35 and 50.

In contrast with the ASD criteria, the diagnostic criteria of Asperger syndrome (AS) require the lack of clinically significant language delay and normal or near-normal cognitive function. Language in AS is not normal, however, and many children have deficits in semantics and verbal pragmatics. Socially, these patients are unable to form friendships and are frequently ridiculed and isolated by their peers.

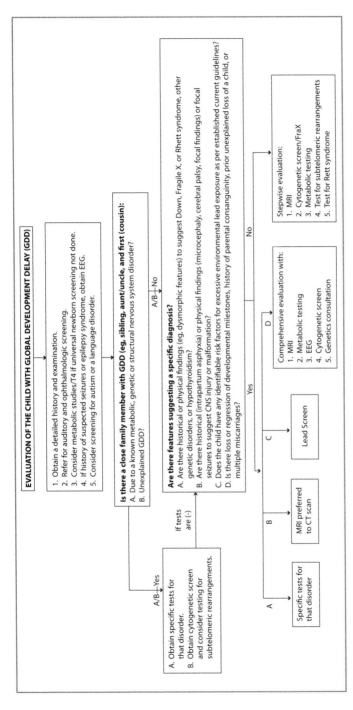

Figure 2-1.

Algorithm for the evaluation of the child with developmental delay. Audiologic and ophthalmologic screening is recommended in all children with global developmental delay. Recommended metabolic studies include a urine organic acid screen, quantitative serum amino acids, serum lactate and ammonia levels, capillary or arterial blood gas, and thyroid function studies. (From Report of the Quality Standards Subcommittee of the American Academy of Neurology and the Practice Committee of the Child Neurology Society. *Neurology.* 2003;60:367–380. Reprinted with permission from Wolters Kluwer Health.)

The most recent criteria for AD and AS are found in the *DSM-IV-TR* (Boxes 2-1 and 2-2 respectively). Pervasive developmental disorders, not otherwise specified, the remaining entity on the autistic spectrum, is described in the *DSM-IV-TR* as a subthreshold diagnostic term used when a child manifests clearly autistic behaviors, but does not meet full criteria for AD or AS. Although Rett syndrome and childhood disintegrative disorder are included in the *DSM-IV-TR* listings, they are not considered ASDs; however, they must be included in the differential diagnosis of each child, depending on the presenting signs and symptoms.

Epidemiology

Some figures in the literature suggest an increase in the incidence of autism from 1 in 10,000 before the 1970s to 1 in 150 in 2008. Although improved recognition of autism, facilitated by greater public awareness, is partially responsible for the higher reported figures, their relative contributions are unknown. On the other hand, the use of different epidemiological methodologies and definitions in determining the frequency of autism is also a factor to take into consideration. The reality is that there seem to be more children with ASDs today than in the past and, therefore, it is important to continue monitoring the incidence and prevalence of this disorder.

All studies have found more boys than girls with autism, with gender rations from 2:1 to 4:1, but as severity of cognitive impairment increases, the male to female ratio deceases to 1.3:1. There does not seem to be a significant difference in ASD between African Americans and whites. The data relating a higher incidence of ASD to higher socioeconomic status and increased maternal age are controversial.

Neurobiology

Genetic studies of concordance in monozygotic twins is 60% for Asperger and 92% for other forms of autism, whereas the concordance in dizygotic twins is 0% for Asperger and 10% for other forms of autism. The epidemiological statistic λ is defined as the rate of recurrence of a condition among siblings divided by the prevalence of that condition in the general population. For ASDs λ is 20, a high figure.

Approximately 25% to 30% of patients with fragile X syndrome have autism, and the prevalence of fragile X among patients with autism is 3%. There are other genetic conditions associated with autism, in particular

Box 2-1. Diagnostic Criteria for 299.00 Autistic Disorder[a]

A. A total of six (or more) items from (1), (2), and (3), with at least two from (1), and one each from (2) and (3):

 (1) qualitative impairment in social interaction, as manifested by at least two of the following:
  (a) marked impairment in the use of multiple nonverbal behaviors such as eye-to-eye gaze, facial expression, body postures, and gestures to regulate social interaction
  (b) failure to develop peer relationships appropriate to developmental level
  (c) a lack of spontaneous seeking to share enjoyment, interests, or achievements with other people (e.g., by a lack of showing, bringing, or pointing out objects of interest)
  (d) lack of social or emotional reciprocity

 (2) qualitative impairments in communication as manifested by at least one of the following:
  (a) delay in, or total lack of, the development of spoken language (not accompanied by an attempt to compensate through alternative modes of communication such as gesture or mime)
  (b) in individuals with adequate speech, marked impairment in the ability to initiate or sustain a conversation with others
  (c) stereotyped and repetitive use of language or idiosyncratic language
  (d) lack of varied, spontaneous make-believe play or social imitative play appropriate to developmental level

 (3) restricted repetitive and stereotyped patterns of behavior, interests, and activities, as manifested by at least one of the following:
  (a) encompassing preoccupation with one or more stereotyped and restricted patterns of interest that is abnormal either in intensity or focus
  (b) apparently inflexible adherence to specific, nonfunctional routines or rituals
  (c) stereotyped and repetitive motor mannerisms (e.g., hand or finger flapping or twisting, or complex whole-body movements)
  (d) persistent preoccupation with parts of objects

B. Delays or abnormal functioning in at least one of the following areas, with onset prior to age 3 years: (1) social interaction, (2) language as used in social communication, or (3) symbolic or imaginative play.

C. The disturbance is not better accounted for by Rett's Disorder or Childhood Disintegrative Disorder.

---

[a]*Reprinted with permission from the* Diagnostic and Statistical Manual of Mental Disorders, Fourth Edition, Text Revision *(copyright 2000). American Psychiatric Association.*

tuberous sclerosis complex and Rett syndrome. The discovery of the *MeCP2* gene in Rett syndrome suggests that mutations of this gene may be as high as 3% to 5% in female autistic populations. Other genetic disorders that are less

---

Box 2-2. Diagnostic Criteria for 299.80 Asperger Syndrome[a]

A. Qualitative impairment in social interaction, as manifested by at least two of the following:
   (1) marked impairment in the use of multiple nonverbal behaviors such as eye-to-eye gaze, facial expression, body postures, and gestures to regulate social interaction
   (2) failure to develop peer relationships appropriate to developmental level
   (3) a lack of spontaneous seeking to share enjoyment, interests, or achievements with other people (e.g., by a lack of showing, bringing, or pointing out objects of interest to other people)
   (4) lack of social or emotional reciprocity
B. Restricted repetitive and stereotyped patterns of behavior, interests, and activities, as manifested by at least one of the following:
   (1) encompassing preoccupation with one or more stereotyped and restricted patterns of interest that is abnormal either in intensity or focus
   (2) apparently inflexible adherence to specific, nonfunctional routines or rituals
   (3) stereotyped and repetitive motor mannerisms (e.g., hand or finger flapping or twisting, or complex whole-body movements)
   (4) persistent preoccupation with parts of objects
C. The disturbance causes clinically significant impairment in social, occupational, or other important areas of functioning.
D. There is no clinically significant general delay in language (e.g., single words used by age 2 years, communicative phrases used by age 3 years).
E. There is no clinically significant delay in cognitive development or in the development of age-appropriate self-help skills, adaptive behavior (other than in social interaction), and curiosity about the environment in childhood.
F. Criteria are not met for another specific Pervasive Developmental Disorder or Schizophrenia

---

[a]Reprinted with permission from the Diagnostic and Statistical Manual of Mental Disorders, Fourth Edition, Text Revision (copyright 2000). American Psychiatric Association.

---

frequently associated with autism include phenylketonuria; neurofibromatosis; and Prader-Willi, Angelman, and Smith-Lemli-Opitz syndromes.

The use of linkage analysis reveals numerous suggestive linkage peaks but with relatively little congruence across them. The most consistent evidence for linkage occurs on 17q11-17q21 and 7q, with 7q22-q32 most strongly implicated by meta-analysis. Genome-wide association studies (GWAS) may provide a powerful alternative approach. Cytogenetic studies in patients with ASDs have also been important in identifying "regions of interest." Candidate gene association studies, although many of them have been unsuccessful because of inadequate sample sizes and sparse geno-typing, have allowed the identification of a few plausible candidate genes. Among them, the following should be highlighted: *MET* (7q31), which encodes a receptor tyrosine kinase involved in neuronal growth and orga-nization; *SLC6A4* (17q11), which encodes the serotonin transporter; and *RELN* or *reelin* (7q22), which encodes a protein controlling intercellular interactions involved in neuronal migration. Of recent interest are also the neuroligin genes *NLG3* (Xq13) and *NLG4* (Xp22.33), which are cell adhe-sion molecules that play a prominent role in synaptic maturation and func-tion, and the genes for the corresponding binding proteins: neurexin genes *CNTNAP2* and *SHANK3*.

In the genetic expression of autism it is important to take into consid-eration the concept of epigenetics. It refers to the stable and potentially heritable changes in gene expression that do not involve a change in DNA sequence. Epigenetic mechanisms may help to explain the onset of symp-toms in autism after a period of apparently normal development and may play a role in how the environment affects phenotypic expression.

Cerebral Dysgenesis

Morphometric neuroimaging studies have shown increases in brain volume, particularly through the first few years of life, involving both gray matter and subcortical white matter in both the cerebrum and the cerebellum. The ver-mis of the cerebellum seems to be diminished in volume, particularly lobules VI and VII.

Neuropathological studies have shown megalencephaly in 20% of brains of patients with ASD. In the cerebral cortex there have been described corti-cal dysgenetic changes, particularly in the frontal and temporal cortex. Also, changes in cortical synaptic density and decreased hippocampal neuronal size have been described. In the cerebellum there are diminished numbers of Purkinje cells, anomalies in the cerebellar nuclei, and corresponding anoma-lies in the olives and other brain stem nuclei that project to the cerebellum.

The anatomical anomalies described previously have functional corre-lates that have been demonstrated with functional neuroimaging studies like functional MRI (fMRI) and positron emission tomography (PET). Patients with ASDs have abnormalities of global attention (superior posterior tem-poral sulcus), social perception/emotional reaction (amygdala), mental function (medial prefrontal region and amygdala), and facial perception (fusiform facial area of the ventral temporal lobe). The dysfunction demonstrated in the amygdala and its importance in emotional processing suggest that deficits in the amygdala-fusiform network may underlie the social cognitive impairments characteristic of individuals who have ASDs.

Neurochemical Dysfunction

The following neurochemical systems have been studied in autism: oxytocin, acetylcholine, glutamate, γ-aminobutyric acid, dopamine, norepinephrine, endogenous opioids, cortisol, and serotonin. The most significant findings are related to the serotoninergic system. Serotonin regulates the development of cerebral cortex and hippocampus, and elevations of its levels in the fetus cause abnormal neuronal development. There is evidence of a higher incidence of autism in fetuses exposed to drugs that increased serotonin. Elevations of whole blood serotonin occur in one-third of patients with ASD, but its function is reduced in the central nervous system. Increased levels are also reported in the parents and siblings of patients. Studies with PET have shown decreased serotonin synthesis in the dentate nucleus of the cerebellum, and it is interesting that the dentato-thalamo-cortical pathway is functionally very important for sensory integration and language. As indicated before, the gene *SLC6A4,* which is the serotonin transporter gene, has been significantly associated with the neurobiological mechanism of autism. Obviously, the relevance of the serotoninergic system in ASD raises therapeutic implications suggesting possible roles for selective serotonin reuptake inhibitors and antipsychotics.

Mitochondrial Dysfunction

In 2002 HEADD (hypotonia, epilepsy, autism, and developmental delay) syndrome was described in 12 children. Seven out of 8 children had mitochondria respiratory chain defects, 4 out of 5 had mitochondrial structural abnormalities, and 5 had mitochondrial DNA deletions. One year later there was a report of 2 patients with autism who had mitochondrial proliferation and decreased complex III. The mitochondrial DNA mutation A3243G, which typically causes MELAS (mitochondrial encephalopathy, lactic acidosis, and stroke-like episodes) syndrome, has been found in patients with autism. Elevated lactate and carnitine deficiency have also been reported in children with autism. Therefore, it has been hypothesized that a subgroup of patients with ASD may have a mitochondrial disorder. The real incidence is unknown, and it is unclear whether the mitochondrial abnormality is pathogenetically related to autism.

Immunological Dysfunction

Recent studies have demonstrated an activation of the immune system in the cerebrospinal fluid (CSF) and the brain of 11 children and adults with autism, with presence of reactive neuroglia and inflammatory response. It has been postulated that such immune reaction can affect the cerebral development of the fetus. However, there was no evidence of T- or B-lymphocytic activation. There are also reports of association of autism with several classes of human leukocyte antigen haplotypes, a higher prevalence of autoimmune disorders in patients with autism, and high levels of brain-specific autoantibodies in the sera of some children with autism. These findings suggest the hypothesis that dysregulation of the immune system could play a role in particular subtypes of autism.

Other Questionable Factors

Some investigators and groups of parents of children with autism believe that there is a relationship between autism and immunizations with vaccines containing the mercury-based preservative thimerosal. Specific accusations have been leveled at the MMR vaccine. Population studies have demonstrated no causal association between childhood immunization and the development of autism.

Similarly, a "gastrointestinal intolerance reaction" to certain food proteins has been hypothesized as a possible pathogenetic mechanism for a subgroup of children with autism. The concept is that an immunologic reaction in the gut involves the brain as a bystander, but there is no substantiating scientific evidence.

Exposure to heavy metals, particularly lead or mercury (mainly through fish consumption) has also been suggested as a possible cause, but no scientific conclusion has been reached.

The effects of birth weight, duration of gestation, and events around the time of birth have been investigated as well, but findings have not been consistent.

Diagnosis

Clinical Evaluation

The diagnosis of autism often is not made until 2 to 3 years after symptoms are recognized, primarily because of concerns about the stigma of a possibly incorrect diagnosis; nevertheless, identifying children with autism and initiating intensive, early intervention during the preschool years results in improved outcomes.

The diagnosis of autism should include the use of a diagnostic instrument with at least moderate sensitivity and good specificity for autism. Recommended instruments include

Diagnostic Parental Interviews

Gilliam Autism Rating Scale

The Parent Interview for Autism

Pervasive Developmental Disorders Screening Test-III

Autism Diagnostic Interview, Revised

Diagnostic Observation Instruments

Childhood Autism Rating Scale

The Screening Tool for Autism in Two-Year-Olds

The Autism Diagnostic Observation Schedule—Generic

In 2000 the AAN Quality Standards Subcommittee and the Child Neurology Society (CNS) established the practice parameter "Screening and Diagnosis of Autism" (Figure 2-2). The information was expanded in 2007 by the AAP Council on Children With Disabilities.

Recommendations

The following are the clinical practice recommendations of the AAN and CNS practice parameter for Level One: Routine Developmental Surveillance:

1) Developmental surveillance should be performed at all well-child visits from infancy through school age, and at any age thereafter if concerns are raised about social acceptance, learning, or behavior.

2) Recommended developmental screening tools include the Ages and Stages Questionnaire, the BRIGANCE Screens, the Child Development Inventories, and the Parents' Evaluations of Developmental Status.

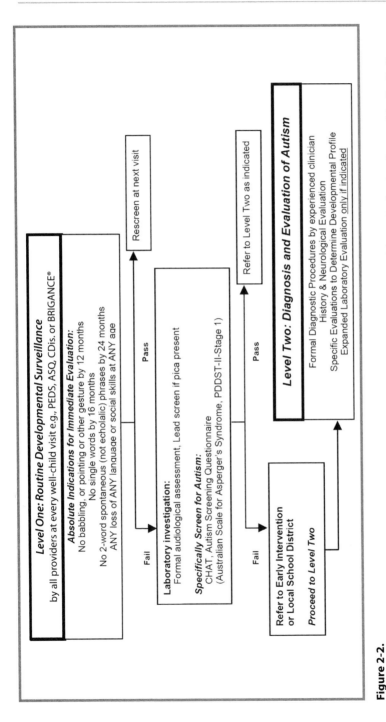

Figure 2-2.
Algorithm for evaluation of the child with suspected autism. (From Practice parameter: screening and diagnosis of autism. Report of the Quality Standards Subcommittee of the American Academy of Neurology and the Practice Committee of the Child Neurology Society. *Neurology.* 2000;55:468–479. Reprinted with permission from Wolters Kluwer Health.)

3) Because of the lack of sensitivity and specificity, the DDST-II, and the Revised Denver Pre-screening Developmental Questionnaire (R-DPDQ) are not recommended for appropriate primary care developmental surveillance.

4) Further developmental evaluation is required whenever a child fails to meet any of the following milestones: babbling by 12 months, gesturing (ie, pointing, waving bye-bye) by 12 months, single words by 16 months, 2-word spontaneous (not echolalic) phrases by 24 months, or loss of any language or social skills at any age.

5) Siblings of children with autism should be carefully monitored for acquisition of social, communication, and play skills, and the occurrence of maladaptive behaviors. Screening should be performed not only for autism-related symptoms, but also for language delays, learning difficulties, social problems, and anxiety or depressive symptoms.

6) Screening specifically for autism should be performed on all children failing routine developmental surveillance procedures using one of the validated instruments: the Checklist for Autism in Toddlers (CHAT) or the Autism Screening Questionnaire.

7) Laboratory investigations recommended for any child with developmental delay and suspected autism should include audiologic assessment and lead screening.

The document by the AAP Council on Children With Disabilities also emphasizes surveillance, screening, and early diagnosis.

Although lack of speech, scripted speech, parroting without communicative intent, and pop-up and giant words are classic presentations, earlier pre-speech deficits often exist that, if detected, can facilitate earlier diagnosis. These deficits include

- Lack of appropriate gaze
- Lack of warm, joyful, expression with gaze
- Lack of the alternating to-and-fro pattern of vocalizations between infant and parent that usually occurs at approximately 6 months of age (ie, infants with ASDs usually continue vocalizing without regard for the parent's speech)
- Lack of recognition of mother's (or father's or consistent caregiver's) voice
- Disregard for vocalization (ie, lack of response to name), yet keen awareness for environmental sounds

- Delayed onset of babbling past 9 months of age
- Decreased or absent use of pre-speech gestures (waving, pointing, showing)
- Lack of expressions such as "oh oh" or "huh"
- Lack of interest or response of any kind to neutral statements (ie, "Oh no, it's raining again!")

The AAP brochure "Is Your One-Year-Old Communicating With You?" was developed to help raise parent and physician awareness of these earlier social communication milestones and to promote recognition of symptoms of ASDs before 18 months of age.

The following are the clinical practice recommendations of the AAN and CNS practice parameter for Level Two: Diagnosis and Evaluation of Autism:

1) Genetic testing in children with autism, specifically high-resolution chromosome studies (karyotype) and DNA analysis for fragile X, should be performed in the presence of mental retardation, if there is a family history of fragile X or undiagnosed mental retardation, or if dysmorphic features are present. (The role of systematic use of microarray gene studies in populations of autistic children is still to be defined.)

2) Selective metabolic testing is indicated by the presence of suggestive clinical and physical findings such as lethargy, cyclic vomiting, early seizures, dysmorphic or coarse features, or evidence of mental retardation, or if newborn screening is questionable.

3) There is inadequate evidence to recommend an EEG study in all individuals with autism. Indications for an adequate sleep-deprived EEG with appropriate sampling of slow-wave sleep include clinical seizures, suspicion of subclinical seizures, or a history of regression (clinically significant loss of social and communicative function) at any age, but especially in toddlers and preschoolers.

4) Recording of event-related potentials and magnetoencephalography are research tools without evidence of routine clinical utility.

5) There is no evidence to support the role of routine clinical neuroimaging in the diagnostic evaluation of autism, even in the presence of megalencephaly.

6) There is inadequate supporting evidence for hair analysis, assay of celiac antibodies, allergy testing (ie, food allergies for gluten, casein, *Candida*, and other molds), testing for immunologic or neurochemical abnormalities, assay of micronutrients such as vitamins, intestinal permeability

studies, stool analysis, measurement of urinary peptides, investigation for mitochondrial disorders, thyroid function tests, or erythrocyte glutathione peroxidase studies.

Treatment

Behavioral Treatments

Nowadays social and functional communication abilities are considered to be a priority in early treatment. Earlier behavioral programs focused on the acquisition of speech in children with autism. There is now a growing interest in developmental-pragmatic approaches in which the focus is not necessarily spoken language but functional communication, like teaching the child to express what he or she wants and feels by diverse means. The Picture Exchange Communication System (PECS) has been developed as an effective method to teach communication to children with autism.

To target skills other than communication, or to change dysfunctional symptoms, strictly structured behavioral interventions are being supplemented with naturalistic behavioral interventions. Applied behavioral methods for teaching skills and facilitating more appropriate and adaptive behaviors have been tested for their effectiveness in children and adults with autism and other developmental disabilities. Other well-established programs combine elements of behavior and developmental orientations in which the effectiveness of the parent-training components have been evaluated.

Pharmacotherapy

Risperidone has been studied in a multisite, prospective, double-blind, randomized trial. It was demonstrated to be beneficial for irritability, repetitive behaviors, and aggression, but a significant effect on social-communicative features was not demonstrated. The maximum dose was 2.5 mg or 3.5 mg, for weight less than or greater than 45 kg, respectively. In open label studies other atypical neuroleptics that have been studied with good results are olanzapine and ziprasidone.

Serotonin transporter inhibitors, like clomipramine, fluoxetine, sertraline, fluvoxamine, and paroxetine improve social interaction, aggression, and irritability. It has been hypothesized that these drugs may modify key neuron-developmental processes in very young children with ASDs, but there is no research substantiation as yet.

Stimulants and non-stimulant medications are used to treat the frequently associated comorbidity of ADHD.

Melatonin is a good initial measure to treat the comorbidity of sleep disturbance, specifically insomnia. Otherwise, a sleep study is indicated to establish a specific diagnosis.

Antiepileptic drugs are indicated to treat the frequent comorbidity of epilepsy. Levetiracetam, valproic acid, and lamotrigine may have some beneficial effect on behavioral manifestations of autism as well.

Complementary and Alternative Medicine

In the United States almost three-quarters of children with ASDs receive complementary and alternative medicine (CAM) in combination with more traditional treatments. Amongst the proposed treatments are elimination diets, dietary supplements and vitamins, treatment targeting the immune system, steroids, antifungal agents to reduce intestinal *Candida* overgrowth, and chelating agents. No well-designed studies have supported the efficacy of these therapies, and for those therapies that have been examined, clinical trials have demonstrated rather a lack of effect. An example is the highly publicized secretin case: The incidental observation that the symptoms of 3 children with autism improved significantly after secretin perfusion was not substantiated in 12 of 13 subsequent placebo-controlled trials. Nevertheless, despite their lack of efficacy, CAM may interact with prescribed conventional therapies, so parents must be questioned specifically about them.

Attention-Deficit/Hyperactivity Disorder

Definition

This term, which includes the concepts of inattention, hyperactivity, and impulsivity, was first established by the American Psychiatric Association in 1980. Previously, different terminologies had been applied to patients with the characteristics of ADHD, including *abnormal defect in moral control in children, minimal cerebral lesion, syndrome of the hyperkinetic child,* and *minimal cerebral dysfunction.*

Attention-deficit/hyperactivity disorder and its subtypes are a group of neurobehavioral disorders characterized by inattention, increased motor activity, and impulsiveness. They are the most common emotional, cognitive, and behavioral disorders treated in children and adolescents. The current prevailing opinion characterizes ADHD as a disorder of executive function attributable to abnormal dopamine transmission in the frontal lobes and frontostriatal circuitry.

Epidemiology

Review of epidemiological studies during the past decade shows a wide range of prevalence estimates, ranging from very low (0.2%–0.9%) to very high (19.8%–27%). Prevalence estimates of childhood ADHD in the United States are between 5% and 8%. There are no differences found between estimates from North America and Europe. Figures are lower in the Middle East and Africa; however, methodological issues may be responsible.

The most consistently reported demographic factor characterizing ADHD samples across epidemiological studies is the higher rates of ADHD among men than among women, averaging 11.3% and 5.4%, respectively (2.4:1 ratio).

The influences of race, ethnicity, and socioeconomic status on the prevalence of ADHD are not well defined, and conflicting results have appeared. However, access to treatment and knowledge about the disorder seems to be better among white, non-Hispanic, higher educated families.

Longitudinal studies have consistently shown that ADHD symptoms tend to decline over time, but a considerable number of affected subjects remain symptomatic and impaired in adulthood, even if the full syndrome has remitted. In a recent study in the Netherlands, the prevalence of ADHD in adulthood was estimated to be 1%.

Neurobiology

Genetics

Twin studies have found an ADHD diagnostic concordance of 51% in monozygotic twins and 33% in dizygotic twins, supporting a genetic basis for the condition. Linkage analysis studies have found chromosome regions of interest, different depending on the geographic regions: United States

(5p12, 10q26, 12q23, 16p), Germany (5p, 6q, 7p13, 9q33, 12q, 15q15, 17p), and Colombia (4q13, 8p23, 8q12, 11q23, 12q23).

A recent international ADHD gene study was IMAGE (International Multisite ADHD Gene). A total of 674 probands and 51 genes were studied. Eighteen genes seemed to be associated with ADHD in this study. The following is a summary of the genes most strongly associated with ADHD, as supported by data in the literature: (1) *DRD4* (Dopamine D4 receptor gene), (2) *DRD5* (Dopamine D5 receptor gene, (3) *SLC6A3* (Dopamine transporter gene), (4) *SNAP25* ("Synaptosome Associated Protein of 25 KD" gene), and (5) *HTR1B* (Serotonin 1B receptor gene).

Brain Size

Overall, volumetric studies using MRI have shown abnormalities in the prefrontal regions, the basal ganglia, and the cerebellum. The following structures have shown to have a lower volume in patients with ADHD compared with controls: total cerebral volume from infancy to adolescence, right cerebral hemisphere, corpus callosum, anterior frontal lobule, caudate and globus pallidum, cerebellar hemisphere and vermis (lobules VIII-X), and white matter tracts. On the other hand, gray matter heterotopias seem more prevalent among subjects with ADHD.

In some studies, total brain volume correlated with the scores of full-scale IQ and attention problems as measured by the Child Behavior Checklist.

These findings suggest that the disorder may result from a disruption in a more distributed circuitry than just the frontostriatal pathway, including the frontal regions, the basal ganglia, the cerebellar hemispheres, and the cerebellar vermis.

Neurotransmitter Systems

The neurotransmitter systems thought to be involved in the pathophysiology of ADHD are the catecholamines dopamine (DA) and norepinephrine (NE). Most of the supporting evidence comes from the catecholamine-releasing effects of the stimulant medications that reduce the symptoms of ADHD. Stimulants, such as methylphenidate (MPH) and amphetamine block the reuptake of both DA and NE and inhibit monoamine oxidase, an enzyme that plays a role in metabolizing catecholamines. The amphetamines also facilitate the release of DA and NE into the synaptic cleft. The modes of action of non-stimulant medications that treat ADHD (atomoxetine, guanfacine, bupropion) are also ultimately based on their effects on the catecholamines. Evidence from genes involved in ADHD inheritance patterns also points toward involvement of the catecholamine neurotransmitter system.

Homovanillic acid levels have been shown to correlate with ADHD symptoms, and high levels are associated with a better response to treatment. Functional studies with single-photon emission computed tomography and PET have demonstrated an increase of the dopamine transporter in the striatum, which normalizes after treatment with MPH.

There is also evidence that the cholinergic system may play a modulatory role in the pathogenesis of ADHD. It is known that nicotinic cholinergic receptors *(alpha 7, alpha 4, beta 2)* participate in the working memory process. Also, the nicotinic system is related to the dopaminergic and glutamatergic systems, which regulate cognitive function. Finally, nicotinic cholinergic drugs are effective in treating ADHD.

Diagnosis

The diagnosis of ADHD is made by careful clinical history. A child with ADHD is characterized by a considerable degree of inattentiveness, distractibility, impulsivity, and often hyperactivity that is inappropriate for the developmental age of the child. Although ADHD is often first observed in early childhood, many overactive toddlers will not develop ADHD. Other common symptoms include low frustration tolerance, shifting activities frequently, difficulty organizing, and daydreaming.

Children with predominantly inattentive symptoms may have more difficulties in school and in completing homework, and fewer difficulties with peers or family. Conversely, children with excessive hyperactive or impulsive symptoms may do relatively well in school but have difficulties at home or in situations with less guidance or structure.

In the United States the basis for the diagnosis of ADHD is the *DSM-IV-TR* criteria set (Box 2-3). It includes 18 criteria, consisting of 9 inattention symptoms and 9 hyperactivity-impulsivity symptoms. Individuals must display, in 2 distinct settings, 6 of 9 inattentions symptoms, or 6 of 9 hyperactive-impulsivity features for at least 6 months to qualify for a diagnosis. Some of the features must be present before the age of 7 years and

Box 2-3. Diagnostic Criteria for Attention-Deficit/ Hyperactivity Disorder[a]

A. Either (1) or (2):

(1) six (or more) of the following symptoms of **inattention** have persisted for at least 6 months to a degree that is maladaptive and inconsistent with developmental level:

Inattention

(a) often fails to give close attention to details or makes careless mistakes in schoolwork, work, or other activities

(b) often has difficulty sustaining attention in tasks or play activities

(c) often does not seem to listen when spoken to directly

(d) often does not follow through on instructions and fails to finish school-work, chores, or duties in the workplace (not due to oppositional behavior or failure to understand instructions)

(e) often has difficulty organizing tasks and activities

(f) often avoids, dislikes, or is reluctant to engage in tasks that require sustained mental effort (such as schoolwork or homework)

(g) often loses things necessary for tasks or activities (e.g., toys, school assignments, pencils, books, or tools)

(h) is often easily distracted by extraneous stimuli

(i) is often forgetful in daily activities

(2) six (or more) of the following symptoms of **hyperactivity-impulsivity** have persisted for at least 6 months to a degree that is maladaptive and inconsistent with developmental level:

Hyperactivity

(a) often fidgets with hands or feet or squirms in seat

(b) often leaves seat in classroom or in other situations in which remaining seated is expected

(c) often runs about or climbs excessively in situations in which it is inappropriate (in adolescents or adults, may be limited to subjective feelings of restlessness)

(d) often has difficulty playing or engaging in leisure activities quietly

(e) is often "on the go" or often acts as if "driven by a motor"

(f) often talks excessively

Impulsivity

(g) often blurts out answers before questions have been completed

(h) often has difficulty awaiting turn

(i) often interrupts or intrudes on others (e.g., butts into conversations or games)

B. Some hyperactive-impulsive or inattentive symptoms that caused impairment were present before age 7 years.

C. Some impairment from the symptoms is present in two or more settings (e.g., at school [or work] and at home).

Box 2-3. Diagnostic Criteria for Attention-Deficit/ Hyperactivity Disorder[a], continued

D. There must be clear evidence of clinically significant impairment in social, academic, or occupational functioning.

E. The symptoms do not occur exclusively during the course of a Pervasive Developmental Disorder, Schizophrenia, or other Psychotic Disorder and are not better accounted for by another mental disorder (e.g., Mood Disorder, Anxiety Disorder, Dissociative Disorder, or a Personality Disorder).

Code based on type:

314.01 Attention-Deficit/Hyperactivity Disorder, Combined Type: if both Criteria A 1 and A2 are met for the past 6 months

314.00 Attention-Deficit/Hyperactivity Disorder, Predominantly Inattentive Type: if Criterion A 1 is met but Criterion A2 is not met for the past 6 months

314.01 Attention-Deficit/Hyperactivity Disorder, Predominantly Hyperactive-Impulsive Type: if Criterion A2 is met but Criterion A 1 is not met for the past 6 months

Coding note: For individuals (especially adolescents and adults) who currently have symptoms that no longer meet full criteria, "In Partial Remission" should be specified.

---

[a]*Reprinted with permission from the* Diagnostic and Statistical Manual of Mental Disorders, Fourth Edition, Text Revision *(copyright 2000). American Psychiatric Association.*

---

they must interfere with developmentally appropriate social, academic, or occupational functioning. The symptoms may not be better accounted for by other psychiatric or physical disorders. The frequency and severity of these features must be more than what is typically seen in developmentally comparable individuals. *DSM-IV-TR* characterizes 3 subtypes of ADHD: (1) predominantly hyperactive, (2) predominantly inattentive, and (3) a combined type based on the predominance of the core symptoms.

Rating scales are extremely helpful in documenting the individual profile of ADHD symptoms as well as assessing the response to treatments (ie, the Conners Rating Scales Revised, the Academic Performance Rating Scale, the ADHD Rating Scale-IV, and others). Rating scales are available for all age groups and can be useful in assessing and monitoring home, academic, and occupational performance.

Differential Diagnosis

Hyperthyroidism, sleep disorders, oppositional defiant disorder and conduct disorder, mood disorders, anxiety disorders, cognitive performance and learning disabilities, school problems, drug abuse, tics, and seizures are all conditions that may be comorbidities in patients with ADHD and therefore should be investigated.

Treatment

Once a diagnosis is made, the management of ADHD must involve patient education, psychosocial interventions, and medication management. All patients diagnosed with ADHD must be educated about the disorder. In children, psychosocial interventions may include parent training and school-based interventions. In adolescents, who may be more likely to present with behavioral problems and conflicts at home, behavioral family therapy can be helpful.

The primary care physician can screen, diagnose, educate, and initiate medication management in patients with uncomplicated ADHD. Because many patients with ADHD have comorbid disorders such as depression and anxiety, adjunctive treatments or referrals are often necessary. Finally, reasonable accommodations are allowable by law for students and employees, and physicians can help their patients with ADHD by documenting the disorder and writing letters on their behalf.

Table 2-2 summarizes the pharmacologic treatment of ADHD.

Some clinicians are reluctant to use stimulant medication because of specific concerns of growth retardation and sudden cardiac death. Overall, the findings confirm that stimulants cause a slowing in growth velocity for weight and height, which can persist, although attenuated, for at least 4 years during continuous treatment. A slight decrease in weight and height velocity also is observed during treatment with atomoxetine. From a clinical perspective, weight and height should be assessed at least semiannually in these patients.

Stimulants and atomoxetine have cardiovascular effects with increases in heart rate and blood pressure. These changes usually are not clinically significant in the short term, but their possible significance for the long term deserves further investigation. Although a causal link between therapeutic stimulant use and sudden cardiac death is not established, there are concerns

Table 2-2. Medications for Attention-Deficit/Hyperactivity Disorder[a]

Medication	Dosage Form	Starting Dose	Final Dose
Amphetamine preparations			
Short-acting			
Adderall	5.0, 7.5, 10.0, 12.5 15.0, 20.0, 30.0 mg	3–5 y: 2.5 mg qd >6 y: 5 mg qd–bid	Lesser of 1 mg/kg per day or 40 mg
Dexedrine	5.0 mg	3–5y: 2.5 mg qd	
Dextrostat	5, 10 mg	>6 y: 5 mg qd–bid	
Long-acting			
Dexedrine	5, 10, 15 mg	>6 y: 5–10 mg	Lesser of 1 mg/kg
Spansule		qd–bid	per day or 40 mg
Adderall XR	5, 10, 15, 20, 25, 30 mg	>6 y: 10 mg qd	Lesser of 1 mg/kg per day or 30 mg
Lisdexam-fetamine	30, 50, 70 mg	30 mg qd	Lesser of 1 mg/kg per day or 70 mg
Methylphenidate preparations			
Short-acting			
Focalin	2.5, 5.0, 10, 0 mg	2.5 mg bid	Lesser of 1.0 mg/kg per day or 20 mg
Methylin	5, 10, 20 mg	5 mg bid	Lesser of 2.0 mg/kg
Ritalin	per day or 60 mg		
Intermediate-acting			
Metadate ER	10, 20 mg	10 mg qam	Lesser of 2.0 mg/kg
Methylin ER	10, 20 mg		per day or 60 mg
Ritalin SR	20 mg		
Metadate CD	10, 20, 30, 40, 50, 60 mg	20 mg qam	Lesser of 2.0 mg/kg per day or 60 mg
Ritalin LA	10, 20, 30, 40, mg		
Long-acting			
Concerta	18, 27, 36, 54 mg	18 mg qam	Lesser of 2.0 mg/kg per day or 72 mg
Daytrana Patch	10, 15, 20, 30 mg patches	10 mg	Lesser of 1.0 mg/kg per day or 30 mg
Focalin XR	5, 10, 15, 20 mg	5 mg qam	Lesser of 1.0 mg/kg per day or 30 mg

Table 2-2. Medications for Attention-Deficit/Hyperactivity Disorder,[a] continued

Medication	Dosage Form	Starting Dose	Final Dose
Selective norepinephrine reuptake inhibitor			
Strattera	10, 18, 25, 40, 60, 80 100 mg	<70 kg: 0.5 mg/kg/d for 4 days; then 1 mg/kg/d for 4 days; then 1.2 mg/kg/d	Lesser of 1.4 mg/kg per day or 100 mg
Antidepressants			
Bupropion			
Wellbutrin	75, 100 mg tablet	Lesser of 3 mg/kg/d	Lesser of 6 mg/kg/d
Wellbutrin SR	100, 150, 200 mg tablet	or 150 mg/d	or 300 mg, with no single dose
Wellbutrin XL	150, 300 mg tablet		>150 mg
Imipramine			
Tofranil	10, 20, 50, 75 mg tablet	1 mg/kg/d	Lesser of 4 mg/kg/d or 200 mg
Nortriptyline			
Pamelor	10, 25, 50, 75 mg	0.5 mg/kg/d	Lesser of 2 mg/kg/d
Aventyl	tablet		or 100 mg
α_2-Adrnergic agonists			
Clonidine			
Catapres	0.1, 0.2, 0.3 mg tablet	<45 kg: 0.05 mg qhs >45 kg: 0.1 mg qhs	27–40.5 kg: 0.2 mg 40.5–45 kg: 0.3 mg >45 kg: 0.4 mg
Guanfacine			
Tenex	1, 2 mg tablet	<45 kg: 0.5 mg qhs >45 kg: 1 mg qhs	27–40.5 kg: 2 mg 40.5–45 kg: 3 mg >45 kg: 4 mg

Abbreviations: qd, every day; bid, twice a day; qam, every morning; qhs, every bedtime.

[a]Data from Pliszka S, AACAP Work Group on Quality Issues. Practice parameter for the assessment and treatment of children and adolescents with attention-deficit/hyperactivity disorder. *J Am Acad Child Adolesc Psychiatry.* 2007;46:894–921. Reprinted with permission from Wolters Kluwer Health.

that treatment may increase the risk for sudden death in patients who have structural cardiac abnormalities, so that careful pretreatment assessment and clinical screening currently is recommended in this subgroup of patients.

Cerebral Palsy

Definition

The concept of cerebral palsy (CP) refers to a group of heterogeneous clinical syndromes characterized by abnormal motor activities and postural mechanisms. These abnormalities are due to isolated or multiple anomalies of the developing brain, and are static. Although the neuropathological lesions and their clinical expression may change with age, there is no progression of the disease. The full extent of motor disability may not be evident until the age of 3 or 4 years. Intellectual, sensory, and/or behavioral difficulties may accompany CP; however, they are not included in the diagnostic criteria. Box 2-4 enumerates a series of genetic and metabolic disorders that may be mistaken for CP, particularly in the initial stages.

Epidemiology

The prevalence of CP in developed countries is 2 to 2.5 per 1,000 live newborns. In developing countries, the prevalence is higher due to a higher incidence of perinatal asphyxia. In Sweden, the prevalence of CP decreased from 2.2 per 1,000 during the period of 1954 to 1962 to 1.4 per 1,000 during 1967 to 1970. The advances in neonatal care during the 1980s increased the survival of very low birth weight newborns, and the prevalence of CP increased to 2.4 per 1,000, as CP in this population is 20 times more prevalent than in normal weight newborns. However, the frequency of CP in very low birth weight newborns decreased from 11.3% in the 1980s to 5.2% in the 1990s. Nevertheless, preterm infants still constitute 50% to 60% of all infants with CP. African Americans have a higher risk of CP, in part related to a higher incidence of prematurity.

Cerebral palsy occurs in 1 in every 500 school-aged children; therefore, it is among the commonest of chronic disabilities of childhood. About 30% of children with CP cannot walk, and nearly 20% walk only with an assistive device. About half of children with CP have one or more additional disabilities (epilepsy, cognitive deficit, visual or hearing impairment).

Box 2-4. Genetic and Metabolic Disorders That May Be Misdiagnosed as Cerebral Palsy[a]

Adrenoleukodystrophy
Adrenomyeloneuropathy
Aicardi-Goutieres syndrome
Allan-Herndon-Dudley syndrome
Angelman syndrome
Argininemia
Ataxia-telangiectasia
Ceroid lipofuscinosis
Duchenne/Becker muscular dystrophy
Glutaconic aciduria (3-methyl)
Glutaric aciduria type I
GM1 gangliosidosis
Hereditary progressive spastic paraplegia
Infantile neuroaxonal dystrophy
Kallmann syndrome with spastic paraplegia
L-dopa sensitive dystonia
Lesch-Nyhan syndrome
MASA syndrome
Menkes disease (mild forms)
Olivopontocerebellar atrophy
Orotic aciduria
Pelizaeus-Merzbacher disease
Pettigrew syndrome
Pontocerebellar atrophy/hypoplasia
Posterior fossa tumor
Type C Niemann-Pick disease
X-linked spinocerebellar ataxia

Abbreviation: MASA: mental retardation, aphasia, shuffling gait, adducted thumbs.
[a]*Translated from Legido A, Katsetos CD. Cerebral palsy: new pathogenetic concepts [in Spanish].* Rev Neurol.
2003;36:157–165.

Pathogenesis

Genetic Factors

The presence of multiple cases of CP in the same family and a higher incidence of CP in children of consanguineous couples suggest the existence of a genetic basis in 1% to 2% of cases.

In patients with spastic diplegia and quadriplegia, the most frequent mechanism of inheritance is autosomal recessive, but there are also cases reported of autosomal dominant and X-linked recessive inheritance. Some cases of athetoid CP have been reported with similar mechanisms of inheritance. Congenital hemiplegia seems to be transmitted as a dominant trait with high penetrance.

There have also been reported cases of chromosome anomalies associated with specific forms of CP. For example, a gene in 2q24-25 has been related to an autosomal recessive form of symmetrical spastic CP in 3 families. Another gene in Xp11.4q21 was related in a family to spastic diplegia, associated also with mental retardation, microcephaly, short stature, and cryptorchidism.

The presence of apolipoprotein E ε4 allele, located in chromosome 19, was found to be a risk factor for the development of CP in a study where the authors compared 40 patients with CP and 40 controls.

A recent population-based case-control study was conducted in Australia in which investigators measured 28 single-nucleotide polymorphisms in newborn screening blood spots. For inducible nitric-oxide synthase, possession of the T allele was more common in all children with CP and for heterozygotes who were born at term. For lymphotoxin alpha, homozygous variant status was associated with risk for CP and with spastic hemiplegic or quadriplegic CP. Among term infants, heterozygosity for the endothelial protein C receptor single-nucleotide polymorphism was more frequent in children with CP. In preterm infants, the variant A allele of interleukin 8 was associated with CP risk. Interleukin 8 heterozygote status was associated with spastic diplegia. Variants of several genes were associated with CP in girls but not in boys. These findings support the concept that there may be a genetic contribution to CP risk, and additional investigation of genes and gene-environment interaction in CP is warranted.

Hematologic Factors

The use of MRI in patients with CP has demonstrated that about 40% of cases are due to vascular factors (ischemia or hemorrhage). In 1997 a paper reported for the first time 3 patients who had CP secondary to perinatal stroke on the basis of a mutation of factor V Leiden. The mutation is inherited as an autosomal dominant trait and replaces arginine for glutamine at the site where activated C protein (ACP) acts to degrade the mutant factor

V, which therefore becomes resistant to ACP and produces more thrombin, inducing a hypercoagulable state. Additional controlled studies of the following coagulation factors have been performed: antithrombin III, protein C, protein S, lupus anticoagulant, and antiphospholipid factor. All of them have been significantly elevated in various patients with CP, confirming the centrality of thrombophilic processes in the pathogenesis of this condition.

Immunologic Factors

Likewise, blood levels of the following immunologic factors—interleukins (IL) IL-1, IL-8, IL-9, alpha tumor necrosis factor (TNFα), and RANTES – have been found to be significantly elevated in the patients with CP with diagnostic sensitivity and specificity of 100%. The levels of IL-6, IL-11, IL-13, and other chemical cytokines (MIP1a, MIP1b, MIP2, CP1, and MCP2) were also associated with CP with a sensitivity and a specificity above 88%. Similarly, 14 of the 31 children with CP had levels of interferon-α, -β, and -γ higher than the controls, and most of these patients had diplegic CP. Those patients without elevation of interferons suffered spastic hemiplegia.

Infectious Factors

There are clinical, epidemiological, neuropathological, and experimental studies that suggest that maternal-fetal infection is related to the pathogenesis of CP, particularly in the preterm newborn with periventricular leukomalacia (PVL). Since the mid-1950s it is known that prenatal exposure to infectious agents can affect brain development negatively and can cause brain lesions, CP, and cognitive deficits. Intrauterine infection is a predictive factor of Apgar scores and may manifest during the neonatal period as a perinatal asphyxia picture with depression and suggestive signs of encephalopathy.

In a population-based study in northern California, evidence of maternal infection or fever during the admission for delivery was associated with risk of CP in infants of normal weight, neonatal seizures, and admission to the neonatal intensive care unit. There are now many other studies regarding term and near-term infants, which have found an association of maternal infection or fever with low Apgar score, neonatal encephalopathy, and seizures, and with CP risk.

The presence of chorioamnionitis and increased interleukins in the amniotic fluid has been related to a high risk of developing PVL and CP in preterm newborns. Neuropathological studies have demonstrated the presence of IL-6 and TNFα in the PVL lesions, supporting the pathogenetic relationship of intrauterine infection, cytokines, and PVL. The periventricular white matter of the premature newborn is particularly vulnerable to develop PVL between gestational weeks 23 and 32, when most oligodendrocyte precursors are late pre-oligodendrocytes, which are particularly vulnerable to damage by oxidative stress.

Birth Asphyxia

In a population-based American study, only 6% of children with CP had had a recognized birth complication capable of causing birth asphyxia or interruption of oxygen supply to the fetus. There are studies that have shown that as the incidence of perinatal asphyxia decreases, the rate of CP has not changed, supporting a lack of direct relationship.

The CP that birth asphyxia causes is spastic quadriplegia, although there are other potential causes of that syndrome. Global hypoxia-ischemia is not likely to cause hemiplegic or spastic diplegic CP. And global hypoxia-ischemia is not a plausible cause of CP in an infant who did not manifest encephalopathy in the newborn period.

Other Factors

The following should be considered risk factors for developing CP: prematurity itself, atypical intrauterine growth, congenital anomalies, and multiple gestation.

Types of Cerebral Palsy

The most frequent classification is clinically based, in relation to the number of limbs involved, the muscle tone, and the associated movement limitation.

Spastic Hemiplegia

There is unilateral motor involvement. It can be congenital or acquired. The congenital form represents 23% to 40% of all cases of CP; therefore, it is the most frequent one. A stroke in the territory of the middle cerebral artery is the most frequent underlying neuropathology. The left cerebral hemisphere is affected in two-thirds of patients. Other neuropathological findings are neuronal migration disorders and unilateral periventricular leukomalacia.

There are also ischemic- or hemorrhagic-associated diencephalic lesions in the thalamus and basal ganglia.

The child exhibits impaired gross and fine motor coordination of the upper extremity, has difficulty moving the hand quickly, and is unable to grasp small objects with a pincer grasp. Facial involvement is unusual. Gait is circumductive with a variable degree of abnormality. Corticosensory impairment and hemineglect of the affected side are common. Mental retardation or epilepsy occurs in about one-third of patients.

Spastic Quadriplegia

It usually affects term newborns of low birth weight. It is the most severe form of CP and its frequency ranges from 10% to 40%. Prenatal causes are most frequent, including infections (TORCH syndrome [toxoplasmosis, other agents, rubella, cytomegalovirus, and herpes simplex]) and cerebral dysgenesis, but perinatal and postnatal causes may be found. The typical neuropathological finding is the cystic degeneration as the final outcome of softening, necrosis, and edema of the central white matter. Mantle sclerosis may be found in patients with mild-to-moderate quadriplegia.

There is generalized spasticity, decreased movement of the extremities, tendency to opisthotonus, diffuse hyperreflexia, Babinski signs and, frequently, clonus. Because of the involvement of the corticobulbar fibers, there is supranuclear bulbar palsy that produces dysphagia, hypersalivation, and dysarthria. The incidence of epilepsy is as high as 90%. These patients also have severe mental retardation, microcephaly, and visual and auditory disturbances.

Spastic Diplegia

This form of CP is typically associated with PVL of the premature newborn. Other neuropathological lesions that can be seen in this type of CP are porencephalic cysts, microgyria, and intraventricular hemorrhage with secondary ventricular dilation.

On physical examination there is spasticity of the lower extremities, with tendency to scissoring, hyperreflexia, clonus, and the Babinski sign. There is commonly some degree of upper extremity impairment, but usually only to a mild degree. Some infants with spastic diplegia manifest ataxia after further maturation, with difficulty in coordination. With time, contractures develop in the lower extremities, maintaining the hips and knees in flexion, and the feet in equinovarus position.

Epilepsy may develop in some patients, but cognitive impairment is not frequent.

Extrapyramidal Cerebral Palsy

In this type of CP there is an abnormal function of the smooth coordination of agonist and antagonist muscles in producing movement. It involves defects of posture and involuntary movements (ie, athetosis, ballismus, chorea, dystonia) and is associated with increased tone.

The extrapyramidal form of CP is often, but not always, preceded by hypoxic-ischemic brain injury (more frequently affecting the thalamus and the putamen) or kernicterus (more frequently involving the globus pallidum and the subthalamic nucleus of Luys).

The choreoathetoid form of extrapyramidal CP is characterized by large amplitude involuntary movements. The most obvious component is athetosis. Chorea is present in variable degree, but tremor, myoclonus, and even some dystonia may be present. Ballismus may be seen in extreme forms of choreoathetoid CP. The purely dystonic form of extrapyramidal CP is uncommon and is characterized by abnormal dystonic posturing, but severely affected children with spastic quadriplegic CP often exhibit variable degrees of dystonia as well.

Atonic Cerebral Palsy

This form is uncommon. There is generalized hypotonia, with hyper-reflexia, and a significant decrease of strength in the lower extremities, compared with the upper extremities. The mechanism seems to be related to the effect that cortical and subcortical cerebral structures exercise on the gamma motor neuron. There is slow attainment of motor milestones. On neurologic examination, when patients are held under the arms, they flex both legs at the hips (Förster sign). In some cases with time there may appear cerebellar and extrapyramidal signs. The hypotonia of the lower extremities usually persists.

Ataxic Cerebral Palsy

This form of CP may be accompanied by other motor abnormalities, including spastic diplegia, but the diagnosis is applied only when there is predominantly cerebellar dysfunction.

Early manifestations include hypotonia, truncal ataxia with sitting, dysmetria, and gross incoordination. But the motor manifestations do not become apparent until late in the first year of life. There is delay in acquisition of motor milestones and involvement of fine motor coordination. There may be associated cognitive deficit, but not severe.

If there is no clear history of a cause for CP, the clinician should rule out other causes of ataxias.

Mixed Cerebral Palsy

Mixed CP includes manifestations of both spastic and extrapyramidal types; often an ataxic component is present. These patterns of motor impairment are the result of compromise of large areas of the brain with sequelae of basal ganglia, cortex, and subcortical disruption.

Diagnosis

Clinical Evaluation

The diagnosis of CP is basically clinical and takes into consideration the description of symptoms and signs described in the preceding section. However, according to Paneth (2008), perhaps the single commonest error in CP assessment is assigning the diagnosis too soon. For reasons as yet poorly understood, many children, especially children from high-risk backgrounds such as prematurity, exhibit a variety of neurologic abnormalities in the first 18 months of life that can suggest the possibility of CP. Sometimes, even quite striking neurologic abnormalities found on examination in the first year or so of life can disappear. This phenomenon is especially common in very premature infants. Therefore, the diagnosis of CP should be assigned very cautiously before the age of 24 months (or 24 months after the expected date of delivery in the case of premature babies), unless the disorder is exceptionally severe.

Assessing the functional impact of the motor impairment is an important component of CP assessment. An excellent system for categorizing degree of ambulatory capacity, the Gross Motor Function Classification

System (GMFCS), has become a well-established tool for describing the degree of activity limitation in CP. The system distinguishes 5 levels of activity limitation. Level 1, the mildest, describes children whose level of function is not too far distant from that of children without CP, whereas Level 5 describes children who cannot walk independently (www.canchild.ca/Portals/0/outcomes/pdf/GMFCS.pdf).

Recommendations

In 2004 the AAN Quality Standards Subcommittee and the CNS Practice Committee established the practice parameter "Diagnostic Assessment of the Child With Cerebral palsy" (Figure 2-3).

The following are the consensus recommendations:

1) All children should undergo a detailed history and physical examination. It is important to determine that the child's condition is due to a static and not to a progressive or degenerative neurologic disorder.

2) It is also important to classify the type of CP as this has diagnostic implications as well as implications regarding associated problems.

3) Because children with CP commonly have associated mental retardation, ophthalmologic abnormalities, hearing impairments, speech and language disorders, and disorders of oral-motor function, screening for these conditions should be part of the initial assessment.

4) An EEG is recommended when there are features suggestive of epilepsy or a specific epileptic syndrome.

5) To establish an etiology and prognosis in children with CP, neuroimaging is recommended, with MRI preferred over CT. However, if neuroimaging performed during the neonatal period provided an etiology of the child's CP, it may obviate the need for later study.

6) Metabolic and genetic studies should not be routinely obtained in the evaluation of the child with CP.

7) If the clinical history or findings on neuroimaging do not determine a specific structural abnormality or if there are additional and atypical features in the history or clinical examination, metabolic and genetic testing should be considered.

8) Because the incidence of cerebral infarction is high in children with hemiplegic CP, diagnostic testing for a coagulation disorder should be considered.

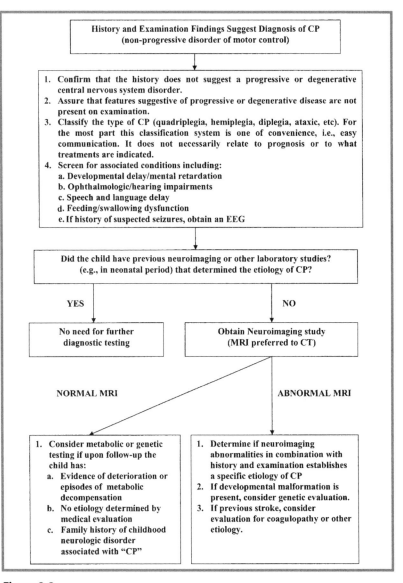

Figure 2-3.

Algorithm for the evaluation of the child with cerebral palsy (CP). Screening for associated conditions (mental retardation, vision/hearing impairments, speech and language delays, oral-motor dysfunction, and epilepsy). Neuroimaging (magnetic resonance imaging preferred to computed tomography) is recommended for further evaluation if the etiology of the child's CP has not been previously determined. In some children additional metabolic or genetic testing may be indicated. (From Report of the Quality Standards Subcommittee of the American Academy of Neurology and the Practice Committee of the Child Neurology Society. *Neurology*. 2004;62:851–863. Reprinted with permission from Wolters Kluwer Health.)

Treatment

The treatment of the patient with CP needs to be multidisciplinary, targeting not only the neurologic and musculoskeletal problems, but all the associated medical problems, including growth and nutrition, vision therapy, oral-motor therapy, dental hygiene, gastrointestinal problems, and psychological support. The best result depends on the participation of a group of professionals.

The goals of rehabilitation are improving mobility, preventing deformity, helping the child to learn the skills of daily living, and educating the parents about the child's condition. Methods used in CP rehabilitation are physiotherapy, occupational therapy, bracing, assistive devices, adaptive technology, and sports and recreation.

Spasticity should be treated when it arrests developmental progress or causes loss of function; produces contractures, deformities, pressure sores, or pain; or causes difficulty in positioning or caring for the child. The treatment of spasticity usually follows a stepwise approach, related to the severity of the condition and the complexity and potential risks of the interventions.

1) Basic measures such as positioning, exercises, and bracing are indicated initially in all cases.

2) Oral antispastic drugs such as baclofen, diazepam, dantrolene, and tizanidine are recommended for severe spasticity, but they must be used with caution in the ambulatory child.

3) Botulinum toxin causes a reversible chemodenervation by inhibiting acetylcholine release. It is very helpful in cases of a dynamic contracture that interferes with function. Because the effects dissipate within a few months, botulinum toxin is commonly administered as an adjunct to an intense course of physical therapy to achieve specific tone reduction and range of motion goals.

4) Abnormalities of tone affecting the balance of agonist and antagonist muscle groups commonly lead to deformities and contractures in the growing child. Periodic orthopedic assessment is an important component of the care of the child with CP, and surgical interventions are frequent.

5) Intrathecal baclofen is administered by a spinal catheter leading from a drug pump implanted in the abdominal wall. It is very useful in patients with severe diffuse spasticity to facilitate aspects of daily care such as

bathing, toileting, dressing, and seating. There are data suggesting that it may be effective in prevention of joint contractures and musculoskeletal deformities as well.

6) Selective dorsal rhizotomy is most commonly indicated for spastic diplegic children who are independently ambulatory or have the potential to become so. Randomized controlled trials have shown that it reduces tone and improves scores on the Gross Motor Function Measure beyond what can be achieved by protracted, intensive physical therapy alone. In highly selected young patients, rhizotomy too may prevent deformity and obviate the need for some orthopedic interventions.

Web Sites

American Association on Intellectual and Developmental Disabilities: www.aaidd.org

Developmental Disabilities Nurses Association: www.ddna.org

Cure Autism Now: www.canfoundation.org

The National Alliance for Autism Research: www.naar.org

Attention Deficit Disorder Resources: www.addresources.org

Children and Adults with Attention Deficit Disorders: www.helpforadhd.org

Attention Deficit Disorder Association: www.add.org

Kennedy Krieger Institute Phelps Center for Cerebral Palsy and Neurodevelopmental Medicine: www.kennedykrieger.org

United Cerebral Palsy Association: www.ucp.org

Bibliography

Abrahams BS, Geschwind DH. Advances in autism genetics: on the threshold of a new neurobiology. *Nat Rev Genet.* 2008;9:341–355

Albright AL, Barron WB, Fasick MP, Polinko P, Janosky J. Continuous intrathecal baclofen infusion for spasticity of cerebral origin. *JAMA.* 1993;270:2475–2477

Albright AL, Barry MJ, Fasick P, Barron W, Shultz B. Continuous intrathecal baclofen infusion for symptomatic generalized dystonia. *Neurosurgery.* 1996;38:934–938

American Academy of Pediatrics. *Is Your One-Year Old Communicating With You* [brochure]? Elk Grove Village, IL: American Academy of Pediatrics; 2004

American Academy of Pediatrics Subcommittee on Attention-Deficit/Hyperactivity Disorder, Committee on Quality Improvement. Clinical practice guideline: treatment of the school-aged child with attention-deficit/hyperactivity disorder. *Pediatrics.* 2001;108:1033–1044

Ashwal S, Russman BS, Blasco PA, et al. Practice parameter: diagnostic assessment of the child with cerebral palsy. Report of the Quality Standards Subcommittee of the American Academy of Neurology and the Practice Committee of the Child Neurology Society. *Neurology.* 2004;62:851–863

Bacchelli E, Maestrini E. Autism spectrum disorders: molecular genetic advances. *Am J Med Genet C Semin Med Genet.* 2006;142:13–23

Bauman ML, Kemper TL. Neuroanatomic observations of the brain in autism: a review and future directions. *Int J Dev Neurosci.* 2005;23:183–187

Berker AN, Yalçin MS. Cerebral palsy: orthopedic aspects and rehabilitation. *Pediatr Clin North Am.* 2008;55:1209–1225

Biederman J, Spencer TJ. Psychopharmacological interventions. *Child Adolesc Psychiatric Clin N Am.* 2008;17:439–458

Bush G. Neuroimaging of attention deficit hyperactivity disorder: can new imaging findings be integrated in clinical practice? *Child Adolesc Psychiatric Clin N Am.* 2008;17:385–404

Chez MG, Chin K, Hung PC. Immunizations, immunology, and autism. *Semin Pediatr Neurol.* 2004;11:214–217

Cohly HH, Panja A. Immunological findings in autism. *Int Rev Neurobiol.* 2005;71:317–341

Collett BR, Ohan JL, Myers KM. Ten-year review of rating scales. V. Scales assessing attention deficit/hyperactivity disorder. *J Am Acad Child Adolesc Psychiatry.* 2003;42:1015–1037

Dodge NN. Cerebral palsy: medical aspects. *Pediatr Clin North Am.* 2008;55:1189–1207

Filipeck PA, Accardo PJ, Ashwal S, et al. Practice parameter: screening and diagnosis of autism. Report of the Quality Subcommittee of the American Academy of Neurology and the Child Neurology Society. *Neurology.* 2000;55:468–479

Gibson CS, Maclennan AH, Dekker GA, et al. Candidate genes and cerebral palsy: a population-based study. *Pediatrics.* 2008;122:1079–1085

Gupta AR, State MW. Recent advances in the genetics of autism. *Biol Psychiatry.* 2007;61: 429–437

Hirtz DG, Wagner A, Filipeck PA. Autistic spectrum disorders. In: Swaiman KF, Ashwal S, Ferriero DM, eds. *Pediatric Neurology. Principles and Practice.* Philadelphia, PA: Mosby and Elsevier; 2006:905–935

Johnson CP, Myers SM, Council on Children with Disabilities. Identification and evaluation of children with autism spectrum disorders. *Pediatrics.* 2007;120:1183–1215

Katragadda S, Schubiner H. ADHD in children, adolescents, and adults. *Prim Care Clin Office Pract.* 2007;34:317–341

Kieling C, Goncalves RRF, Tannock R, Castellanos FX. Neurobiology of attention deficit hyperactivity disorder. *Child Adolesc Psychiatric Clin N Am.* 2008;17:285–307

Lainhart JE. Advances in autism neuroimaging research for the clinician and geneticist. *Am J Med Genet C Semin Med Genet.* 2006;142:33–39

Lam KS, Aman MG, Arnold LE. Neurochemical correlates of autistic disorder: a review of the literature. *Res Dev Disabil.* 2006;27:254–289

Legido A, Katsetos CD. Cerebral palsy: new pathogenetic concepts [in Spanish]. *Rev Neurol.* 2003;36:157–165

Losh M, Sullivan PF, Trembath D, Piven J. Current developments in the genetics of autism: from phenome to genome. *J Neuropathol Exp Neurol.* 2008;67:829–837

Madsen KM, Hviid A, Vestergaard M, et al. A population-based study of measles, mumps, and rubella vaccination and autism. *N Engl J Med.* 2002;347:1477–1482

Mandelbaum DE. Attention-deficit-hyperactivity disorder. In: Swaiman KF, Ashwal S, Ferriero DM, eds. *Pediatric Neurology. Principles and Practice.* Philadelphia, PA: Mosby and Elsevier; 2006:871–886

McDougle CJ, Erickson CA, Stigler KA, Posey DJ. Neurochemistry in the pathophysiology of autism. *J Clin Psychiatry.* 2005;66(suppl 10):9–18

McLaughlin JF, Bjornson KF, Astley SJ, et al. Selective dorsal rhizotomy: efficacy and safety in an investigator-masked randomized clinical trial. *Dev Med Child Neurol.* 1998;40:220–232

Mick E, Faraone SV. Genetics of attention deficit hyperactivity disorder. *Child Adolesc Psychiatric Clin N Am.* 2008;17:261–284

Nelson KB. Causative factors in cerebral palsy. *Clin Obstet Gynecol.* 2008;51:749–762

Nelson KB, Dambrosia JM, Grether JK, Phillips TM. Neonatal cytokines and coagulation factors in children with cerebral palsy. *Ann Neurol.* 1998;44:665–675

Paneth N. Establishing the diagnosis of cerebral palsy. *Clin Obstet Gynecol.* 2008;51:742–748

Pardo CA, Vargas DL, Zimmerman AW. Immunity, neuroglia and neuroinflammation in autism. *Int Rev Psychiatry.* 2005;17:485–495

Pliszka S, AACAP Work Group on Quality Issues. Practice parameter for the assessment and treatment of children and adolescents with attention-deficit/hyperactivity disorder. *J Am Acad Child Adolesc Psychiatry.* 2007;46:894–921

Polanczyk G, Jensen P. Epidemiologic considerations in attention deficit hyperactivity disorder: a review and update. *Child Adolesc Psychiatric Clin N Am.* 2008;17:245–260

Rapin I, Tuchman RF. Autism: definition, neurobiology, screening, diagnosis. *Pediatr Clin North Am.* 2008;55:1129–1146

Sherr EH, Shevell MI. Mental retardation and global developmental delay. In: Swaiman KF, Ashwal S, Ferriero DM, eds. *Pediatric Neurology. Principles and Practice.* Philadelphia, PA: Mosby and Elsevier; 2006:799–820

Shevell M. Global developmental delay and mental retardation or intellectual disability: conceptualization, evaluation, and etiology. *Pediatr Clin North Am.* 2008;55:1071–1084

Shevell M, Ashwal S, Donley D, et al. Practice parameter: evaluation of the child with global developmental delay. Report of the Quality Standards Subcommittee of the American Academy of Neurology and the Practice Committee of the Child Neurology Society. *Neurology.* 2003;60:367–380

Spencer TJ, Biederman J, Mick E. Attention-deficit/hyperactivity disorder: diagnosis, lifespan, comorbidities, and neurobiology. *Ambul Pediatr.* 2007;7:73–81

Stein MA, McGough JJ. The pharmacogenomic era: promise for personalizing attention deficit hyperactivity disorder therapy. *Child Adolesc Psychiatric Clin N Am.* 2008;17:475–490

Steinbok P, Reiner AM, Beauchamp R, Armstrong RW, Cochrane DD, Kestle J. A randomized clinical trial to compare selective posterior rhizotomy plus physiotherapy with physiotherapy alone in children with spastic diplegic cerebral palsy. *Dev Med Child Neurol.* 1997;39:178–184

Steyaert JG, De La Marche W. What's new in autism? *Eur J Pediatr.* 2008;167:1091–1101

Swaiman KF, Wu Y. Cerebral palsy. In: Swaiman KF, Ashwal S, Ferriero DM, eds. *Pediatric Neurology. Principles and Practice.* Philadelphia, PA: Mosby and Elsevier; 2006:491–504

Tuchman R. Autism. *Neurol Clin.* 2003;21:915–932

Tuchman R, Rapin I, eds. *Autism: A Neurological Disorder of Early Brain Development.* London, UK: MacKeith Press; 2006:1–354

Vitiello B. Understanding the risk of using medications for attention deficit hyperactivity disorder with respect to physical growth and cardiovascular function. *Child Adolesc Psychiatric Clin N Am.* 2008;17:459–474

Wright FV, Sheil EM, Drake JM, Wedge JH, Naumann S. Evaluation of selective dorsal rhizotomy for the reduction of spasticity in cerebral palsy: a randomized controlled trial. *Dev Med Child Neurol.* 1998;40:239–247

Chapter 3

Chronic Progressive Encephalopathies: Inborn Errors of Metabolism

Joseph J. Melvin, DO
Harold G. Marks, MD

Introduction

Inborn errors of metabolism (IEMs) were first recognized in the early twentieth century. An IEM is a biochemical disorder that causes a defect in a protein molecule. The IEM is usually due to mutations in a gene that encodes a defective protein. Gene products in IEMs are most commonly enzymes, but they may also be receptors, transport proteins, or regulators of other genes.

Most IEMs are individually rare, but cumulatively they represent a significant problem, and overall they are the most frequent cause of chronic progressive encephalopathies: Children present progressive loss of milestones and developmental or cognitive deterioration.

It is important to be aware of these diseases, as some are treatable, and a diagnosis allows genetic counseling and a chance for prevention of recurrence. Diagnosing individual disorders is often extremely difficult given the expanding number of genotypes described, as well as the diversity of clinical phenotypes that may be associated with a specific genotype. However, recent technological advancements such as tandem mass spectrometry have made the diagnosis of metabolic diseases much easier. This chapter will concentrate on the clinical approach, as well as the most useful laboratory tests, in the diagnosis of metabolic diseases for the general practitioner. Treatment options will be discussed briefly, because most patients will be managed at a specialized center.

Clinical Classification of Inborn Errors of Metabolism

The classification of IEMs has always been difficult. Classification schemas have been based variably on pathoanatomical or pathophysiological considerations, on symptomatic presentation, or even on age of clinical presentation.

An easy way to subdivide the IEMs clinically is based on the type of the accumulating substance or deficient product. Thus IEMs can be classified into disorders of small and large molecules. Examples of small molecule disorders include amino acid disorders, organic acid disorders, urea cycle defects, fatty acid oxidation defects, and other defects of energy generation, including mitochondrial disorders and neurotransmitter disorders. The small molecule disorders may present as life-threatening intoxication in the neonatal period or as episodic dysfunction often related to catabolic stress later in life depending on the amount of enzyme activity. Large molecule disorders are the "storage diseases" in which proteins, lipids, or carbohydrates accumulate within cellular organelles, disrupt cellular function, and lead to cell death. Large molecule diseases typically present as progressive degenerative disorders.

One may further define IEMs based on their symptomatic presentation into 3 broad clinical categories: acute intoxication (vomiting, lethargy, coma, and seizures), problems of energy metabolism (hypoglycemia, lactic acidosis, hypotonia, myopathy, cardiomyopathy, cardiac failure, seizures, choreoathetosis, dystonia, myoclonus, ataxia, mental retardation, and loss of auditory and visual function), and defective degradation of complex molecules (progressive dysfunction of multiple organs causing mental retardation, developmental regression, liver and spleen dysfunction, and renal dysfunction). Although fairly simplistic, this approach combined with the small versus large molecule disorders classification provides a good starting point for a clinical approach to the diagnosis of IEMs (Box 3-1).

Evaluation of Inborn Errors of Metabolism

The basis of the diagnosis of IEMs is a high index of suspicion triggered by the recognition of key findings in the history or physical examination.

History

Family history. The presence of parental consanguinity is obviously important. The caveat is that most IEMs are autosomal recessive and, thus, most newborns that have proven IEMs have a negative family history. A history of frequent miscarriages or of unexplained death of siblings (including sudden infant death syndrome [SIDS]) is more frequent in autosomal recessive

---

Box 3-1. Classification and Examples of Inborn Errors of Metabolism (IEMs)

Small molecule IEMs with a clinical presentation of acute intoxication
   Amino acid disorders: phenylketonuria, maple syrup urine disease, tyrosinemia type I
   Organic acid disorders: isovaleric acidemia, propionic acidemia
   Urea cycle defects: citrullinemia, ornithine transcarbamylase deficiency
   Carbohydrate metabolism disorders: galactosemia, hereditary fructose intolerance
Small molecule IEMs with a clinical presentation of defects in energy metabolism
   Glycogenoses: glycogen storage disease Ia and Ib)
   Defects of gluconeogenesis
   Fatty acid oxidation defects: Medium chain acyl-CoA dehydrogenase deficiency)
   Pyruvate metabolism disorders: pyruvate dehydrogenase deficiency)
   Mitochondrial defects: lactic acidosis, and stroke-like episodes; complex I dysfunction
   Creatine deficiency syndromes
Large molecule IEMs with storage of the breakdown of complex molecules material in cellular organelles causing cell dysfunction and death
   Lysosomal disorders: Tay-Sachs disease, Gaucher disease, mucopolysaccharidoses
   Peroxisomal disorders: adrenoleukodystrophy
   Carbohydrate-deficiency glycoprotein syndromes
   Disorders of copper metabolism
   Cholesterol synthesis disorder: Smith-Lemli-Opitz syndrome

---

disorders. However, patterns of inheritance of IEMs include X-linked recessive, X-linked dominant, autosomal dominant, and mitochondrial. Therefore, a careful genetic family history is still very important.

Prenatal history. It is often helpful. A history of neonatal deaths, the presence of the maternal HELLP syndrome (hemolytic anemia, elevated liver enzymes, and low platelet count) may be associated with infant beta oxidation defects. Fetal ascites is present in a number of inborn errors. Unexplained neonatal seizures, particularly those that are intractable to standard antiepileptic therapy, may be due to an IEM. Neonatal jaundice, sepsis, hypoglycemia, and acidosis can all be associated with small molecule disorders. Sepsis is by far the most common cause of these findings in otherwise normal newborns. However, sepsis can still coexist with or precipitate the presentation of IEMs. An important point to remember is that IEMs in the neonatal period usually present with a symptom-free period as the intoxication associated with small molecule diseases gradually builds over a 48- to 72-hour period.

Dietary history. In older children the dietary history may be helpful. Asking about food preferences and aversions, as well as the presence of unusual odors associated with body fluids, is an important part of the history (ie, patients with amino acid disorders tend to reject protein-containing foods).

Medical history. The presence of recurrent encephalopathy with illness, fever, fasting, or the ingestion of specific foods suggests a small molecule disorder with intoxication resulting from a partial enzyme deficiency. The history of slowly progressive neurologic deterioration is more consistent with a large molecule storage disease. In certain circumstances, such as the metabolic myopathies or neurotransmitter diseases, variation in symptoms during the day or after exercise is a key finding in the history.

A history of cardiomyopathy has been recognized as the chief clinical manifestation of a variety of inherited disorders of cardiac energy metabolism including storage diseases, fatty acid disorders, and mitochondrial respiratory chain disorders. Also, a history of any of the following abnormalities in the neonatal period should raise the suspicion of metabolic disease: hypoglycemia, hypotonia, hyperammonemia (>200 µmol/L), metabolic acidosis, refractory seizures, burst suppression electroencephalogram, or dysmorphic features in combination with the above factors.

Physical Examination

Certain aspects of the physical examination are important in patients with suspected IEMs. Special attention should be directed toward the hair, skin, nails, eyes, and abdomen. Particularly suggestive are broken, twisted, or absent hair; rashes; nail dystrophy; and specific lesions such as the angiokeratomas of Fabry disease. Biotinidase deficiency is frequently associated with seborrheic or atopic dermatitis and partial or complete alopecia. These findings are more suspicious in the presence of neurologic abnormalities.

Any patient with a suspected IEM should have a formal ophthalmologic evaluation including a dilated direct funduscopic examination and a slit lamp examination. Eye movement abnormalities are often supportive of a particular diagnosis. Examples include horizontal supranuclear gaze palsy in type 3 Gaucher disease, and chronic progressive external ophthalmoplegia in mitochondrial cytopathies, abetalipoproteinemia, or Refsum disease.

Other physical findings suggestive of metabolic disease, especially in the newborn period, are displayed in Box 3-2.

Neonatal Screening

In many cases the diagnosis is established through the newborn screening programs for IEMs, which are expanding in the United States. In the past, each IEM required a separate test with associated costs and a requirement for a portion of the dried blood spot specimen from a heel stick. This limitation was partially responsible for the limited number of mandated newborn screening tests available, usually 7 or less, depending on the state. The development and application of automated electrospray ionization (ESI) tandem mass spectrometry (MS) has made high-volume screening for amino acid, organic acid, and fatty acid metabolic disorders practical.

Automated ESI tandem MS newborn screening of amino acids and acylcarnitines extracted from dried blood spot filter papers is capable of detecting more than 30 inherited metabolic disorders. The number of IEMs detectable in the newborn period due to tandem MS screening greatly

---

Box 3-2. Clinical Findings Suggestive of Inborn Errors of Metabolism

Dysmorphism
  Glutaric aciduria type II, storage diseases, Zellweger, Smith-Lemli-Opitz CDGS, Pyruvate dehydrogenase deficiency, and pyruvate carboxylase deficiency
Liver Disease
  Galactosemia, Niemann-Pick C, fatty acid oxidation disorders, tyrosinemia type 1, and mitochondrial disorders
Cardiac Disorders
  Fatty acid oxidation disorders, mitochondrial disease, Pompe disease, and CDGS
Hydrops Fetalis
  Lysosomal disorders
Renal Cysts
  Mitochondrial disease, Zellweger disease

Abbreviation: CDGS, carbohydrate-deficient glycoprotein syndromes.

extends the possibilities of early, generally presymptomatic diagnosis, which allows for more effective treatment options. In addition, tandem MS using dried blood spots may be applied for newborn screening of lysosomal diseases such as Fabry, Gaucher, Hurler, Krabbe, Hunter, Niemann-Pick A/B, and Pompe diseases.

The recent development of treatment via enzyme replacement therapy has made early detection of lysosomal diseases through newborn screening a new consideration in many states. The results of the expanded newborn screening are often readily available to the private physician and can provide a good source of information on metabolic disorders that already have been assayed in a particular patient.

Laboratory Investigation

If the patient presents without a previous diagnosis through a newborn screening program, the initial laboratory evaluation of a possible metabolic disease should begin with basic laboratory tests (Box 3-3).

Small Molecule Metabolic Diseases

A complete blood count, chemistry panel (including electrolytes, glucose, ketones, creatinine, total protein, albumin, ammonia, and uric acid), and transaminases are the basics of an initial evaluation. A gapped acidosis and elevated ammonia are often seen in a variety of small molecule disorders. Neutropenia and thrombocytopenia are commonly seen in a variety of organic acidemias. Pancytopenia may occur in large molecule disorders, secondary to hypersplenism and/or marrow replacement. The presence of abnormalities in preliminary testing may suggest more specific tests (Box 3-3).

The second tier of tests should include plasma amino acids, ammonia, lactate, and pyruvate and urine organic acids, which will detect abnormalities in most symptomatic individuals with small molecule disorders For example, dicarboxylic aciduria in a child with weakness and episodic symptoms suggestive of hypoglycemia should lead to plasma carnitine and acylcarnitine assays looking for disorders of beta-oxidation and oxidative phosphorylation defects.

Figures 3-1 and 3-2 show a logical approach to the differential diagnosis of these disorders depending on the presence of acidosis or ketosis.

Box 3-3. Laboratory Workup of Inborn Errors of Metabolism

Small Molecule Metabolic Diseases
  Initial Evaluation
        Blood: acid-base status, electrolytes, liver function tests, ammonia glucose,
              free fatty acids, complete blood count, and platelets
        Urine: uric acid, ketones
  Second-Tier Evaluation
        Blood: plasma amino acids (quantitative), carnitine, and acylcarnitine profile,
              serum lactate, and pyruvate (and ratio)
        Urine: organic acids (quantitative)
        CSF: lactate, amino acids, and neurotransmitters

Large Molecule Metabolic Diseases
        Blood: Specific enzyme assay, gene DNA testing
        Urine: Oligosaccharides and glycosaminoglycans

Other Tests
        Neuroimaging studies: MRI, MRS, PET
        Neurophysiological tests: EEG, ERG, EMG/NCV
        Skin biopsy: OM, EM, fibroblasts culture (enzyme assay)
        Muscle biopsy (OM, EM, mitochondrial studies)
        Ophthalmological evaluation (retinal changes)
        Bone radiographs

Abbreviations: CSF, cerebrospinal fluid; MRI, magnetic resonance imaging; MRS, magnetic resonance spectroscopy; PET, positron emission tomography; EEG, electroencephalogram; ERG, electroretinogram; EMG, electromyogram; NCV, nerve conduction velocity; OM, optical microscopy; EM, electron microscopy.

The timing of samples is often critical, particularly in patients with intermittent manifestations. The ideal time to obtain samples of blood, urine, and cerebrospinal fluid (CSF) is during episodes of active symptomatology. Because immediate analysis of the samples may not be possible, appropriate collection, storage, and shipment of the samples must be undertaken. Samples should be flash frozen immediately and stored in liquid nitrogen.

Large Molecule Metabolic Diseases

They require a different approach (Box 3-3). Patients with suspected mucopolysaccharidosis, mucolipidoses, and glycoproteinoses and related disorders often excrete abnormal oligosaccharides in the urine. Qualitative screening or quantitative thin layer chromatography of urine may be diagnostic in such cases. A specific enzyme assay with or without DNA diagnosis

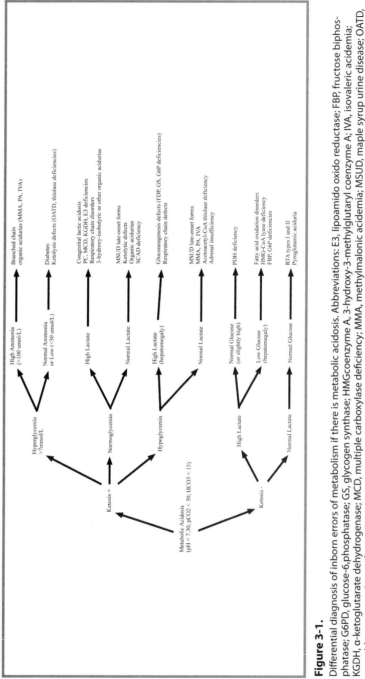

Figure 3-1.

Differential diagnosis of inborn errors of metabolism if there is metabolic acidosis. Abbreviations: E3, lipoamido oxido reductase; FBP, fructose biphosphatase; G6PD, glucose-6,phosphatase; GS, glycogen synthase; HMGcoenzyme A, 3-hydroxy-3-methylglutaryl coenzyme A; IVA, isovaleric acidemia; KGDH, α-ketoglutarate dehydrogenase; MCD, multiple carboxylase deficiency; MMA, methylmalonic acidemia; MSUD, maple syrup urine disease; OATD, oxoacid coenzyme-A transferase; PA, proprionic acidemia; PC, pyruvate carboxylase; PDH, pyruvate dehydrogenase, RTA, renal tubular acidosis; SCAD, short-chain acyl-coenzyme A dehydrogenase. (From Fernandes J, Saudubray JM, van den Berghe G, eds. *Inborn Metabolic Diseases*. Berlin: Springer-Verlag; 2000:7. Reprinted with kind permission of Springer Science & Business Media.)

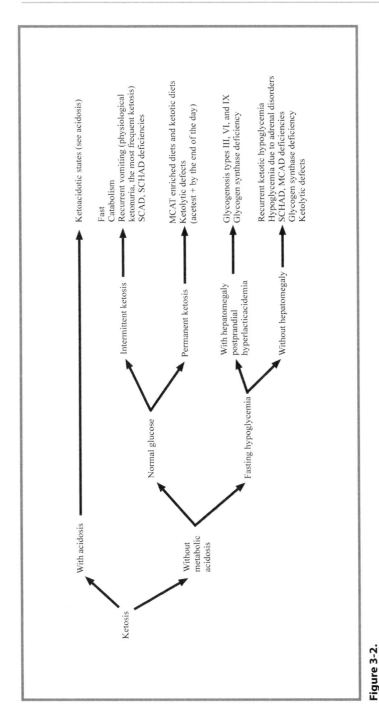

Figure 3-2.
Differential diagnosis of inborn errors of metabolism if there is ketosis. Abbreviations: MCAD, medium-chain acyl-coenzyme A dehydrogenase; MCT, medium-chain triglycerides; SCAD, short-chain acyl coenzyme A dehydrogenase; SCHAD, hydroxyl short-chain acyl-coenzyme-A dehydrogenase. (From Fernandes J, Saudubray JM, van den Berghe G, eds. *Inborn Metabolic Diseases.* Berlin: Springer-Verlag; 2000:18. Reprinted with kind permission of Springer Science & Business Media.)

may be performed for confirmation. The sphingolipidoses do not provide clues in most cases on examination of plasma or urine.

Other studies necessary to be performed in the evaluation of patients with suspected inborn errors of metabolism are enumerated in Box 3-3. All patients with abnormal neurologic signs require an imaging study, preferably magnetic resonance imaging (MRI) of the head (and spine in selected cases). Unfortunately, imaging studies may be normal in many cases until late in the illness. However, an MRI may demonstrate cerebral dysgenesis, cerebral atrophy, basal ganglia abnormalities, and white or gray matter changes in many small and large molecule metabolic disorders. In some cases, the pattern of abnormalities may allow identification of the disorder. The value of MR spectroscopy is being increasingly recognized, and it is now the imaging modality of choice for primary creatine deficiency syndromes.

Tissue biopsies for morphological study and enzyme analysis are still necessary in some cases. However, advances in DNA technology are reducing the number of cases in which this is necessary. Direct DNA diagnosis is now possible for a number of disorders. However, in most cases, it is still essential to establish the diagnosis on a biochemical basis before proceeding to DNA analysis.

Specific Small Molecule Metabolic Disorders

Amino Acid Disorders

Hereditary disorders of amino acid processing are the result of defects either in the breakdown of amino acids or the inability to get amino acids into the cells. Because these disorders produce symptoms early in life and are often treatable, newborns are routinely screened in the United States for several common ones, including phenylketonuria (PKU), maple syrup urine disease (MSUD), homocystinuria, and tyrosinemia.

Phenylketonuria

Phenylketonuria is an autosomal recessive disease caused by mutations in the gene coding for phenylalanine hydroxylase (chromosome 12q). Phenylketonuria is one of the most common IEMs, affecting 1 in 10,000 live births in whites. The inability to convert phenylalanine to tyrosine due to the deficiency of the enzyme phenylalanine hydroxylase causes an accumulation of phenylalanine. Phenylalanine is an essential amino acid that cannot be synthesized in the body but is present in a variety of foods. Phenylalanine is normally converted to tyrosine and eliminated from the body.

Clinical Characteristics

Untreated PKU produces the gradual onset of profound mental retardation in most, but not all, patients. Other clinical features in untreated patients include fair pigmentation for ethnicity, eczema, microcephaly, autistic behaviors, and stereotyped hand movements. Children often give off a mousey body and urine odor as a result of a by-product of phenylalanine (phenylacetic acid) in their urine and sweat. Neurologic signs include seizures, spasticity, hyperreflexia, and tremors.

Diagnosis

It is usually made through newborn screening with blood levels of phenylalanine in excess of 2 mg/dL or a phenylalanine to tyrosine ratio of greater than 2.5. Further diagnosis requires amino acid quantification to confirm elevated phenylalanine levels. In addition, studies for biopterin metabolism should be performed to rule out a biopterin-deficient hyperphenylalaninemia. White matter abnormalities can be seen on brain MRI.

Treatment

A low protein, phenylalanine-restricted diet with supplemental protein supplied via a medical phenylalanine formula is still the treatment of choice. Newer therapies include using a second enzyme, phenylalanine ammonia lyase to promote phenylalanine degradation through an alternative pathway, the use of large neutral amino acid supplements to block phenylalanine uptake by the carrier into the brain, and the use of biopterin (cofactor) supplementation.

Because natural sources of protein contain too much phenylalanine, children with PKU cannot have meat, milk, or other common foods that contain protein. Instead, they must eat a variety of phenylalanine-free processed foods, which are specially manufactured. They are allowed to have low-protein natural foods, such as fruits, vegetables, and restricted amounts of certain grain cereals.

A phenylalanine-restricted diet should continue for life or intelligence may decrease and neurologic and psychiatric problems may ensue.

Maple Syrup Urine Disease

Children with MSUD are unable to metabolize branched-chain amino acids
(BCAA) (leucine, isoleucine, and valine). Maple syrup urine disease is an
autosomal recessive disease caused by abnormalities in genes that code for
proteins in the branched-chain alpha-ketoacid dehydrogenase. The incidence in all newborns is 1 in 216,000. However, it is more common in the
Mennonite population, with an incidence of 1 in 760.

Clinical Characteristics

Classical MSUD in untreated neonates presents with ketonuria, irritability,
and poor feeding progressing to encephalopathy with lethargy, intermittent
apnea, opisthotonus, and stereotyped movements. Coma, central respiratory
failure, and death may occur secondary to cerebral edema within the first
week of life.

Rarely, affected individuals have a partial enzyme deficiency that only
manifests intermittently. These patients can experience severe encephalopathy and intermittent ataxia under catabolic stress such as infection or
surgery. This form of MSUD can respond to thiamine therapy.

Diagnosis

The first clinical sign of MSUD may be the sweet-smelling diaper or ceru-
min. A bedside diagnosis can be made using the dinitrophenylhydrazine
reaction on urine, which produces a yellow-white precipitate. An MRI
demonstrating localization of edema only to the cerebellum and posterior
internal capsule may be pathognomonic.

Confirmation of the diagnosis is based on the presence of increased
levels of leucine, valine, and isoleucine in plasma amino acids. Quantitative analysis of these amino acids in plasma and urine is performed by ion
exchange or high-performance liquid chromatography. In classic MSUD,
plasma leucine concentration will be greater than 400 μM at 48 hours, and
often may be well above 2,000 μM. Alloisoleucine is the pathognomonic
amino acid in MSUD. In some states, newborns are routinely screened for
MSUD. Molecular genetic testing is also available

Treatment

It includes dietary leucine restriction, high-calorie BCAA-free formulas, and
frequent monitoring. Metabolic decompensation is corrected by treating

the precipitating stress while delivering sufficient calories, insulin, free amino acids, isoleucine, and valine, and in some centers, hemodialysis/hemofiltration. Cerebral edema is a common complication of metabolic decompensation. Liver transplantation is an effective therapy for classic MSUD.

Homocystinuria

The disorder is biochemically characterized by the inability to metabolize the amino acid homocysteine due to cystathionine β-synthase deficiency. As a consequence, there is accumulation of homocysteine, methionine, and a variety of other metabolites of homocysteine in the body which, ultimately, are excreted in the urine.

Clinical Characteristics

Cystathionine β-synthase deficiency represents a multisystem disorder that affects the eyes, integument, skeleton, vascular system, and nervous system. Homocystinuria is usually asymptomatic in the neonate. If untreated, these children eventually develop mental retardation, ectopia lentis, a marfanoid appearance, osteoporosis, other skeletal deformities, and thromboembolism. The first symptoms usually involve the eyes. Ectopia lentis is the most readily recognizable manifestation of the disease. It may be the only manifestation. Dislocation is usually present by 10 years of age. The dislocation is usually downward as opposed to the upward dislocation usually seen in Marfan syndrome. The body type is classically tall and thin with a curved spine, elongated limbs, and long fingers. Osteoporosis is the most common skeletal finding, and half of all patients will have osteoporotic changes of the spine by the age of 16 years. A number of other skeletal abnormalities including, genu valgum, everted feet, pectus excavatum or carinatum, and scoliosis may also be seen. Psychiatric and behavioral disorders and mental retardation are common. Thromboembolism is the major cause of morbidity and the most frequent cause of death. High homocysteine concentrations adversely affect collagen metabolism and are responsible for intimal thickening of blood vessel walls leading to arterial and venous thromboembolic disease. Vascular occlusion can occur in any vessel and at any age, including infancy.

Diagnosis

Diagnostic confirmation is made through newborn screening or quantitative plasma amino acids demonstrating increased homcysteine and methionine in classical homocystinuria. Cystathionine β-synthase enzyme activity is decreased. Molecular genetic diagnosis is available.

Treatment

Almost half of all patients with cystathionine β-synthase deficiency are responsive to vitamin B_6 (200 mg/d), and this treatment alone will often reduce plasma homocysteine levels. With treatment, all of these patients will eventually become folate and B_{12} depleted and will need supplementation. Most pyridoxine-responsive patients cannot achieve a normal level of homocysteine on pyridoxine, folate, and B_{12} treatment alone. The addition of a protein-restricted diet and methionine-free amino acid supplement will result in near-normal total homocysteine levels in most patients. Treatment with betaine, 5 to 10 g/d in 2 divided doses, provides an alternate remethylation pathway to convert excess homocysteine to methionine and may help prevent thrombosis.

Tyrosinemia

Children with tyrosinemia are unable to completely metabolize the amino acid tyrosine.

There are 2 main types of tyrosinemia: I and II. Type I tyrosinemia is most common in children of French-Canadian or Scandinavian descent. Tyrosinemia type I results from deficiency of the enzyme fumarylaceto-acetate hydrolase (FAH). Typical biochemical findings include increased succinylacetone concentration in the blood and urine and elevated plasma concentrations of tyrosine, methionine, and phenylalanine.

Clinical Characteristics

Untreated tyrosinemia type I usually presents either in young infants with severe liver involvement or later in the first year of life with liver dysfunction and renal tubular dysfunction associated with growth failure and rickets. Patients may have episodes of change in mental status, abdominal pain, peripheral neuropathy, and respiratory failure. If untreated, death usually occurs before the age of 10 years from liver failure, neurologic crisis, or hepatocellular carcinoma.

Type II tyrosinemia is less common. Affected children may have mental retardation and hyperkeratosis of the skin, and corneal ulcers.

Diagnosis

It is made through newborn screening or quantitative plasma amino acids. Elevated plasma concentrations of tyrosine, methionine, and phenylalanine are present. However, elevated urinary succinylacetone concentration is a key finding. Elevated concentration of tyrosine or methionine in the blood suggests tryrosinemia type I and should be further evaluated by the quantification of urinary succinylacetone. Molecular genetic testing by targeted mutation analysis for the 4 common FAH mutations and sequence analysis are clinically available and can detect mutations in more than 95% of affected individuals.

Unfortunately, infants with tyrosinemia type I may have only modestly elevated or even normal blood concentrations of tyrosine and methionine when the first newborn screening sample is collected. Increases in serum concentration of alpha fetoprotein (AFP) and prothrombin time/partial thromboplastin time (PT/PTT) are more severe in tyrosinemia type I than in nonspecific liver disease and are often the presenting findings in tyrosinemia type I. Transaminases and bilirubin may only be slightly elevated, if at all. The presence of a normal serum concentration of AFP and a normal PT/PTT makes the diagnosis of tyrosinemia type I extremely unlikely.

Treatment

Combined treatment with nitisinone (Orfadin), 2-(2-nitro-4-trifluoro-methylbenzoyl)-1,3 cyclohexanedione, and a low-tyrosine diet has resulted in a greater than 90% survival rate, with normal growth and improved liver function. Often, children with type I tyrosinemia require a liver transplant. Type II tyrosinemia is less common. Affected children may have mental retardation and hyperkeratosis of the skin, and corneal ulcers. In type II tyrosinemia, unlike in type I tyrosinemia, restriction of dietary tyrosine alone can prevent the development of clinical symptoms.

Organic Acid Disorders

The term *organic aciduria* (OA) applies to a group of disorders characterized by the excretion of organic acids in the urine. Most organic acid disorders result from dysfunction of amino acid catabolism, usually the result of deficient enzyme activity. Most classic organic acid disorders are caused by abnormal amino acid catabolism of BCAA (Box 3-4).

Box 3-4. Organic Acid Disorders

Propionic academia
Methylmalonic acidemia
3-methylcrotonyl-CoA carboxylase deficiency
3-hydroxy-3-methylglutaryl-CoA lyase deficiency
Ketothiolase deficiency
Glutaric aciduria type I

Neonates affected with an OA are usually well at birth and for the first few days of life. The clinical presentation includes vomiting, poor feeding, seizures, abnormal muscle tone, and lethargy progressing to coma. In older children or adolescents, variant forms of the OAs can present as loss of intellectual function, ataxia or other focal neurologic signs, Reye syndrome, recurrent ketoacidosis, or psychiatric symptoms. A variety of MRI abnormalities have been described in the OAs, including distinctive atrophy with wide opening of the Sylvian fissures and basal ganglia lesions in glutaric aciduria type I (Figure 3-3) and abnormalities of the globus pallidus in methylmalonic acidemia. Isolated biotin-resistant 3-methylcrotonyl-CoA carboxylase deficiency is an autosomal recessive disorder of leucine catabolism that seems to be the most frequent OA detected in tandem MS–based neonatal screening programs. The phenotype is variable, ranging from neonatal onset with severe neurologic involvement to asymptomatic adults.

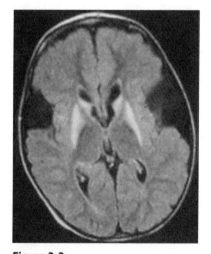

Figure 3-3.
Glutaric aciduria type I. Axial FLAIR (fluid attenuation inversion recovery) image shows large Sylvian fissures and abnormal hyperintense signal in the basal ganglia. (From Faerber EN, Poussaint TY. Magnetic resonance of metabolic and degenerative diseases in children. *Top Magn Reson Imaging.* 2002;13:3–21. Reprinted with permission from Wolters Kluwer Health.)

Diagnosis

Clinical laboratory findings that suggest an organic acid disorder in the neonatal period include acidosis, positive urine ketones (rarely seen in neonates), hyperammonemia, abnormal liver function tests, hypoglycemia, and neutropenia. First-line diagnosis in the OA disorders is urine organic acid analysis using gas chromatography with mass spectrometry. The urinary organic acid profile is usually abnormal in the face of acute illness with decompensation. However, in some organic acid disorders laboratory testing may be normal if an individual is not acutely ill. Depending on the specific disorder, plasma amino acid analysis can also be helpful. Confirmation of the OA disorders can be done by measuring the activity of the deficient enzyme in lymphocytes or cultured fibroblasts. Molecular genetic testing is clinically available for proprionic acidemia, methylmalonic acidemia, biotin-unresponsive 3-methylcrotonyl-CoA carboxylase deficiency, isovaleric acidemia, and glutaric aciduria type I.

Treatment

Neonates demand emergency diagnosis and treatment depending on the specific biochemical defect. Treatment strategies include dietary restriction of the precursor amino acids and the use of adjunctive compounds to dispose of toxic metabolites or increase activity of deficient enzymes. Metabolic decompensation caused by catabolic stress, such as vomiting, diarrhea, febrile illness, and decreased oral intake, requires aggressive intervention, which may include hemodialysis.

Urea Cycle Defects

The urea cycle disorders result from defects in the metabolism of nitrogen produced by the breakdown of protein and other nitrogen-containing molecules. Severe deficiency of activity of any of the first 4 enzymes (carbamyl phosphate synthase I [CPSI], ornithine transcarbamylase [OTC], argininosuccinate synthase [ASS], and argininosuccinate lyase [ASL]) in the urea cycle or the cofactor (N-acetylglutamate synthase [NAGS]) results in the accumulation of ammonia and other precursor metabolites.

Clinical Characteristics

Infants with a urea cycle disorder appear normal initially, but over 48 to 72 hours develop cerebral edema leading to lethargy, hyperventilation or hypoventilation, hypothermia, seizures, and coma. In milder urea cycle enzyme deficiencies, increases in plasma ammonia may be triggered by illness or stress at almost any time of life. The hyperammonemia is less severe and the symptoms may be more subtle in terms of the change in mental status. In individuals with partial enzyme deficiencies, the clinical episodes may be delayed for years and be triggered by illness or a high-protein meal.

Diagnosis

Mental status changes with a plasma ammonia concentration of 200 μmol/L or greater associated with a respiratory alkalosis or a normal anion gap and a normal serum glucose concentration support a diagnosis of a urea cycle disorder. Plasma quantitative amino acid analysis can be used to diagnose a specific urea cycle disorder. The plasma concentration of citrulline helps differentiate proximal and distal urea cycle defects. Citrulline is elevated with defects of the distal enzymes (ASS, ASL, and arginase [ARG]). Urinary orotic acid is needed to distinguish CPSI deficiency and NAGS deficiency from OTC deficiency; it is elevated in OTC deficiency. The definitive diagnosis of CPSI deficiency, OTC deficiency, or NAGS deficiency depends on determination of enzyme activity from a liver biopsy specimen. Molecular genetic testing for OTC deficiency is clinically available in the United States. Molecular genetic testing for CPSI deficiency, NAGS deficiency, citrullinemia type I, ARG deficiency, and argininosuccinic aciduria is clinically available. Deficiencies of CPSI, ASS, ASL, NAGS, and ARG are inherited in an autosomal recessive manner. Ornithine transcarbamylase deficiency is inherited in an X-linked manner.

Treatment

Emergency treatment regimens for urea cycle disorders include dialysis to reduce plasma ammonia concentration, intravenous administration of arginine chloride, and nitrogen scavenger drugs to allow alternative pathway excretion of excess nitrogen, and restriction of protein for 24 to 48 hours. However, calories must be provided in the form of intravenous glucose and intralipids with protein-free formula to reduce catabolism.

Long-term treatment requires special diet and scavenger compounds that decrease ammonia levels by stimulating alternative pathways for waste nitrogen excretion (phenylbutyrate or Buphenyl). Patients require a careful monitoring of growth and development.

Fatty Acid Oxidation Defects

Fatty acid oxidation disorders are a group of inherited metabolic conditions resulting from enzyme defects affecting the ability of the body to oxidize fatty acids to produce energy within muscles, liver, and other cell types. Each fatty acid oxidation disorder is associated with a specific enzyme defect in the metabolic pathway that affects use of stored fat (Box 3-5). During fasting states, free fatty acids are released into the blood, where they are taken up by the liver and muscle cells and activated to coenzyme-A esters. They are transported into the mitochondria and oxidized by sequential reactions that are each catalyzed by one of multiple enzymes.

The acyl-CoA dehydrogenases are chain-length specific enzymes. Deficiencies or abnormalities in these result in very-long-chain acyl-CoA dehydrogenase deficiency (VLCAD), long-chain acyl-CoA dehydrogenase deficiency (LCAD), medium-chain acyl-CoA dehydrogenase deficiency (MCAD), short-chain acyl-CoA dehydrogenase deficiency (SCAD), and long-chain 3-hydroxyl acyl-CoA dehydrogenase. Illness may lead to a fasting state that depletes glucose stores. Once this occurs, fatty acid metabolism becomes the dominant energy source. If there is an abnormality in fatty acid metabolism, life-threatening episodes of metabolic decompensation and encephalopathy can occur.

Medium-chain acyl-CoA dehydrogenase deficiency is the most common of the fatty acid oxidation disorders, with an incidence of approximately one in 10,000 to 20,000 births. Long-chain 3-hydroxyl acyl-CoA dehydrogenase deficiency and VLCAD are rare disorders with an estimated incidence of 1

Box 3-5. Fatty Oxidation Disorders

LCAD, VLCAD, MCAD, and SCAD
Multiple acyl-CoA dehydrogenase deficiency (glutaric aciduria type II)
Trifunctional enzyme deficiency
CPT I (uptake defect) and CPT II (translocase)
Acetoacetyl-CoA thiolase
LC 3-hydroxyacyl-CoA dehydrogenase
LCHAD

Abbreviations: LC, long chain; AD, acyl-CoA dehydrogenase; VLC, very long chain; MC, medium chain; SC, small chain; CPT, carnitine palmityl transferase; LCH, long chain hydroxyl.

in 100,000 births. There is a mild form of SCAD deficiency that seems to be quite common, but the clinical significance of this condition is unclear.

Clinical Characteristics

Patients with fatty acid oxidation disorders may present with hypoketotic hypoglycemia, liver disease, near SIDS, encephalopathy, myopathy, cardiomyopathy, or sudden death. Symptoms may appear at any age from birth to adult life. It is important to note that fatty acid oxidation defects are very often associated with cardiomyopathy. Children with the most common fatty acid oxidation disorder, MCAD, are typically normal at birth and develop episodes of hypoketotic hypoglycemia, vomiting, lethargy, and seizures associated with fasting. Very-long-chain acyl-CoA dehydrogenase deficiency and LCAD are very similar clinically and can present with SIDS, hypoglycemia, hepatomegaly, myopathy, Reye syndrome, and cardiomyopathy.

Diagnosis

Diagnosis is made by obtaining a plasma acylcarnitine profile. Urine organic acids in these patients typically show elevations of dicarboxylic acids. Diagnosis may be confirmed by enzyme assay in fibroblasts. Gene mutation analysis is available.

Short-chain acyl-CoA dehydrogenase deficiency does not present with deficits in energy metabolism, but rather may present in the neonatal period with failure to thrive and hypotonia. Hypoglycemia is not a common feature. Urine organic acids in SCAD reveal increased excretion of ethylmalonic acid and butyrylcarnitine. Diagnosis is confirmed by enzyme assay in fibroblasts.

Most of these conditions are chronic, with lifelong episodes of hypoglycemia. In some of the more severe infantile forms, there is a very poor prognosis.

Treatment

For most fatty acid oxidation disorders, including MCAD, management involves avoidance of fasting in addition to dietary management. During illness, aggressive management is necessary: The patient should be admitted for intravenous dextrose (at least 10%) and normal saline at 1.5 maintenance to prevent hypoglycemia. Supplemental carnitine, a low-fat diet, and home glucose monitoring are often part of daily management. Current standard of care seems to focus on fat restriction and increased meal frequency, with the increasing use of cornstarch and/or carnitine supplementation. The clinical efficacy of medium-chain triglyceride oil, lipid substrates, and special medical foods requires further study before being recommended as a standard treatment.

Mitochondrial Disorders

Mitochondrial diseases represent an extremely diverse group of inherited disorders of energy metabolism that encompass a wide range of symptoms and presentations, severity, and outcome. They form one of the most prevalent groups of inherited metabolic diseases. However, given the diversity of clinical presentations and due to the difficulty in establishing a diagnosis, they must be considered in the differential diagnosis of a variety of clinical symptoms and signs.

The terms *mitochondrial cytopathies* and *mitochondrial diseases* are usually reserved for disorders of oxidative phosphorylation (OXPHOS). A series of chemical reactions result in the phosphorylation of adenosine diphosphate to adenosine triphosphate (ATP) by the process of OXPHOS, which occurs in enzyme complexes imbedded in the inner mitochondrial membrane that make up the electron transport chain. The mitochondria also play important roles in the generation of free radicals and apoptosis.

Mitochondria are a fundamental component of cellular metabolism and, thus, any organ can be involved in mitochondrial disease. Mitochondrial disorders are not diseases of specific organs, but rather a disease of an organelle supplying energy to a variety of organs. Therefore, symptoms of altered energy production are more severe in organs and tissues with high-energy requirements such as muscle, heart, and brain.

There are many mitochondrial cytopathies with overlapping clinical features. A useful way to divide these diseases is according to type of mutation and gene product that is affected. Box 3-6 shows a list of possible mutations in mitochondrial DNA (mtDNA) or nuclear DNA and a representative selection of the abnormal phenotypes that can occur. It is important to point out that in mitochondrial cytopathies, mutations in different genes can lead to the same phenotype.

Box 3-6. Mitochondrial Disorders

Mutations in mitochondrial DNA
  Point mutations: MERRF, MELAS, LHON, NARP
  Large-scale deletions: KSS, Pearson syndrome, progressive external
    ophthalmoplegia
  Polypeptide subunits of OXPHOS: MELAS, LHON, Leigh syndrome

Mutations in nuclear DNA
  Mitochondrial biogenesis disorders
    DDP1 mutations: X-linked deafness-dystonia syndrome
    ABC7 mutations: X-linked ataxia and sideroblastic anemia
    TAZ mutations: Barth syndrome
  Polypeptide subunits of OXPHOS: Leigh syndrome, cardiomyopathy,
    paraganglioma, pheochromocytoma
  Assembly proteins disorders
    SURF1 mutations: Leigh syndrome
    COX15 mutations: hypertrophic cardiomyopathy

Proteins for mitochondrial DNA maintenance disorders
  Multiple mitochondrial DNA deletions
    Twinkle mutations: PEO
  Mitochondrial DNA depletion syndromes
    TK2 mutations: SMA-like syndrome

Abbreviations: MERRF, myoencephalopathy, ragged red fibers; MELAS, myoencephalopathy, lactic acidosis, and stroke-like episodes; LHON, Leber hereditary optic neuropathy; NARP, neurogenic ataxia and retinitis pigmentosa; KSS, Kearns-Sayre syndrome; OXPHOS, oxidative phosphorylation; PEO, progressive external ophthalmoplegia; SMA, spinal muscular atrophy.

Clinical Characteristics

The most common central nervous system findings of mitochondrial diseases are chronic encephalopathy, seizures, dementia, migraine, stroke-like episodes, ataxia, and spasticity. Chorea and dementia may also be prominent features. Other clinical symptoms include ptosis, external ophthalmoplegia, proximal myopathy and exercise intolerance, cardiomyopathy, sensorineural deafness, optic atrophy, pigmentary retinopathy, and diabetes mellitus. Diabetes mellitus and deafness are also well-recognized clinical phenotypes (including DIDMOAD or Wolfram syndrome). Recent literature has focused on the association of autism with mitochondrial disease.

Examples of classic mitochondrial diseases include Kearns-Sayre syndrome, which usually presents with ophthalmoplegia, retinopathy, cardiac conduction defects, ataxia, and short stature. Symptoms of episodic vomiting, lactic acidosis, myopathy, seizures, stroke-like events, and short stature characterize mitochondrial myoencephalopathy, lactic acidosis, and stroke-like episodes. Myoclonic epilepsy with ragged red fibers is characterized by myoclonus, epilepsy, ataxia, and myopathy with ragged red fibers. Leber hereditary optic neuropathy typically presents with blindness in men. Respiratory irregularities and myopathic weakness with visual and hearing impairments often signal Leigh syndrome.

Magnetic resonance imaging frequently shows typical abnormalities of the basal ganglia (Figure 3-4), and white matter changes. Magnetic resonance spectroscopy demonstrates elevated lactate levels.

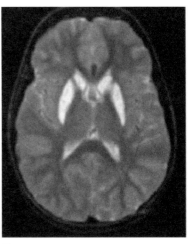

Figure 3-4.
Mitochondrial disorder. Leigh disease due to complex I deficiency. T2-weighted imaging shows abnormal hyperintense signal bilaterally within the caudate and globus pallidus. (From Cecil KM. MR spectroscopy of metabolic disorders. *Neuroimaging Clin N Am.* 2006;16:87–116 with permission from Elsevier.)

Diagnosis

The diagnosis of mitochondrial disease can be done on the basis of genetics; biochemical defects found in serum, CSF, or muscle; or clinical symptomatology. Pathogenic mtDNA mutations are found in many adults with a suspected mitochondrial defect. Unfortunately, mtDNA mutations are usually identified in only a small proportion of pediatric patients. In pediatric mitochondrial disorders, the diagnosis relies mostly on muscle biopsy and enzymatic investigations, which are often difficult to interpret. Therefore, establishing a reliable diagnosis is more difficult in the pediatric population. Diagnostic clinical criteria for mitochondrial disorders in children have been modified from an adult classification system referred to as the *modified Walker criteria,* which focuses on clinical symptoms, histology, enzymology, and molecular studies.

The genetics of mitochondrial disorders are different from most metabolic disorders. Oxidative phosphorylation disorders can be due to mutations in both nuclear and mtDNA. Most disorders express an autosomal recessive or mitochondrial inheritance pattern. Except for rare occasions, all mitochondria are inherited from the maternal line. Mitochondria in sperm are not viable. Therefore, mutations in mtDNA can only be inherited through the maternal lineage. However, some OXPHOS disorders are inherited in an autosomal dominant or X-linked pattern because other parts of the mitochondria are determined via nuclear DNA. Another important factor is that the number of mtDNA can range from hundreds to thousands in a single cell. There can be up to 5 different mtDNA sequences per cell (polyplasmy). The mtDNA genomes of a particular cell can contain all normal genomes or all mutated genomes (homoplasmy). However, there can be a mixture of normal and mutated genomes within a cell (heteroplasmy). A single mitochondrion can have both normal and mutated genomes.

Treatment

Due to the diversity of biochemical and genetic defects, there are limited data regarding proven effective therapies. Treatments for mitochondrial disorders are intended to increase energy production and reduce the production of toxic metabolites that may damage cellular energy production. Treatment is usually focused on increasing respiratory chain activity by various dietary manipulations and vitamins as well as supplementation with cofactors required for proper functioning. Patients should avoid prolonged periods without a meal. Frequent small meals should be given to maintain normoglycemia. Patients may be unable to tolerate overnight fasting. A bedtime snack consisting of complex carbohydrates may stave off clinical problems. Uncooked cornstarch is a good source of complex carbohydrates, but is often unpalatable to children.

Coenzyme Q10 (CoQ10) is the most widely recognized supplement used in the treatment of mitochondrial disorders. There are anecdotal reports of decreased serum lactate, improved exercise tolerance, and increased muscle strength. As an antioxidant, it has a role in limiting free radical production, which is known to increase in mitochondrial disease. It is the therapy for patients with CoQ10 deficiency.

The role of carnitine therapy in mitochondrial disease is varied. Carnitine plays a role in reestablishing homeostasis of acyl groups. In addition, secondary carnitine deficiency exists in the setting of mitochondrial cytopathies. Therefore, carnitine replacement may be helpful. Finally, carnitine may provide improved integrity of the mitochondrial membrane.

Patients with a suspected mitochondrial disease are often placed on a combination of coQ10, carnitine, vitamin E, and a balanced B vitamin supplement. The use of creatine as a supplement for energy production is now gaining support in the literature. Other vitamin supplements are also used; however, the evidence to support vitamin and supplement therapy remains largely anecdotal.

The risk for malignant hyperthermia may be a consideration in mitochondrial dysfunction, especially if myopathy is present.

Neurotransmitter Metabolism Disorders

Neurotransmitter metabolic disorders involve problems with the synthesis of the biogenic amines (dopamine, norepinephrine, epinephrine), serotonin, and γ-aminobutyric acid. The neurotransmitter defects also include defects in the synthesis and recycling of tetrahydrobiopterin, a cofactor for the enzymes tyrosine hydroxylase, phenylalanine hydroxylase, and tryptophan hydroxylase. Box 3-7 shows a list of the known disorders in this category of metabolic diseases. The biogenic amine synthesis disorders are usually divided into 2 categories: diseases usually associated with hyperphenylalaninemia and diseases not associated with hyperphenylalaninemia.

Clinical Characteristics

The clinical presentation of these disorders usually begins in infancy or childhood. Neurologic signs and symptoms include trunkal hypotonia, choreoathetosis, ptosis, hypokinetic parkinsonism, tremor, oculogyric crises, and developmental delay or mental retardation. A prominent symptom is often lower extremity dystonia that can be mistaken for spastic cerebral palsy. Other clinical features may include hypersalivation, temperature instability, and excessive sweating. A key finding that suggests the possibility of the neurotransmitter disorders is the presence of diurnal fluctuation in symptoms.

Diagnosis

Because none of the above symptoms is pathognomonic for the neurotransmitter disorders and the diseases can cause multiple neurologic symptoms,

---

Box 3-7. Neurotrasmitter Disorders

Disorders of Biogenic Amine Synthesis With Hyperphenylalaninemia
    GTP cyclohydrolase deficiency
    6-pyruvoyl-tetrahydropterin synthase
    Dihydropteridine reductase deficiency
    Pterin carbinolamine-4alpha-dehydratase

Disorders of Biogenic Amine Synthesis With Hyperphenylalaninemia
    Dopa-responsive dystonia or autosomal dominant GTPCH deficiency
    Sepiapterin reductase deficiency
    Tyrosine hydroxylase deficiency (see below)
    Aromatic L-amino acid decarboxylase
    Dopamine β-hydroxylase deficiency
    MAO-A deficiency
    3-phosphoglycerate dehydrogenase deficiency
    Pyrroline-5-carboxylate synthase deficiency

GABA Metabolism Disorders
    GABA transaminase deficiency
    Succinic semialdehyde dehydrogenase deficiency

Abbreviations: GTP, guanosine triphosphate; GTPCH, guanosine triphosphate cyclohydrolase; MAO, monoamine oxidase; GABA, γ-aminobutyric acid.

---

it is important to consider neurotransmitter disorders when evaluating a patient with a neurologic disease whose etiology is unknown. The diagnostic confirmation of neurotransmitter disorders requires the examination of the CSF for neurotransmitter metabolite analysis. Unfortunately, CSF collection for the evaluation of neurotransmitter diseases requires specialized tubes supplied by the very few laboratories that perform the necessary analysis.

Treatment

Treatment depends on the specific defect, but can involve supplementation with L-dopa, dopamine agonists, tetrahydrobiopterin, and serotonin.

Disorders of Carbohydrate Metabolism

Galactosemia

Galactosemia is an autosomal recessive disorder of galactose metabolism due to a deficiency of galactose-1-phosphate uridyltransferase (GALT).

Clinical Characteristics

Clinical symptoms of classic galactosemia include feeding problems, hypoglycemia, failure to thrive, hepatocellular damage manifested as bleeding, and prolonged jaundice. If not promptly treated, hyperammonemia, sepsis due to *Escherichia coli*, and shock develop. Cataracts are present in10% of patients, even in the neonatal period.

Even with treatment, children with galactosemia remain at increased risk for developmental delays, speech problems, and abnormalities of motor function. Females with galactosemia are at increased risk for premature ovarian failure.

Diagnosis

The diagnosis of galactosemia is established by measurement of GALT enzymatic activity. In classic (G/G) galactosemia, GALT enzyme activity is less than 5% of control values; in Duarte variant (D/G) galactosemia, GALT enzyme activity is between 5% and 20% of control values. Genetic testing is clinically available (gene map locus is 9p13). Virtually all affected infants are detected in newborn screening programs.

Treatment

A lactose-galactose–restricted diet is the treatment of choice and, if provided early on, the neonatal symptoms quickly resolve. Lactose should be removed from the diet of an infant suspected of having galactosemia while results of biochemical and molecular testing are pending. Immediate dietary intervention is needed in infants with GALT enzyme activity less than 10% of control activity. Milk products should be replaced immediately with formulas containing sucrose, fructose, and non-galactose polycarbohydrates without any bioavailable lactose (eg, Isomil or Prosobee). Infants who survive the newborn period with classical galactosemia who continue to drink milk that contains galactose develop mental retardation and ataxia. There is debate whether galactose intake should be restricted in infants and children with

5% to 20% of control GALT enzyme activity. Referral to an endocrinologist or a metabolic center should be done as early as possible.

Fructose 1-Phosphate Aldolase Deficiency (Hereditary Fructose Intolerance)

Hereditary fructose intolerance is a rare autosomal recessive disorder of fructose metabolism due to a deficiency of fructose-1-phosphate aldolase activity. As a result, there is an accumulation of fructose-1-phosphate in the liver, kidneys, and small intestine. In infants, there is marked intolerance to fruits and vegetables. The fructose-1-phospate blocks the formation of glycogen and its conversion to glucose, resulting in hypoglycemia.

Clinical Characteristics

Acutely ill children are usually tachypneic due to a metabolic acidosis with a renal Fanconi syndrome. Patients will often have enlarged liver with coagulopathy and may be icteric. The hypoglycemia is associated with sweating, confusion, and sometimes seizures and coma. Children who continue to eat foods containing fructose develop kidney and liver damage, resulting in jaundice, vomiting, mental deterioration, and seizures. Chronic symptoms include cachexia, failure to thrive, liver failure, and kidney damage.

Diagnosis

Clinical diagnosis is usually based on the patient's dietary history. The presence of a non–glucose-reducing sugar in the urine will often confirm the diagnosis during an acute illness. This is readily accomplished with Clinitest. Confirmatory diagnosis of hereditary fructose intolerance relies on the fructose tolerance test that measures clinical symptoms on intravenous fructose challenge and direct assay of aldolase activity in liver biopsy samples.

Treatment

Definitive treatment consists of eliminating fructose from the diet. Eliminating fructose early in the disease course results in a good long-term outcome. Prolonged delay in diagnosis may result in cirrhotic liver changes with subsequent degeneration of hepatic function.

Specific Large Molecule Metabolic Disorders

Peroxisomal Disorders

The different types of peroxisomal disorders are enumerated in Box 3-8. In peroxisomal disorders, such as Zellweger syndrome, neonatal adrenoleukodystrophy (ALD), and infantile Refsum disease, peroxisomes are absent, decreased in number, or severely abnormal, resulting in defects in the multiple metabolic pathways. In contrast, in a subgroup of peroxisomal disorders due to single enzyme defects, the organelles are present but distinct peroxisomal enzymes are absent or defective.

Clinical Characteristics

Individuals with Zellweger syndrome usually present in the newborn period or later in childhood. Newborns have profound hypotonia and poor feeding. Neonatal seizures are a frequent complication. Liver dysfunction may present as neonatal jaundice with elevation in liver enzymes. Dysmorphic features include flattened facies, large anterior fontanelle, widely split sutures, and a broad nasal bridge. In severely affected children, bony stippling (chondrodysplasia punctata) at the patellae is often seen.

In older children, retinal dystrophy, sensorineural hearing loss, developmental delay, and liver dysfunction are the presenting symptoms. Children who present with both sensorineural hearing loss and visual problems should be considered at risk for peroxisomal disorders. Older children may develop adrenal insufficiency.

Box 3-8. Peroxisomal Disorders

Disorders of peroxisomal biogenesis and maintenance
    Zellweger syndrome
    Neonatal adrenoleukodystrophy (ALD)

Multiple peroxisomal enzyme deficiency
    Rhizomelic chondrodysplasia punctata

Single peroxisomal enzyme deficiency
    X-linked ALD
    Classic Refsum disease
    Hyperoxaluria type I
    Acatalasemia

The course of neonatal ALD and infantile Refsum disease is clinically variable and may include nonspecific developmental delays, hearing loss, vision impairment, liver dysfunction, episodes of hemorrhage, and intracranial bleeding. While some children can be very hypotonic, others may walk and talk. The condition may be slowly progressive in these children.

Childhood cerebral X-linked ALD is the most severe type of ALD. Patients usually show normal development until they reach 4 to 10 years of age, at which time behavioral changes including memory impairment and emotional instability. Progressive deterioration of vision, hearing, and motor function rapidly follow. In addition, adrenal dysfunction or gonadal insufficiency may be seen. The average time between the initial symptoms and a vegetative state or death is approximately 2 years, although it can range anywhere from 6 months to 20 years. A small number of patients with X-linked ALD will present between the ages of 11 and 21 years. The symptoms are similar to those of childhood cerebral ALD, but progression of the disease is often slower.

Diagnosis

The diagnosis of peroxisomal disorders is usually made via measurement of plasma very-long-chain fatty acid levels. There is elevation of C26:0 and C26:1 and the ratios C24/C22 and C26/C22. Adrenal function is abnormal in 90% of neurologically symptomatic patients with childhood cerebral X-linked ALD. Genetic testing via DNA linkage analysis has been used primarily to determine carrier status in at-risk female relatives and for prenatal diagnosis when the nature of the familial mutation is known. In Zellweger syndrome, MRI studies may reveal hypomyelination, cortical gyral abnormalities, and cysts. Diffusion weighted imaging and diffusion tensor imaging may show white matter changes not detected by standard MRI. In neonatal ALD, children may develop progressive degeneration of the myelin on MRI, which correlates with loss of previously acquired milestones. In childhood X-linked ALD, MRI findings usually demonstrate bilateral symmetrical involvement of the parieto-occipital white matter.

Treatment

At present, there is no therapy offering complete cure. However, dietary modifications with Lorenzo's oil, medications, or bone marrow transplantation often can modify the clinical course.

Lysosomal Storage Disorders

The lysosomal storage disorders are a group of more than 40 conditions resulting from defects in lysosomal function. Lysosomes are cytoplasmic organelles containing enzymes that break down macromolecules to peptides, amino acids, monosaccharides, nucleic acids, and fatty acids. In lysosomal storage disorders, the activity of one or more of the lysosomal enzymes is deficient. Deposition of the non-degraded substrate within the organelles interferes with cell function. The lysosomal storage disorders can be grossly subdivided into 5 categories depending on the class of substance stored (Box 3-9).

Clinical Characteristics

It is difficult to generalize the symptoms of lysosomal storage disorders. Although the diseases share a common pathogenesis, the different types of substrate stored and locations of storage lead to tremendous clinical variability. These disorders should be considered in the differential diagnosis of patients having developmental delay, loss of learned skills or dementia,

---

Box 3-9. Lysosomal Storage Disorders

Sphingolipidoses
  GM1 and GM2 gangliosidoses
  Pompe disease (also glycogen storage disease)
  Fabry disease
  Niemann-Pick (types A, B, and C)
  Krabbe disease
  Gaucher disease
  Metachromatic leukodystrophy
Mucopolysaccharidoses
  Hurler disease
  Scheie disease
  Hunter disease
  Sanfilippo disease
  Morquio disease
  Marotaux Lamy disease
  Sly disease
Mucolipidoses
Neuronal ceroid lipofuscinosis
Glycoproteinoses
Fucosidosis

ataxia, seizures, or weakness. This is especially true if the individual is regressing after a period of relatively normal development and the condition seems progressive. Overall, all clinical manifestations worsen over time, as more substrate continues to accumulate.

As a group, lysosomal storage disorders affect nearly every body system, and symptoms can vary in severity from relatively mild somatic manifestations to severe and rapidly progressing degenerative neurologic disorders. While no single symptom defines these disorders there are some symptoms or signs that can be considered red flags (Box 3-10).

Diagnosis

The diagnosis should be suspected in the presence of clinical features with degenerative signs, like loss of motor skills, increasing dementia or behavioral abnormalities, and muscular or neurologic deterioration. In suspected cases, purely neurologic symptoms in the absence of findings, such as coarse facial features, bone abnormalities, and hepatosplenomegaly, should lead to testing for GM1 and GM2 gangliosidoses, metachromatic leukodystrophy, and Krabbe disease. Patients with mild to severe neurologic symptoms who also have evidence of suggestive clinical features (Box 3-10) usually require extensive testing to arrive at a definitive diagnosis. About 10% of infants born with nonimmune fetal hydrops have a lysosomal storage disorder.

Box 3-10. Clinical Findings Suspicious of Lysosomal Storage Disease

Coarse facial features (sometimes with macroglossia)
Corneal clouding or related ocular abnormalities
Angiokeratoma
Umbilical/inguinal hernias
Short stature
Joint or skeletal deformities
Organomegaly (especially liver and spleen)
Hypotonia
Ataxia
Developmental delay
Loss of developmental milestones

While studies of oligosaccharides and glycosaminoglycans (mucopoly-saccharides) in urine are often performed as screening, there are frequent false-negative and false-positive results.

The confirmatory diagnosis for most lysosomal storage disorders is established via specific enzymatic assays. The tests compare enzyme levels in a patient sample (usually blood, but urine or skin fibroblasts may also be used) against normal benchmarks. Prenatal testing is often possible but is most reliably conducted through amniocentesis. The tests must be performed at a specialized laboratory.

Treatment

Treatment options vary for the lysosomal storage disorders, and patients often undergo a variety of therapies and care. For most of them only palliative care can address clinical symptoms. However, some others have disease-specific therapies. The 3 approaches to address lysosomal storage enzymatic deficit include the following.

Hematopoietic stem cell transplant (HSCT). Stem cells from bone marrow or cord blood are transplanted intravenously to produce the enzyme as well as new healthy cells. Bone marrow transplant has been most used to treat mucopolysaccharidosis type I (MPS I), and has had positive results when performed early in a disease's course.

Results of a very small clinical trial of patients with infantile Krabbe disease found that children who received umbilical cord blood stem cells from unrelated donors prior to symptom onset developed with little neurologic impairment. Results also showed that disease progression stabilized faster in patients who receive cord blood compared with those who receive adult bone marrow.

Enzyme replacement therapy (ERT). A recombinant form of the deficient enzyme is administered intravenously.

The first ERT for Gaucher type I went on the market in 1991. Enzyme replacement therapy is a treatment option for Gaucher type I, Fabry disease, MPS I, and Pompe disease, with clinical investigations underway for MPS II, and MPS VI.

Enzyme replacement therapy and HSCT can result in a significant improvement in the clinical course if treatment is started when the individual is presymptomatic or only mildly affected. Therefore, it is important to establish a diagnosis as early as possible. Unfortunately, ERT and HSCT have had very limited effects on central nervous system symptoms, since the large enzyme molecules introduced intravenously cannot penetrate the blood-brain barrier.

Substrate inhibition. The rate of production of the substrate is slowed by drug therapy. Substrate inhibition has recently been introduced in 2002 for patients with Gaucher type I patients where ERT is not an option. Further clinical studies for substrate inhibition in Gaucher disease, Fabry disease, GM2-gangliosidoses (Tay-Sachs disease, Sandhoff disease, GM2 activator disease), and Niemann-Pick type C are in progress.

Neuronal Ceroid Lipofuscinosis (NCLs)

The NCLs are a group of severe autosomal recessive inherited diseases characterized by progressive blindness and neurodegeneration, and the accumulation of autofluorescent lipofuscin-like (age pigment) material in the lysosomes of neurons and other cell types.

The NCLs were originally classified according to the clinical onset of symptoms as infantile, late-infantile, juvenile, and adult forms, but now several variant forms are recognized. Seven human disease gene loci have been identified. The function of most of the encoded proteins is unknown. The underlying genes for some NCL types have not yet been identified. Phenotypes have been characterized clinically by age of onset and order of appearance of the clinical features: infantile neuronal ceroid-lipofuscinosis (INCL, Santavuori-Haltia), late-infantile (LINCL, Jansky-Bielschowsky), juvenile (JNCL, Batten disease, Spielmeyer-Vogt), adult (ANCL, Kuf disease), and Northern epilepsy (progressive epilepsy with mental retardation).

Clinical Characteristics

Children with INCL are normal at birth, with symptoms usually appearing between 6 and 24 months of age. Clinical signs include delayed development, myoclonic jerks and seizures, deceleration of head growth, and electroencephalographic changes. Infants develop blindness and seizures by 2 years of age, followed by progressive mental deterioration.

The first symptoms of LINCL typically appear between 2 and 4 years of age, usually starting with seizures, followed by regression of developmental milestones, cognitive impairment, ataxia, and extrapyramidal movements and spasticity. Visual impairment appears at age 4 to 6 years and rapidly progresses to blindness. Life expectancy ranges from 6 years to older than 40 years.

The onset of JNCL is usually between ages 4 and 10 years. Rapidly progressing visual loss resulting in total blindness within 2 to 4 years is often the first clinical sign. Epilepsy with generalized tonic-clonic seizures, complex-partial seizures, or myoclonic seizures typically appears between ages 5 and 18 years. Life expectancy ranges from the late teens to the 30s.

Initial signs and symptoms of ANCL usually appear around 30 years of age, with death occurring about 10 years later. Affected individuals have either progressive myoclonic epilepsy or behavior abnormalities, and all have dementia, ataxia, and late-occurring pyramidal and extrapyramidal signs. Northern epilepsy is characterized by tonic-clonic or complex-partial seizures, mental retardation, and motor dysfunction. Onset occurs between ages 2 and 10 years.

Diagnosis

The diagnosis of NCL is often based on assay of enzyme activity or molecular genetic testing. Clinical findings and electron microscopy of biopsied tissues are also useful. Magnetic resonance imaging may show marked cerebral and cerebellar atrophy (Figure 3-5). Testing depends on the age of onset. Six genes, *CLN1, CNL2, CLN3, CLN5, CLN6,* and *CLN8,* are known to be associated with NCL. Assays of the enzymatic activity of palmitoyl-protein thioesterase 1 (PPT1), the protein

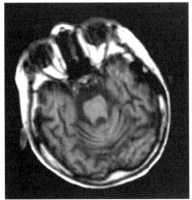

Figure 3-5.
Neuronal ceroid lipofuscinosis. T1-weighted magnetic resonance imaging shows marked cerebral and cerebellar atrophy. (Courtesy of Harold G. Marks, MD, St Christopher's Hospital for Children.)

product of the gene *CLN1,* and tripeptidyl-peptidase 1 (TPP-1), the protein product of the gene *CLN2,* are clinically available. Molecular genetic testing of the *CLN1, CLN3, CLN5, CLN6,* and *CLN8* genes is now possible as is the measurement of the enzyme activities of the CLN1/PPT1, CLN2/TPP-1, and

CLN10/CTSD enzymes. Low levels are definitive diagnostic of NCL caused by mutations in these genes, even in cases of adult onset. Enzyme tests can be carried out using blood, skin biopsy, or saliva as the source of cells, and care must be taken to use the most specific assays possible, especially for cases of later onset.

Treatment

Seizures are usually refractory and require the combination of several antiepileptic drugs. No treatment is available for the underlying metabolic defect.

Carbohydrate-deficient Glycoprotein Syndromes

The carbohydrate deficient glycoprotein syndromes (CDGS) are a group of disorders of abnormal glycosylation of N-linked oligosaccharides. Thirteen different enzymes are currently recognized to be defective in individual types of CDGS.

Clinical Characteristics

The symptoms and signs of these CDGS most commonly begin in infancy and range from severe developmental delay and hypotonia with multiple organ system involvement to hypoglycemia and protein-losing enteropathy with normal development.

Typical clinical findings are esotropia or roving eye movements, inverted nipples, long fingers and toes, joint restriction at knees and hips, fat pads in the pubic area and above the gluteal region, and lipodystrophic changes in the buttocks. Neurologic symptoms include, in addition to developmental delay and hypotonia, poor sucking, failure to thrive, hyperreflexia, seizures, and stroke-like episodes. Other systemic features include renal cysts, bone abnormalities, hypogonadism, cataracts, and deafness.

CDG-Ia is the most common type of CDGS and is associated with cerebellar hypoplasia. The clinical course CDG-Ia has been divided into infantile, late-infantile, and childhood ataxia-mental retardation types.

Diagnosis

It should be suspected on the basis of the clinical features described above. Neuroimaging may detect an enlarged cisterna magna, cerebellar atrophy,

Dandy-Walker malformations, and small white matter cysts. The confirmatory diagnostic test for all types of CDGS is the analysis of serum transferrin.

Disorders of Copper Metabolism

Menkes Disease

Menkes disease is an X-linked genetic disorder of copper metabolism caused by mutations in the *ATP7A* gene that is responsible for the production of the ATPase enzyme that regulates copper levels in the body. The copper transport systems both within the cell and across the cell membrane are dysfunctional.

Clinical Characteristics

The clinical features are attributable to the deficiency of one or more important copper requiring enzymes, such as cytochrome c oxidase, superoxide dismutase, dopamine B hydroxylase (catecholamine production), and lysyl oxidase (cross linking of collagen and elastin).

Menkes disease is a progressive degenerative condition involving several organ systems. Newborns with the classic form of the disease appear normal at birth, including their hair. At 2 to 3 months of age developmental delay, failure to thrive, hypotonia, and seizures appear. Other clinical features are unstable body temperature, connective tissue symptoms including tortuous vessels, skeletal changes, bladder diverticulae, loose skin, and loose joints. Patients also develop typical dysmorphic features including short, sparse, sagging cheeks with pronounced jowls. The pathognomonic finding is the presence of sparse, coarse, and depigmented hair, which gives the name to the disease of *kinky or steely hair disease.*

Though most patients (90%–95%) have a severe clinical course, there are clinical variants that result in less severe symptoms, including mild Menkes disease and occipital horn syndrome. In these forms, symptoms may not appear until the child is older.

Diagnosis

The clinical symptoms and signs described above should raise the diagnostic suspicion. Head computed tomography or MRI may show extra-axial collections, which raises the differential diagnosis with subdural hematoma due to child abuse (Figure 3-6). The confirmation is established by the presence of low copper and ceruloplasmin levels in blood after the child is 6 weeks old (low levels are not diagnostic before then), high copper levels in the placenta, abnormal catechol levels in blood and CSF even in a newborn, and microscopic examination of hair demonstrating typical abnormalities.

Treatment

The objective of treatment is to provide copper to the intracellular compartments where the copper enzymes are synthesized. However, parenteral administration of various copper preparations (as copper sulphate or copper-ethylenediamineteraacetic acid) does not produce substantial clinical improvement. There are reports of copper-histidine, the physiological copper complex found

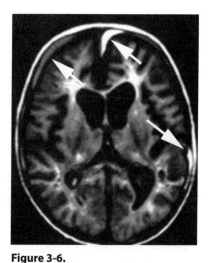

Figure 3-6.
Menkes syndrome. T1-weighted magnetic resonance imaging shows cortical and subcortical atrophy with cystic changes in the white matter. There are subdural hematomas of different signal intensities, perhaps reflecting different ages (white arrows). Subdural hemorrhage in Menkes syndrome is a complication of brain atrophy, but it can be confused with abusive head injury. (From Sfaello I, Castelnau P, Blanc N, Ogier H, Evrard P, Arzimanoglou A. Infantile spasms and Menkes disease. *Epileptic Disord.* 2000;2:227–230. Reprinted by permission.)

in human serum, having a positive effect in some patients, especially in seizure control. However, patients receiving copper-histidine after the first few months of age do not benefit in the same way, although survival may be prolonged. This suggests that copper therapy should be initiated very early to observe any possible benefits.

Wilson Disease

Wilson disease is an autosomal recessive disorder of copper transport. The gene has been mapped to chromosome 13 q14.3. The defect results in impaired biliary excretion of copper and impaired incorporation of copper into ceruloplasmin, resulting in the toxic accumulation of copper in the liver and other tissues, such as kidney, brain, and cornea (Kayser-Fleischer rings).

Clinical Characteristics

The clinical presentation involves different degrees of liver disease and neurologic or psychiatric symptoms. Wilson disease manifests as liver disease in children and adolescents, peaking at ages 10 to 13 years, and as neuropsychiatric illness in young adults aged 19 to 20 years.

Hepatic dysfunction is the presenting feature in more than half of patients. The most common presenting neurologic feature is an asymmetrical tremor. The tremor may be predominantly resting, postural, or kinetic. Other symptoms include dysarthria, excessive salivation, ataxia, and personality changes. Late neurologic manifestations are dystonia, choreoathetoid movements, spasticity, and generalized seizures. Psychiatric features include emotional lability, impulsiveness, disinhibition, and self-injurious behavior.

Diagnosis

Wilson disease should be considered in the differential diagnosis of any unexplained chronic liver disease, especially in patients younger than 40 years. The presence of Kayser-Fleischer rings and ceruloplasmin levels of less than 20 mg/dL in a patient with neurologic symptoms suggests Wilson disease. Kayser-Fleischer rings are formed by the deposition of copper in the Descemet membrane of the cornea. They may be visible to the naked eye, but identification using slit-lamp examination is best. Kayser-Fleischer rings are almost invariably present in patients with neurologic symptoms. However, they are no longer considered pathognomonic of Wilson disease unless accompanied by neurologic manifestations because they may be seen in patients with chronic cholestatic disorders. In addition to decreased ceruloplasmin levels, there is an increase in urinary copper concentration. The gold standard for diagnosis remains the evaluation of copper concentration in liver biopsy.

Treatment

The mainstay of treatment is pharmacologic therapy with chelating agents such as penicillamine. Oral administration of zinc interferes with absorption of copper and is useful after decoppering with a chelating agent. Antioxidants, such as vitamin E, help to prevent tissue damage. Orthotopic liver transplantation is a potentially curative treatment for Wilson disease. Transplantation is usually reserved for patients with liver failure despite chelation therapy.

Web Sites

Climb: www.climb.org.uk

Organic Acidemia Association: www.oaanews.org

International Organization for Glutaric Aciduria, Type I:
www.glutaricacidemia.org

National MPS Society: www.mpssociety.org

National Gaucher Foundation: www.gaucherdisease.org

National Niemann-Pick Disease Foundation, Inc.: www.nnpdf.org

Batten Disease Support and Research Association: www.bdsra.org

Association for Glycogen Storage Disease: www.agsdus.org

Acid Maltase Deficiency Association: www.amda-pompe.org

United Leukodystrophy Foundation: www.ulf.org

United Mitochondrial Disease Foundation: www.umdf.org

Pediatric Neurotransmitter Disease Association: www.pndaassoc.org

Bibliography

Andersson H, Kaplan P, Kacena K, Yee J. Eight-year clinical outcomes of long-term enzyme replacement therapy for 884 children with Gaucher disease type 1. *Pediatrics.* 2008;122:1182–1190

Babovic-Vuksanovic D, Patterson MC, et al. Severe hypoglycemia as a presenting symptom of carbohydrate-deficient glycoprotein syndrome. *J Pediatr.* 1999;135:775–781

Barone R, Nigro F, Triulzi F, Musumeci S, Fiumara A, Pavone L. Clinical and neuroradiological follow-up in mucopolysaccharidosis type III (Sanfilippo syndrome). *Neuropediatrics.* 1999;30:270–274

Bax MC, Colville GA. Behaviour in mucopolysaccharide disorders. *Arch Dis Child.* 1995;73: 77–81

Beaudet AL, Scriver CR, Sly WS, Valle D. Genetics, biochemistry, and molecular bases of variant phenotypes. In: Scriver CR, Beaudet AL, Sly WS, Valle D, eds. *The Metabolic and Molecular Bases of Inherited Disease.* 8th ed. New York, NY: McGraw-Hill; 2001:3–45

Bertini I, Rosato A. Menkes disease. *Cell Mol Life Sci.* 2008;65:89–91

Bijarnia S, Wiley V, Carpenter K, Christodoulou J, Ellaway CJ, Wilcken B. Glutaric aciduria type I: outcome following detection by newborn screening. *J Inherit Metab Dis.* 2008;31:503–507

Blau N, Thony, B, Cotton RGH, Hyland K. Disorders of tetrahydrobiopterin and related biogenic amines. In: Scriver CR, Beaudet AL, Sly WS, Valle D, eds. *The Metabolic and Molecular Bases of Inherited Disease.* 8th ed. New York, NY: McGraw-Hill; 2001:1725–1776

Brusilow SW, Horwich AL. Urea cycle enzymes. In: Scriver CR, Beaudet AL, Sly WS, Valle D, eds. *The Metabolic and Molecular Bases of Inherited Disease.* 8th ed. New York, NY: McGraw-Hill; 2001:1909–1963

Burlina AB, Bonafé L, Zacchello F. Clinical and biochemical approach to the neonate with a suspected inborn error of amino acid and organic acid metabolism. *Semin Perinatol.* 1999;23:162–173

Carchon H, Van Schaftingen E, Matthijs G, Jaeken J. Carbohydrate-deficient glycoprotein syndrome type IA (phosphomannomutase-deficiency). *Biochim Biophys Acta.* 1999;1455:155–165

Carstea ED, Morris JA, Coleman KG, et al. Niemann-Pick C1 disease gene: homology to mediators of cholesterol homeostasis. *Science.* 1997;277:228–231

Cartier N, Aubourg P. Hematopoietic stem cell gene therapy in Hurler syndrome, globoid cell leukodystrophy, metachromatic leukodystrophy and X-adrenoleukodystrophy. *Curr Opin Mol Ther.* 2008;10:471–478

Cecil KM. MR spectroscopy of metabolic disorders. *Neuroimaging Clin N Am.* 2006;16:87–116

Cecil KM, Faerber EN. Inherited metabolic and neurodegenerative brain disorders. In: Slovis TL, Bulas D, Faerber E, et al, eds. *Caffey's Pediatric Diagnostic Imaging.* Philadelphia, PA: Mosby Elsevier; 2008:688–725

Childs B. A logic of disease. In: Scriver CR, Beaudet AL, Sly WS, Valle D, eds. *The Metabolic and Molecular Bases of Inherited Disease.* 8th ed. New York, NY: McGraw-Hill; 2001:129–153

Clarke JTR. *A Clinical Guide to Inherited Metabolic Diseases.* 2nd ed. Cambridge, UK: Cambridge University Press; 2002

Copeland S. A review of newborn screening in the era of tandem mass spectrometry: what's new for the pediatric neurologist? *Semin Pediatr Neurol.* 2008;15:110–116

de Baulny HO, Benoist JF, Rigal O, Touati G, Rabier D, Saudubray JM. Methylmalonic and propionic acidaemias: management and outcome. *J Inherit Metab Dis.* 2005;28:415–423

de Lonlay P, Seta N, Barrot S, et al. A broad spectrum of clinical presentations in congenital disorders of glycosylation I: a series of 26 cases. *J Med Genet.* 2001;38:14–19

De Vivo DC, Trifiletti RR, Jacobson RI, Ronen GM, Behmand RA, Harik SI. Defective glucose transport across the blood-brain barrier as a cause of persistent hypoglycorrhachia, seizures, and developmental delay. *N Engl J Med.* 1991;325:703–709

Debray FG, Lambert M, Mitchell GA. Disorders of mitochondrial function. *Curr Opin Pediatr.* 2008;20:471–482

Deodato F, Boenzi S, Santorelli FM, Dionisi-Vici C. Methylmalonic and propionic aciduria. *Am J Med Genet C Semin Med Genet.* 2006;142C:104–112

Dionisi-Vici C, Deodato F, Röschinger W, Rhead W, Wilcken B. 'Classical' organic acidurias, propionic aciduria, methylmalonic aciduria and isovaleric aciduria: long-term outcome and effects of expanded newborn screening using tandem mass spectrometry. *J Inherit Metab Dis.* 2006;29:383–389

Endo F, Matsuura T, Yanagita K, Matsuda I. Clinical manifestations of inborn errors of the urea cycle and related metabolic disorders during childhood. *J Nutr.* 2004;134(6 suppl):1605S–1609S

Enns GM. Neurologic damage and neurocognitive dysfunction in urea cycle disorders. *Semin Pediatr Neurol.* 2008;15:132–139

Faerber EN, Poussaint TY. Magnetic resonance of metabolic and degenerative diseases in children. *Top Magn Reson Imaging.* 2002;13:3–21

Fernandes J, Saudubray JM, van den Berghe G, eds. *Inborn Metabolic Diseases.* Berlin: Springer-Verlag; 2000

Gibson K, Halliday JL, Kirby DM, Yaplito-Lee J, Thorburn DR, Boneh A. Mitochondrial oxidative phosphorylation disorders presenting in neonates: clinical manifestations and enzymatic and molecular diagnoses. *Pediatrics.* 2008;122:1003–1008

Gillan JE, Lowden JA, Gaskin K, Cutz E. Congenital ascites as a presenting sign of lysosomal storage disease. *J Pediatr.* 1984;104:225–231

Gospe SM. Current perspectives on pyridoxine-dependent seizures. *J Pediatr.* 1998;132:919–923

Gropman AL, Batshaw ML. Cognitive outcome in urea cycle disorders. *Mol Genet Metab.* 2004;81(suppl 1):S58–S62

Haltia M. The neuronal ceroid-lipofuscinoses: from past to present. *Biochim Biophys Acta.* 2006;1762:850–856

Harmanci O, Bayraktar Y. Gaucher disease: new developments in treatment and etiology. *World J Gastroenterol.* 2008;14:3968–3973

Heese BA. Current strategies in the management of lysosomal storage diseases. *Semin Pediatr Neurol.* 2008;15:119–126

Huster D, Lutsenko S. Wilson disease: not just a copper disorder. Analysis of a Wilson disease model demonstrates the link between copper and lipid metabolism. *Mol Biosyst.* 2007;3:816–824

Hyland K, Buist NR, Powell BR, et al. Folinic acid responsive seizures: a new syndrome? *J Inherit Metab Dis.* 1995;18:177–181

Ibdah JA, Bennett MJ, Rinaldo P, et al. A fetal fatty-acid oxidation disorder as a cause of liver disease in pregnant women. *N Engl J Med.* 1999;340:1723–1731

Jaeken J, Detheux M, Van Maldergem L, Foulon M, Carchon H, Van Schaftingen E. 3-Phosphoglycerate dehydrogenase deficiency: an inborn error of serine biosynthesis. *Arch Dis Child.* 1996;74:542–545

Kang PB, Hunter JV, Melvin JJ, Selak MA, Faerber EN, Kaye EM. Infantile leukodystrophy owing to mitochondrial enzyme dysfunction. *Pediatr Neurol.* 2002;17:421–428

Katzin LW, Amato AA. Pompe disease: a review of the current diagnosis and treatment recommendations in the era of enzyme replacement therapy. *J Clin Neuromuscul Dis.* 2008;9:421–431

Kayser MA. Inherited metabolic diseases in neurodevelopmental and neurobehavioral disorders. *Semin Pediatr Neurol.* 2008;15:127–131

Keutzer J, Yee J. Enzyme replacement therapy for lysosomal storage disorders. *Hum Gene Ther.* 2008;19:857; author reply 858

Kompare M, Rizzo WB. Mitochondrial fatty-acid oxidation disorders. *Semin Pediatr Neurol.* 2008;15:140–149

Loes DJ, Hite S, Moser H, et al. Adrenoleukodystrophy: a scoring method for brain MR observations. *AJNR Am J Neuroradiol.* 1994;15:1761–1766

Lyon G, Adams RD, Kolodny EH. *Neurology of Hereditary Metabolic Diseases of Children.* 2nd ed. New York, NY: McGraw-Hill;1996

Machin GA. Diseases causing fetal and neonatal ascites. *Pediatr Pathol.* 1985;4:195–211

Mathias D, Gebhard J, Wilhelm L, Schmidt-Gayk H, Mathias IN. 26 years of external quality controls for the screening of congenital metabolic disorders in newborns—a summary of the results. *C Med J.* 2008;69:92–97

Moser HW, Bezman L, Lu SE, Raymond GV. Therapy of X-linked adrenoleukodystrophy: prognosis based upon age and MRI abnormality and plans for placebo-controlled trials. *J Inherit Metab Dis.* 2000;23:273–277

Moser HW, Mahmood A, Raymond GV. X-linked adrenoleukodystrophy. *Nat Clin Pract Neurol.* 2007;3:140–151

Moyer VA, Calonge N, Teutsch SM, Botkin JR. Expanding newborn screening: process, policy, and priorities. United States Preventive Services Task Force. *Hastings Cent Rep.* 2008;38:32–39

Muravchick S. Clinical implications of mitochondrial disease. *Adv Drug Deliv Rev.* 2008; 60:1553–1560

Nassogne MC, Héron B, Touati G, Rabier D, Saudubray JM. Urea cycle defects: management and outcome. *J Inherit Metab Dis.* 2005;28:407–414

Neufeld EF, Muenzer J. The mucopolysaccharidoses. In: Scriver CR, Beaudet AL, Sly WS, Valle D, eds. *The Metabolic and Molecular Bases of Inherited Disease.* 8th ed. New York, NY: McGraw-Hill; 2001:3421–3452

Ogier de Baulny H. Management and emergency treatments of neonates with a suspicion of inborn errors of metabolism. *Semin Neonatol.* 2002;7:17–26

Ogier de Baulny H, Saudubray JM. Branched-chain organic acidurias. *Semin Neonatol.* 2002;7:65–74

Orchard PJ, Blazar BR, Wagner J, Charnas L, Krivit W, Tolar J. Hematopoietic cell therapy for metabolic disease. *J Pediatr.* 2007;151:340–346

Patterson MC. Screening for "prelysosomal disorders": carbohydrate-deficient glycoprotein syndromes. *J Child Neurol.* 1999;14(suppl 1):S16–S22

Patterson MC, Vanier MT, Suzuki K, et al. Niemann-Pick disease type C: a lipid trafficking disorder. In: Scriver CR, Beaudet AL, Sly WS, Valle D, eds. *The Metabolic and Molecular Bases of Inherited Disease.* 8th ed. New York, NY: McGraw-Hill; 2001:3611–3633

Saudubray JM, Charpentier C. Clinical phenotypes: diagnosis/algorithms. In: Scriver CR, Beaudet AL, Sly WS, Valle D, eds. *The Metabolic and Molecular Bases of Inherited Disease.* 8th ed. New York, NY: McGraw-Hill; 2001:1327–1403

Saudubray JM, Nassogne MC, de Lonlay P, Touati G. Clinical approach to inherited metabolic disorders in neonates: an overview. *Semin Neonatol.* 2002;7:3–15

Saudubray JM, Sedel F, Walter JH. Clinical approach to treatable inborn metabolic diseases: an introduction. *J Inherit Metab Dis.* 2006;29:261–274

Sedel F, Tourbah A, Fontaine B, et al. Leukoencephalopathies associated with inborn errors of metabolism in adults. *J Inherit Metab Dis.* 2008;31:295–307

Shimozawa N. Molecular and clinical aspects of peroxisomal diseases. *J Inherit Metab Dis.* 2007;30:193–197

Shroff RC, Patil A, Merchant RH, Udani VP, Colaco MP, Prabhu S. Hematopoietic stem cell gene therapy in Hurler syndrome, globoid cell leukodystrophy, metachromatic leukodystrophy and X-adrenoleukodystrophy. *Curr Opin Mol Ther.* 2008;10:471–478

Siintola E, Lehesjoki AE, Mole SE. Molecular genetics of the NCLs—status and perspectives. *Biochim Biophys Acta.* 2006;1762:857–864

Spitzer AR, Chace D. Proteomics- and metabolomics-based neonatal diagnostics in assessing and managing the critically ill neonate. *Clin Perinatol.* 2008;35:695–716

Stone DL, Sidransky E. Hydrops fetalis: lysosomal storage disorders in extremis. *Adv Pediatr.* 1999;46:409–440

Torres OA, Miller VS, Buist NM, Hyland K. Folinic acid-responsive neonatal seizures. *J Child Neurol.* 1999;14:529–532

Tuchman M, Yudkoff M. Blood levels of ammonia and nitrogen scavenging amino acids in patients with inherited hyperammonemia. *Mol Genet Metab.* 1999;66:10–15

van der Knaap MS, Leegwater PA, Konst AA, et al. Mutations in each of the five subunits of translation initiation factor eIF2B can cause leukoencephalopathy with vanishing white matter. *Ann Neurol.* 2002;51:264–270

van der Ploeg AT, Reuser AJ. Pompe's disease. *Lancet.* 2008;372:1342–1353

Varki A. Biological roles of oligosaccharides: all of the theories are correct. *Glycobiology.* 1993;3:97–139

Widhalm K, Koch S, Scheibenreiter S, et al. Long-term follow-up of 12 patients with the late-onset variant of argininosuccinic acid lyase deficiency: no impairment of intellectual and psychomotor development during therapy. *Pediatrics.* 1992;89:1182–1184

Williams RE, Aberg L, Autti T, Goebel HH, Kohlschütter A, Lönnqvist T. Diagnosis of the neuronal ceroid lipofuscinoses: an update. *Biochim Biophys Acta.* 2006;1762:865–872

Wolf B. Disorders of biotin metabolism. In: Scriver CR, Beaudet AL, Sly WS, Valle D, eds. *The Metabolic and Molecular Bases of Inherited Disease.* 8 ed. New York, NY: McGraw-Hill; 2001:3935–3962

Zatta P, Frank A. Copper deficiency and neurological disorders in man and animals. *Brain Res Rev.* 2007;54:19–33

Chapter 4

Acute Encephalopathy

Jatinder S. Goraya, MD
Ignacio Valencia, MD
Agustín Legido, MD, PhD, MBA

Introduction

Not infrequently, pediatricians and pediatric neurologists are asked to evaluate a child who presents alterations in alertness or awareness. Usually referred to as *change in mental status,* changes in consciousness encompass a spectrum that ranges from minimally reduced consciousness—called *clouding of consciousness*—through lethargy, confusion, delirium obtundation, and stupor to profound reduction in consciousness, or coma (Table 4-1). Though these terms continue to be used in clinical practice, it is to be noted that the definitions are less than precise and subject to various interpretations throughout the medical community. Instead, it is more relevant to record and monitor a patient's responses to specific stimuli.

Chronic states of impaired consciousness also need to be differentiated from acute alterations of consciousness defined above, particularly the vegetative state, which may be encountered during worsening of or recovery from coma. In the vegetative state, the patient lacks environmental awareness, although respiratory and sleep-wake cycles are maintained. A vegetative state is considered persistent if it lasts longer than 12 months after traumatic brain injury or more than 3 months after non-traumatic brain injury.

Acute alteration of consciousness in children can result from diverse etiologies and may be accompanied by other neurologic phenomena such as seizures, focal motor deficits, and increased intracranial pressure (ICP). It is potentially life-threatening, requiring prompt intervention to preserve life and brain function.

Table 4-1. Definitions of Altered States of Consciousness	
Term	**Definition**
Clouding of consciousness	Minimally decreased wakefulness or awareness characterized clinically by reduced attention span. Patients are easily distracted and may startle to stimuli. Patient may misjudge sensory perceptions. They do not think quickly and clearly.
Lethargy	Decreased wakefulness or drowsiness in which patients are able to engage in activity but tend to fall asleep.
Confusion	More advanced state of clouded consciousness in which stimuli are more consistently misjudged. Patients may be disoriented and appear bewildered. They have difficulty following commands.
Delirium	More advanced state of reduced consciousness with activated mental state, presenting as disorientation, irritability, misperception of sensory stimuli, and visual hallucination. Patients are commonly loud, talkative, offensive, suspicious, and agitated.
Stupor	State of unresponsiveness from which patients can be aroused only by vigorous and repeated stimuli. Patients lapse back into the stupor state as soon as the stimulus ceases.
Coma	This is a state of unarousability, and patients do not manifest any clearly discernible psychological, motor, or vocal response to external stimuli. These patients are completely unaware of self or surroundings.

Etiology

The most common causes of acute global neurologic dysfunction in children are head trauma, hypoxia-ischemia, central nervous system (CNS) infections, toxic and metabolic disorders, and seizures. It is, however, not unusual to see focal brain lesions such as a brain tumor or abscess presenting with changed mental status. Although traumatic and non-traumatic causes have equal incidence, the relative frequency of various etiologies varies with age (Table 4-2).

Pathophysiology

Consciousness is a physiologic state of being awake and aware of the self and the environment. Wakefulness refers to a state in which the eyes are open and there is a degree of motor arousal; it contrasts with sleep, a state of eye closure and motor quiescence. Awareness refers to the ability to have, and the having of, experience of any kind. We are typically aware of our

Table 4-2. Etiology of Altered Consciousness in Children	
Category	**Examples**

Trauma
  Non-accidental
  or accidental
	Subdural and epidural hematomas, intracerebral hemorrhages, skull fractures

Hypoxia-ischemia	Near-drowning or foreign body aspiration leading to cardiac arrest
CNS Infections	Meningitis, encephalitis, sepsis, typhoid fever, malaria
Metabolic	Electrolyte imbalance (hypo-/hypernatremia, hypo-/hypercalcemia, hypermagnesemia), hypoglycemia, DKA, non-ketotic hyperglycemic coma Hypo/hyperthermia, Reye encephalopathy Inborn errors of metabolism Organ failure (renal, hepatic, heart, respiratory failure) Endocrine (hypo-/hyperthyroidism, Addison crisis, pituitary apoplexy) Others (porphyria, Wernicke encephalopathy, dialysis encephalopathy)
Toxic	Lead, ethanol, ethylene glycol, carbon monoxide, cyanide
Drugs	Sedatives and hypnotics, barbiturates, phenothiazines, phenytoin, SSRIs, anticholinergics, phencyclidine, monoamine oxidase inhibitors, lithium
Seizures	Postictal state, non-convulsive status epilepticus
Focal lesions	Stroke (ischemic and hemorrhagic), tumor, abscess, subdural hematoma and empyema, and other mass lesions
Psychiatric	Conversion reaction, psychiatric medications
Miscellaneous	Cardiac arrhythmias, Hashimoto encephalopathy, ADEM

Abbreviations: CNS, central nervous system; DKA, diabetic ketoacidosis; SSRI, slow serotonin reuptake inhibitor; ADEM: acute disseminated encephalomyelitis.

surroundings and of bodily sensations, but the contents of awareness can also include our memories, thoughts, emotions, and intentions.

A human being's state of consciousness reflects both his level of arousal and the sum of the cognitive functions of his brain. Arousal depends on the integrity of physiological mechanisms that take their origin from the reticular activating system and other structures that lie in the upper brain stem extending from the level of the middle pons forward into the hypothalamus. Conscious behavior depends on the presence in the cerebral hemispheres of relatively intact functional areas that interact extensively with each other as well as with the deeper activating systems of the upper brain stem, hypothalamus, and thalamus. Any disruption of these neural circuits interferes with arousal leading to variable degrees of decrease in consciousness.

Evaluation

Approach to a child with altered consciousness is essentially the same irrespective of the degree of impairment. Altered consciousness constitutes an acute life-threatening medical emergency requiring prompt and expedited evaluation. Efforts are directed at early identification of the underlying cause, prompt institution of specific interventions, and provision of supportive care. Since long-term neurologic disability remains a possibility in those who survive, it is important that measures necessary to arrest and reverse the ongoing neurologic insult are instituted at the earliest. For this reason, assessment and treatment of a child with change in mental status must take place concurrently. For the matter of convenience, the description of evaluation of the child will proceed through history, physical examination, and laboratory workup.

History

As with any other non-emergent clinical encounter with patient, history is the most important initial component of evaluation of a child with an altered level of consciousness.

An abrupt onset of change in mental status is seen with seizures, intracranial bleeding, trauma, or cardiac arrhythmia. A relatively gradual onset of coma may be seen in infectious or metabolic etiologies. Insidious onset of altered consciousness may complicate slowly growing intracranial masses such as brain tumors. Recurrent episodes of coma may be a manifestation of inborn errors of metabolism. Onset of neurologic symptoms, including alterations in consciousness a few days after the upper respiratory tract or gastrointestinal infections, suggests acute demyelinating encephalomyelitis. Presence of fever points to the possibility of underlying infectious etiologies (such as meningitis, encephalitis, brain abscess, subdural empyema), though other disorders such as malignant hyperthermia, neuroleptic malignant syndrome, hyperserotoninergic syndrome, and anticholinergic drug overdose are also accompanied with very high elevations of temperature.

Hyperthyroidism can also be associated with temperature elevations. Fever may also complicate a prolonged seizure or be associated with a febrile seizure in an infant or young child. Systemic infections such as typhoid fever may result in febrile encephalopathy without directly causing intracranial infection. Malaria is not an uncommon cause of acute encephalopathy in endemic areas, though occasional cases may be encountered in the United States after travel to such areas or among immigrant individuals. Urinary tract infections in infants may result in systemic toxicity and encephalopathy. Rarely, fever may be of central origin by itself. Heat stroke in children exposed to hot and humid climates can also be associated with coma. Hypothermia and coma can be seen together in exposure to cold environmental temperatures, certain drug intoxications, or in hypothyroidism. Very young infants, especially neonates, may have hypothermia with systemic infections.

A history of rash can be an important clue to underlying infectious or collagen vascular diseases, but can also be associated with bleeding disorders causing intracranial hemorrhage. A history of headache, vomiting, or other neurologic symptoms suggests intracranial mass lesion. Intractable vomiting preceding the onset of coma is seen in Reye syndrome and in some inborn errors of metabolism. History of abnormal smell of the body, breath, or urine is described with certain inborn errors of metabolism such as maple syrup urine disease, but can also be seen in hepatic failure (fetor hepaticus) or renal failure (an ammoniacal smell) as well as in diabetic ketoacidosis (the fruity smell of ketones).

Accidental drug ingestion, particularly unwitnessed among young infants, or intentional or recreational drug ingestion in adolescents must always be kept in mind.

Trauma deserves special mention not only because it is one of the most common causes of coma in children, but also because of the fact that abusive head trauma among infants typically presents with no relevant history or with a misleading history. Inconsistencies in history and unusual pattern of injuries must alert the physician to the possibility of abusive head trauma.

Seizure disorders are also commonly associated with loss of consciousness, but the problem arises when the seizure has not been observed and the child is seen in the state of postictal unconsciousness. A history of seizures in the past is helpful but it is not always available. Fortunately, most of the children will wake up during the period of initial evaluation and observation. Children with non-convulsive status epilepticus present with altered mental status but have no or little motor manifestations of seizures, and the diagnosis may be difficult on clinical grounds without having an electroencephalogram (EEG) available.

Psychiatric illnesses such as conversion disorders may present with altered consciousness. Adolescents are particularly vulnerable. A high index of suspicion is required and diagnosis must only be made when organic disorders have been excluded with certainty.

A history of underlying cardiac, respiratory, renal, or endocrine disorders (diabetes, thyroid, parathyroid, or pituitary problems) may provide vital evidence to the possible ongoing pathophysiological process in a child with altered consciousness. A history of similar episodes of change in mental status may suggest a seizure disorder, cardiac arrhythmia, or inborn error of metabolism. Family history of epilepsy, sudden infant deaths, inherited metabolic disorders, or other neurologic disorders may hold the key in some cases.

Physical Examination

While completeness of physical examination in patients with derangement of consciousness cannot be overemphasized, certain parameters of physical examination are more important for initial assessment as well as for monitoring the response to treatment than other interventions.

Evaluation of a patient in coma starts with assessment of ABC (airway patency, adequacy of breathing, and circulation) and vital signs (temperature, heart rate, breathing rate, and blood pressure). It is useful to add pulse oximetry to vital signs in the initial and ongoing assessment. All of these parameters are important in initial stabilization of the patient but may also provide critical information on the etiology (Box 4-1).

Temperature

Derangements of temperature in a child with altered consciousness have been discussed previously under history.

Box 4-1. Cardiovascular Abnormalities and Specific Causes of Coma[a]

Hypertension
Increased intracranial pressure
Subarachnoid hemorrhage
Toxic ingestion
   Amphetamines
   Anticholinergics
   Sympathomimetics

Tachycardia
Alcohol
Amphetamines
Theophylline
Sympathomimetics

Arrhythmia
Amphetamines
Anticholinergics
Tricyclics
Digitalis

Hypotension
Spinal shock
Adrenal insufficiency
Toxic ingestion
   Narcotics
   Cyanide
   Sedatives/hypnotics

Bradycardia
Beta-blockers
Narcotics

[a]*Modified from Bunch ST, Goodwin SR. Altered states of consciousness. In: Maria BL, ed.* Current Management in Child Neurology. *Hamilton, Ontario: B. C. Decker, Inc.; 1999:321.*

Heart Rate

Commonly, tachycardia in a child with decreased level of consciousness is a nonspecific finding related to fever or pain. However, tachycardia associated with supraventricular arrhythmias such as supraventricular tachycardia may impair cardiac output and hence cerebral perfusion. Tachycardia may also be a manifestation of underlying cardiac disorders associated with decreased cardiac output. Bradycardia is usually more ominous and may result from raised ICP (the Cushing triad of bradycardia, hypertension, and slow breathing) or may be agonal. Complete heart block may be associated with bradycardia and reduced cerebral perfusion secondary to reduced cardiac output.

Blood Pressure

Hypotension in a patient with altered mental status suggests hypovolemia, sepsis, cardiogenic, or distributive (anaphylactic or neurogenic) shock. It can also result from drug overdose and adrenal failure. Hypertension may be a manifestation of pain or caused by underlying etiology such as renal failure or intoxication (ie, cocaine abuse). It can also result from elevated ICP as a compensatory mechanism to maintain cerebral perfusion (the Cushing triad). Extreme elevations in blood pressure can be associated with altered mental status secondary to hypertensive encephalopathy, hypertensive intracranial bleeding, or posterior reversible leukoencephalopathy.

Breathing

Breathing rate and pattern of breathing in particular must be carefully observed and recorded. Specific breathing patterns have a great value in localization of lesions along the neuraxis. Kussmaul breathing (fast and deep breathing) is typically associated diabetic ketoacidosis but can result from metabolic acidosis from other etiologies. Abnormal breathing patterns such as periodic breathing; Cheyne-Stokes breathing; ataxic breathing; or slow, irregular breathing indicate deeper levels of coma and result from brain stem lesions (Figure 4-1).

General Examination

The patient must be completely exposed and examined. Focus must be a close look at skin and mucous membranes. Helpful clinical signs are cyanosis (hypoxia, cyanotic congenital heart disease), pallor (anemia, shock), jaundice (liver disease, hemolytic disorder), and cherry red color of skin and mucous membranes (carbon monoxide poisoning). Bruising around the eyes (raccoon eyes) and mastoid process (battle sign) suggests head injury as does the leakage of cerebrospinal fluid (CSF) from the nose (rhinorrhea) or ears (otorrhea). Skin rashes indicate the possibility of infectious etiology or a collagen vascular disorder. Old scars, skin bruises, or burns (thermal or otherwise) of different ages at anatomically inexplicable sites and fractures unexplained by the degree and type of trauma must raise the suspicion of child abuse.

Funduscopic examination in an unconscious child must not be overlooked, and preferably must be done without using mydriatics, which may interfere with monitoring of pupillary size. Papilledema indicates presence of raised ICP. Retinal hemorrhages in an infant or young child strongly suggest abusive head trauma.

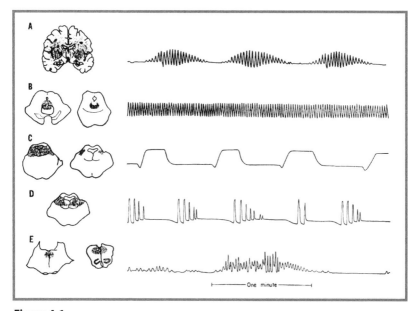

Figure 4-1.
Abnormal respiratory patterns associated with pathologic lesions at various levels of the brain in unconscious patients. Tracings by chest-abdomen pneumograph, inspiration reads up: (A) Cheyne-Stokes respiration, (B) central neurogenic hyperventilation, (C) apneusis, (D) cluster breathing, (E) ataxic breathing. (From Plum F, Posner J. *The Diagnosis of Stupor and Coma.* 3rd ed. Philadelphia, PA: FA Davis; 1982:34.)

All children with depressed mental status must specifically be examined for signs of meningeal irritation. These signs include neck stiffness (nuchal rigidity) and the Kernig and Brudzinski signs. They are present in children with meningitis or subarachnoid hemorrhage, though these signs may be absent in infants and young children.

Neurologic Examination

The neurologic examination in patients with altered consciousness aims to help differentiate structural from nonstructural causes, as well as provide a baseline for monitoring the effects of therapeutic interventions. Emphasis must be focused on the level of alertness, motor responses, and ocular findings.

Assessment of level of consciousness starts with the observation of the patient's spontaneous behavior (in terms of eye opening, motor movements, and vocal responses) as well as his or her responses to verbal commands and physical stimuli. The patient may then be assigned a level of consciousness

(Table 4-1), and recording and quantifying the response allows a global evaluation of the patient's mental status (Glasgow Coma Scale [GCS]), which can be monitored over time (Table 4-3).

Motor responses are assessed by observing the patient's ability to respond to simple commands. In patients who are unable to follow verbal instructions, spontaneous motor movements are observed. In patients who do not spontaneously move their extremities, movements may be induced by a physical stimulus such as supraorbital pressure, squeezing of nail bed, or scratching the sole of the foot. Patients may respond by withdrawing from or pushing off the stimulus (Table 4-3). Whether observed movements are spontaneous or stimulus provoked, it is very important to note any asymmetry between the sides.

Motor evaluation also includes muscle tone and deep tendon reflexes and any abnormalities and asymmetries recorded. Presence of decerebrate

Table 4-3. Glasgow Coma Scale for Children[a]			
Sign	**Glasgow Coma Scale (GCS) for Children >5 years**	**GCS–Modified for Children <5 years**	**Score**
Eye opening	Spontaneous	Spontaneous	4
	To command	To sound	3
	To pain	To pain	2
	None	None	1
Verbal response	Oriented	Alert, babbles, coos, words or sentences normal for age	5
	Confused	Less than usual ability, irritable cry	4
	Inappropriate words	Cries to pain	3
	Incomprehensible sounds	Moans to pain	2
	None	None	1
Motor response	Obeys commands	Normal spontaneous movements	6
	Localizes pain	Localizes pain	5
	Withdraws	Withdraws	4
	Abnormal flexion to pain	Abnormal flexion to pain	3
	Abnormal extension to pain	Abnormal extension to pain	2
	None	None	1

[a]Modified from Kirkham FJ, Newton CR, Whitehouse W. Pediatric coma scales. *Dev Med Child Neurol.* 2008;50:267–274. Reproduced with permission of Blackwell Publishing Ltd.

and decorticate posturing, either spontaneously or in response to physical stimulus must be noted and recorded. Decerebrate posture consists of extension and internal rotation of arms and legs and its presence indicates structural lesions at the brain stem level. Decorticate posturing, which suggests a more rostral lesion in the neuraxis results in adduction and flexion at elbows, wrists, and fingers with extension and rotation of lower extremities.

Ocular examination must focus on pupils (pupillary size, symmetry, and light reflex), extraocular movements, and corneal reflex. Small and reactive pupils can be seen with metabolic disorders and certain intoxications such as opioid and cholinergic drugs, and hypnotics-sedatives. Pinpoint pupils point to structural pontine lesions. Pupillary dilation or mydriasis can result from sympathomimetic or anticholinergic drugs. Dilated and fixed pupils (unreactive to light) indicate a brain stem insult. Anisocoria (inequality of pupillary size) suggests a structural lesion of the third nerve or its brain stem connections (Figure 4-2).

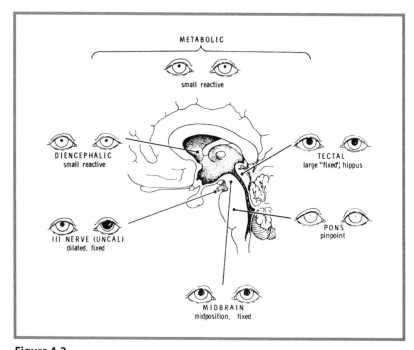

Figure 4-2.
Type of pupillary abnormalities in unconscious patients depending on the anatomical level of neurologic dysfunction. (From Plum F, Posner J. *The Diagnosis of Stupor and Coma.* 3rd ed. Philadelphia, PA: FA Davis; 1982:46.)

Deviation of the eyes to one side indicates an ipsilateral cerebral or a contralateral pontine lesion. Limitation of eye movements in one direction indicates structural lesions of cranial nerves (III, IV, VI) or their central connections in the brain stem. Spontaneous roving eye movements indicate that the brain stem is intact. Eye movements in comatose children can be induced by rotating the head in either direction (oculocephalic reflex). Eyes should turn in the opposite direction, indicating an intact brain stem. Absent oculocephalic reflexes indicate a profound degree of coma with loss of brain stem reflexes, and these patients may be evaluated further by cold caloric (oculovestibular) testing (Figure 4-3). Testing of the oculocephalic reflex must not be done in a patient with suspected cervical spine injury or instability. The corneal reflex, which reflects the function of the trigeminal and facial nerves, is assessed by lightly touching the patient's cornea with a fine wisp of cotton, and it should produce bilateral eye blink.

The gag reflex must be tested to evaluate the function of the glossopharyngeal and vagus nerves. An absent gag reflex is indicative of very deep levels of coma.

Patients must also be observed for any abnormal involuntary movements. Focal seizures indicate a structural lesion. Presence of multifocal myoclonus points to a metabolic etiology.

A vital objective in the initial clinical assessment of the child with acute encephalopathy is to determine whether ICP is elevated and whether, therefore, urgent neurosurgical attention may be required. Papilledema, retinal hemorrhages, and bradycardia in young children are examples of observations that emphasize the possibility of elevated ICP, but much more important than isolated observations at a single point in time are the pattern and the tempo of the evolution of neurologic findings over time. What signifies critically elevated ICP is change. The GCS can serve as a guide for assessment and an instrument for measurement of change. Sequential deterioration in pupillary reactivity, ocular motility, motor responses, and breathing patterns may be indicative of a herniation syndrome. Clinical recognition of elevated ICP therefore requires a careful initial evaluation and deliberate, frequent reassessments over time.

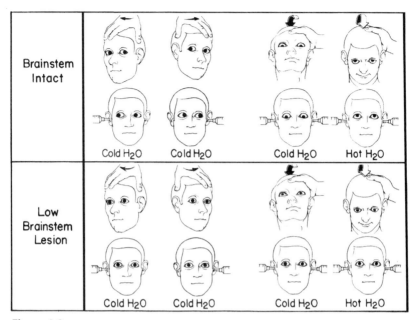

Figure 4-3.

Ocular reflexes in unconscious patients. The upper section illustrates the oculocephalic (above) and oculovestibular (below) reflexes in an unconscious patient whose brain stem ocular pathways are intact. Horizontal eye movements are illustrated on the left and vertical eye movements on the right: lateral conjugate eye movements (upper left) to head turning are full and opposite in direction to the movement of the face. A stronger stimulus to lateral deviation is achieved by irrigating cold water against the tympanic membrane. There is a tonic conjugate deviation of both eyes toward the stimulus; the eyes usually remain tonically deviated for 1 or more minutes before slowly returning to the midline. Because the patient is unconscious, there is no nystagmus. Extension of the neck in a patient with an intact brain stem produces conjugate eye deviation of the eyes in the downward direction, and flexion of the neck produces deviation of the eyes upward. Bilateral cold water irrigation against the tympanic membrane likewise produces conjugate downward deviation of the eyes, whereas hot water (no warmer than 44°C) causes conjugate upward deviation of the eyes. The lower portion of the drawing illustrates the effects of a low brain stem lesion. On the left, neither oculovestibular nor oculocephalic movements cause lateral deviation of the eyes because the pathways are interrupted between the vestibular nucleus and the abducens nucleus. Likewise, in the right portion of the drawing, neither oculovestibular nor oculocephalic stimulation causes vertical deviation of the eyes. (From Plum F, Posner J. *The Diagnosis of Stupor and Coma*. 3rd ed. Philadelphia, PA: FA Davis; 1982:55.)

Laboratory Evaluation

Laboratory workup in most cases will be guided by the findings of history and physical examination. A rapid bedside glucose measurement must precede any other testing. In a patient for whom etiology of coma remains unknown after initial clinical evaluation, serum electrolytes, blood urea nitrogen, creatinine, calcium, magnesium, glucose, liver function tests, ammonia, complete blood count, arterial blood gas, and urine drug screen must be determined. Fever must prompt blood culture and culture of other appropriate sites including urine for bacterial, viral, or other pathogens based on clinical presentation.

Suspicion of a metabolic disorder indicates testing for serum lactate, pyruvate, amino acids, creatine kinase, carnitine, plasma-free fatty acids, urine ketone bodies, urine organic acids, and thyroid function testing. Extended drug screening is indicated to detect drugs/toxins not tested by urine drug screen. More sophisticated testing may be indicated if the cause of coma still remains unknown.

Diagnosis

By following the algorithm presented in Figure 4-4, the ABCs of emergency management have been completed, and the immediate concerns are being addressed. It is important to reassess the initial unanswered questions throughout the evaluation. Repeated neurologic examinations, imaging studies, and electrophysiological studies may reveal dynamic processes that often are not obvious on initial studies.

Neuroimaging Studies

Brain evaluation by computed tomography (CT) or magnetic resonance imaging (MRI) scan is most useful for evaluating patients with acute encephalopathy caused by structural lesions. Computed tomography is usually the initial choice because of easy availability and short scanning times. It also quickly identifies surgically treatable causes like hydrocephalus and masses secondary to tumors or infections. It is superior to MRI in detecting hemorrhages and bony integrity, and therefore it is the imaging modality of choice in evaluating trauma patients. It is also the preferred modality to rule out raised ICP quickly when lumbar puncture is indicated.

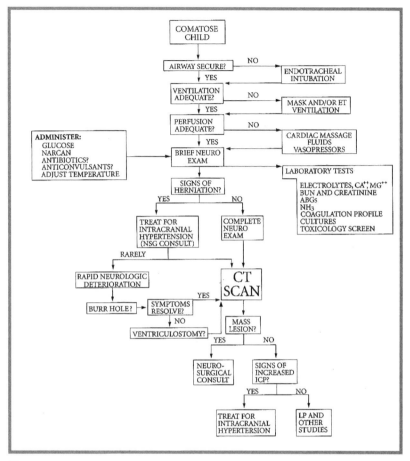

Figure 4-4.
Algorithm for management of children with altered consciousness or coma. Abbreviations: ABG, arterial blood gas; CT, computerized tomography; ET, endotracheal; LP, lumbar puncture; NSG, neurosurgery. (From Bunch ST, Goodwin SR. Altered states of consciousness. In: Maria BL, ed. *Current Management in Child Neurology.* Shelton, CT: PMPH-USA; 1999:318. Reprinted by permission.)

Magnetic resonance imaging provides more structural details and is more sensitive than CT for detecting anoxia, stroke, demyelination, encephalitis, diffuse axonal injury from head trauma, petechial hemorrhages, and cerebral venous thrombosis. Mass lesions caused by tumors and infections are also better delineated by MRI. Magnetic resonance imaging is also superior to CT in evaluating posterior fossa anatomical structures.

Lumbar Puncture

When infection of the central nervous system is suspected in a child with altered consciousness, CSF must be obtained promptly by means of a lumbar puncture. Usually CT of the head is required beforehand to exclude an intracranial mass to minimize the danger of herniation. Treatment with antimicrobials must, however, never be delayed if a lumbar puncture cannot be immediately performed. Lumbar puncture is also indicated in patients with suspected acute demyelinating encephalomyelitis. Cytological examination of CSF for malignant cells may be requested when intracranial involvement by a malignant process is suspected.

Electroencephalography

Electroencephalography is indicated in all children with coma of unknown etiology. Patients with nonconvulsive status epilepticus need an EEG for the diagnosis of ongoing electroencephalographic seizure activity in the absence of external motor convulsive movements. Specific patterns of EEG may suggest the underlying diagnosis. Periodic lateralizing epileptiform discharges (PLEDs) point to underlying herpes encephalitis, infarction, abscess, or other acute structural lesion. Subacute sclerosing panencephalitis is associated with generalized high-voltage periodic discharges. Diffuse slowing with triphasic waves is seen with metabolic encephalopathies like hepatic failure. Continuous EEG monitoring is used to assess and to titrate the effect of medications in patients treated with anesthesia for control of status epilepticus. Finally EEG is helpful in the diagnosis of brain death in patients with irreversible coma.

Differential Diagnosis

There are several conditions that need to be differentiated from coma in the patient with depressed level of consciousness (Figure 4-5). The distinction is important for treatment decisions, prognosis, resource allocation, and medicolegal judgments. Some studies suggest a high rate of misdiagnosis (false-positives and false-negatives) among disorders of consciousness.

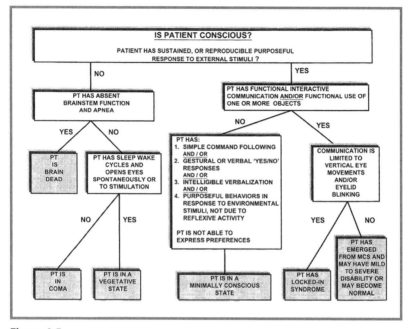

Figure 4-5.
Approach to the differential diagnosis of the unconscious patient. (From Ashwal S. Medical aspects of the minimally conscious state in children. *Brain Dev.* 2003;25:535–545, with permission from Elsevier.)

Vegetative State

The vegetative state (VS) is a condition of complete unawareness of the self and the environment accompanied by sleep-wake cycles with either complete or partial preservation of hypothalamic and brain stem autonomic functions. A patient in the VS appears at times to be wakeful, with cycles of eye closure and eye opening resembling those of sleep and waking. However, close observation reveals no sign of awareness or of a "functional mind." Specifically, there is no evidence that the patient can perceive the environment or his or her own body, communicate with others, or form intentions. The diagnostic criteria are enumerated in Box 4-2.

It has been estimated that there are between 14,000 and 35,000 patients in VS in the United States (4,000 to 10,000 of them children). Vegetative state can follow a variety of severe insults to the brain, most commonly traumatic or hypoxic-ischemic brain injuries, but also metabolic and neurodegenerative conditions, and congenital or developmental disorders. The

---

Box 4-2. Diagnostic Criteria for the Vegetative State[a]

No evidence of awareness of self or environment; no interaction with others

No evidence of sustained, reproducible, purposeful, or voluntary behavioral responses to visual, auditory, tactile, or noxious stimuli

No evidence of language comprehension or expression

Intermittent wakefulness manifested by the presence of sleep-wake cycles

Sufficiently preserved hypothalamic and brain stem autonomic functions to survive if given medical and nursing care

Bowel and bladder incontinence

Variably preserved cranial nerve (papillary, oculocephalic, corneal, vestibulo-ocular, and gag) and spinal reflexes

---

[a]From Practice parameters: assessment and management of patients in the persistent vegetative state (summary statement). The Quality Standards Subcommittee of the American Academy of Neurology. Neurology. 1995;45:1016. Reprinted with permission from Wolters Kluwer Health.

VS may be a transient one, or it may persist until death. According to the Multi-Society Task Force on PVS, the term *persistent* should only be used to describe a condition of past and continuing disability with an uncertain future; *permanent* should be used to imply an irreversible state.

Minimally Conscious State

The minimally conscious state (MCS) is a condition of severely altered consciousness in which minimal but definite behavioral evidence of self or environmental awareness is demonstrated. These patients demonstrate discernible behavioral evidence of consciousness but remain unable to reproduce this behavior consistently. The diagnostic criteria are enumerated in Box 4-3.

Some patients with severe alteration in consciousness have neurologic findings that do not meet criteria for VS. Children in a VS have no evidence of language comprehension or expression using verbal or nonverbal signals. Children in an MCS may show a limited capacity for communication and are also more likely to experience pain and suffering in contrast to children in a VS, who by definition are unable to do so.

It has been estimated that there are between 14,000 and 35,000 adult and pediatric MCS patients.

> **Box 4-3. Diagnostic Criteria for the Minimally Conscious State[a]**
>
> Following simple commands
>
> Gestural or verbal yes/no responses (regardless of accuracy)
>
> Intelligible verbalization
>
> Purposeful behavior, including movements or affective behaviors, that occur in contingent relation to relevant environmental stimuli and are not due to reflexive activity. Some examples of qualifying purposeful behavior include
>
> — Appropriate smiling or crying in response to the linguistic or visual content of emotional but not to neutral topics or stimuli
>
> — Vocalizations or gestures that occur in direct response to the linguistic content of questions
>
> — Reaching for objects that demonstrates a clear relationship between object location and direction of reach
>
> — Touching or holding objects in a manner that accommodates the size and the shape of the object
>
> — Pursuit eye movement or sustained fixation that occurs in direct response to moving or salient stimuli
>
> ---
> *[a]From Giacino JT Ashwal S, Childs N, et al. The minimally conscious state: definition and diagnostic criteria. Neurology. 2002;58:351. Reprinted with permission from Wolters Kluwer Health.*

The causes are similar to the causes of VS. It is thought that MCS requires bilateral multifocal or diffuse injury to cortical or subcortical structures similar to patients in a VS. This would include subcortical white matter injury, diffuse axonal injury particularly in the thalamus, ischemic injury in the neocortex, and focal injury to brain stem or diencephalic structures.

Locked-In Syndrome

This syndrome is most commonly due to acute ventral pontine lesions. Patients with such brain stem lesions often remain comatose for some days or weeks, needing artificial respiration, but gradually wake up, remaining paralyzed and voiceless, superficially resembling patients in a VS or akinetic mutism. Patients with locked-in syndrome are awake and conscious, but selectively deefferented (ie, have no means of producing speech, limb, or facial movements). Eye-coded communication and evaluation of cognitive and emotional functioning is very limited because vigilance is fluctuating and eye movements may be inconsistent, very small, and easily exhausted. Recent reports indicate that on average it takes more than 2.5 months to establish the diagnosis, which is more frequently suspected by the family than by the doctor. However, in some cases, it has taken 4 to 6 years before aware and sensitive patients, locked in an immobile body, were recognized as being conscious.

Akinetic Mutism

This condition is rare, and characteristically accompanies gradually developing or subacute, bilateral damage to the paramedian mesencephalon, basal diencephalon, or inferior frontal lobes. Patients have pathologically slowed or nearly absent body movements, accompanied by loss of speech. Wakefulness and self-awareness are usually present, but the level of mental function is reduced.

Brain Death

The term *brain death* is used to describe irreversible cessation of all functions of the brain, including the brain stem. Traditionally, and in most cases even now, death is diagnosed on the basis of the irreversible cessation of circulatory and respiratory functions. But with advancing science and increasing technological sophistications, it has been possible to sustain cardiorespiratory functions even in patients whose brain has suffered profound and irreversible damage with loss of all its functions. The concept of death in these situations has been replaced with brain death. The cultural, legal, and medical controversies that surround the concept of brain death are beyond the scope of this chapter; however, the usefulness of the concept lies in its application in decision making with regard to withdrawal of life support and organ donation for transplantation.

Patients who are brain dead differ from patients who are in a persistent VS, because the latter have preserved sleep-wake cycles, brain stem functions, and some degree of respiratory drive (Figure 4-4).

The declaration of brain death requires a careful neurologic examination to document irreversible loss of all brain functions (coma, absence of brain stem reflexes, and apnea). Severe electrolyte, acid-base or endocrine disturbances, hypothermia (a core temperature of 32°C or lower), hypotension, drug intoxication, poisoning, or neuromuscular blocking agents must be excluded as these conditions can confound the findings of neurologic examination. Confirmatory laboratory tests, which are optional in adults, are recommended in children younger than 1 year (Box 4-4).

Practitioners are advised to consult the policies of their medical centers and, in some states, the requirements of statutory law in the determination of brain death.

Treatment

The treatment of patients with altered consciousness or who are comatose has the following objectives: (1) maintenance of vital support, (2) management of complications, and (3) specific treatment of the underlying cause.

Vital Support

Maintenance of an adequate airway remains one of the most important principles in the management of these patients. The second important principle is to maintain cardiovascular function. Glucose is the essential source of adenosine triphosphate for cerebral metabolism; glucose administration

---

Box 4-4. Guidelines for the Determination of Brain Death in Children[a]

Neurologic Examination
1. Coma and apnea requiring mechanical ventilation
2. Absence of motor responses
3. Absence of brain stem function
   a. Mid-position dilated pupils without light reflexes
   b. Absent oculocephalic, oculovestibular (caloric), corneal, nasopharyngeal, gag, cough, sucking, and rooting reflexes
   c. Absent respiratory effort with standardized apnea testing

Diagnosis is independently confirmed after a period of observation determined by age:
1. Under 2 months: 48 hours with electroencephalogram (EEG) confirmation at each examination
2. 2 months to 1 year: 24 hours with EEG confirmation (or less time with both EEG and cerebral blood flow confirmation)
3. Over 1 year: 12 to 24 hours with confirmatory tests optional

---

[a]*Adapted from Michelson DJ, Ashwal S. Evaluation of coma and brain death. Sem Pediatr Neurol. 2004;11:105–118, with permission from Elsevier; Wijdicks EFM. The diagnosis of brain death. N Engl J Med. 2001;344:1201–1221.*

is essential if blood levels are low. Correction of acid-base and electrolyte imbalance is paramount in comatose patients because acidosis, alkalosis, or electrolyte imbalance, in many cases related to abnormal antidiuretic hormone function, are frequent and complicate the clinical picture. Fever must be aggressively treated.

Treatment of Complications

Increased ICP may be the primary cause of coma and is a frequent complication of several of its causes that must be treated effectively. Hyperventilation or pharmacologic therapies (osmotic agents such as hypertonic saline and mannitol, diuretics, corticosteroids, barbiturates) may be employed while ICP is being monitored. In extreme cases, unresponsive to medical treatment, decompressive craniectomy may be considered. Seizures may also be a complication of certain causes of coma or its complications (ie, electrolyte or metabolic imbalance) and must be treated aggressively, ideally with simultaneous continuous EEG monitoring, because recent clinical research has emphasized the risk of subclinical seizures in comatose patients. Agitation is a frequent complication in patients with altered mental status and may interfere with ventilatory support and may increase the ICP; however, the physician must consider that the medications used to treat agitation may interfere with the neurologic monitoring of the patient.

Etiological Treatment

In cases of CNS infection, suspected clinically or confirmed with CSF studies, specific antibiotic therapy should be initiated as soon as possible. In patients with toxic ingestion, specific antidotes should be administered (ie, naloxone for opiates, physostigmine for anticholinergic drugs, etc).

Hypothermia is currently under controversial discussion for the treatment of patients with different causes of coma (ie, sudden cardiac arrest, hypoxia-ischemia, trauma).

Prognosis

The most important factors directly related to the prognosis of children with impairment of consciousness or coma are the etiology (Table 4-4) and the rapid identification and treatment of the underlying cause.

Table 4-4. Etiology and Prognosis of Coma in Children[a]		
Etiology	Dead (%)	Intact (%)
Accident (eg, drowning)	84.2	10.5
Congenital (eg, congenital heart disease, including complication of the surgical repair)	72.7	9.1
Infection (with *Neisseria meningitidis* being the most prevalent pathogen)	60.0	26.4
Others (eg, coma as a complication of asthma or complication of a malignancy)	47.6	28.6
Unknown	30.0	47.5
Metabolic (eg, diabetic ketoacidosis, medium-chain acyl-CoA dehydrogenase deficiency, etc)	26.7	60.0
Epilepsy	17.9	71.9
Intoxication (accidental and intentional)	3.4	48.3

[a]Adapted from Wong CP, Forsyth RJ, Kelly TP, Eire JA. Incidence, aetiology, and outcome of non-traumatic coma: a population based study. *Arch Dis Child*. 2001;84:193–199, with permission from BMJ Publishing Group Ltd.

Outcome studies in childhood coma are available for traumatic and non-traumatic causes and typically emphasize the predictive value of signs and symptoms at the time of initial medical intervention. The GCS is widely accepted as a predictor of survival after severe traumatic brain injury. Prognostication about degrees of disability, however, is much more challenging. Simply describing disability is difficult. A companion instrument to the GCS, the 5-point Glasgow Outcome Scale, has been employed for many clinical research purposes; however, it is limited in its ability to measure social, emotional, and cognitive dysfunction. Specific pediatric outcome scales have been developed, such as the Disability Rating Scale, the Wee Functional Independence Measure, and the Pediatric Evaluation of Disability Inventory.

Multimodality evoked potentials (EPs) are helpful in establishing the prognosis of comatose patients. The absence of brain stem auditory evoked potentials (BAEPs) with an intact wave I is predictive of brain death. However, patients with normal BAEPs may often die or survive in a chronic VS. Absent somatosensory evoked potentials with abnormal BAEPs are associated with death or survival in a chronic VS. In a review of 1,000 comatose patients compiled from 15 studies, the use of multimodality EPs to predict the outcome showed no false pessimism. The acceptable error of false optimism occurs relatively frequently because many comatose patients die from causes that are not neurologic, and many neurologic problems are not static.

Bibliography

Abbruzzi G, Stork CM. Pediatric toxicologic concerns. *Emerg Med Clin North Am.* 2002;20: 223–247

Ashwal S. Medical aspects of the minimally conscious state in children. *Brain Dev.* 2003;25: 535–545

Ashwal S. Pediatric vegetative state: epidemiological and clinical issues. *NeuroRehabilitation.* 2004;19:349–360

Ashwal S. Recovery of consciousness and life expectancy of children in a vegetative state. *Neuropsychol Rehabil.* 2005;15:190–197

Ashwal S. The persistent vegetative state. *Adv Pediatr.* 1994;41:195–222

Bunch ST, Goodwin SR. Altered states of consciousness. In: Maria BL, ed. *Current Management in Child Neurology.* Hamilton, Ontario: B. C. Decker, Inc. 1999:317–324

Fenichel GM. Altered states of consciousness. In: Fenichel GM, ed. *Clinical Pediatric Neurology. A Signs and Symptoms Approach.* Philadelphia, PA: Elsevier; 2005:47–75

Giacino JT, Ashwal S, Childs N, et al. The minimally conscious state: definition and diagnostic criteria. *Neurology.* 2002;58:349–353

Kirkham FJ, Newton CR, Whitehouse W. Pediatric coma scales. *Dev Med Child Neurol.* 2008; 50:267–274

Laureys S, Pellas F, Van Eeckhout P, et al. The locked-in syndrome: what is it like to be conscious but paralyzed and voiceless? *Prog Brain Res.* 2005;150:495–511

Medical aspects of the persistent vegetative state (1). The Multi-Society Task Force on PVS. *N Engl J Med.* 1994;330:1499–1508, 1572–1579

Michelson DJ, Ashwal S. Evaluation of coma and brain death. *Semin Pediatr Neurol.* 2004;11: 105–118

Nelson DS. Coma and altered level of consciousness. In: Fleisher GR, Ludwing S, Henretig FM, Ruddy RM, Silverman BK, eds. *Textbook of Pediatric Emergency Medicine.* Philadelphia, PA: Lippincott Williams & Wilkins; 2006:201–212

Plum F, Posner JB. *The Diagnosis of Stupor and Coma.* 3rd ed. Philadelphia, PA: F.A. Davis; 1982

Practice parameters: assessment and management of patients in the persistent vegetative state (summary statement). The Quality Standards Subcommittee of the American Academy of Neurology. *Neurology.* 1995;45:1015–1018

Report of special Task Force. Guidelines for the determination of brain death in children. American Academy of Pediatrics Task Force on Brain Death in Children. *Pediatrics.* 1987;80:298–300

Royal College of Physicians. A working party report. The vegetative state: guidance on diagnosis and management. *Clin Med.* 2003;3:249–254

Taylor DA, Ashwal S. Impairment of consciousness and coma. In: Swaiman KF, Ashwal S, Ferriero DM, eds. *Pediatric Neurology. Principles & Practice.* Philadelphia, PA: Mosby Elsevier; 2006:1377–1400

Trübel HK, Novotny E, Lister G. Outcome of coma in children. *Curr Opin Pediatr.* 2003;15: 283–287

Wijdicks EFM. The diagnosis of brain death. *N Engl J Med.* 2001;344:1201–1221

Wong CP, Forsyth RJ, Kelly TP, Eyre JA. Incidence, aetiology, and outcome of non-traumatic coma: a population based study. *Arch Dis Child.* 2001;84:193–199

Young GB. The EEG in coma. *J Clin Neurophysiol.* 2000;17:473–485

Zeman A. Consciousness. *Brain.* 2001;124(Pt 7):1263–1289

Zeman A. Persistent vegetative state. *Lancet.* 1997;350:795–799

Chapter 5

Traumatic Brain Injury

Joseph H. Piatt Jr, MD

Introduction and Definitions

Traumatic brain injury (TBI) is a major public health problem. Trauma is the leading cause of death from the end of the first year of life, through childhood and adolescence, and well into young adulthood. Brain injury is the leading cause of traumatic death in childhood and is responsible for the preponderance of the long-term disability associated with trauma. The Centers for Disease Control and Prevention reports that from 1995 through 2001 among children up through 19 years of age there were annual averages of 564,000 emergency department visits, 62,000 hospitalizations, and 7,440 deaths due to TBI. The costs of health care services and lost productivity and the personal cost to patients and families are enormous burdens on society.

For didactic and investigative purposes, TBI must be categorized both qualitatively and quantitatively. Neurosurgeons and pathologists tend to think of TBI in qualitative terms: skull fractures at various anatomical sites, brain contusion and laceration, subarachnoid hemorrhage, hematomas in various compartments, diffuse axonal injury, and secondary brain ischemia, because these factors reflect mechanism and determine surgical intervention. Other physicians engaged in the care of TBI are often more concerned with quantitative characterizations: Is the injury severe enough to justify brain imaging, admission to hospital, or intubation? The framework of this chapter is predominantly quantitative.

The internationally accepted metric for quantity of injury is the Glasgow Coma Scale (GCS, Box 5-1). The GCS was developed more than 30 years ago for use among adults. Limitations in its applicability to children were recognized very early. As a simple example, an adult with a normal level of responsiveness will earn 4 points for spontaneous eye opening, but an infant with normal responsiveness who is screaming with her eyes shut and who closes her eyes even tighter when stimulated will earn only 1 point. Many modifications of the GCS have been proposed to extend its applicability to infants and young children, but none has attained wide acceptance. Another

Box 5-1. The Glasgow Coma Scale

Motor

	Following of commands	6
	Localization of painful stimuli	5
	Normal withdrawal	4
	Flexion posturing	3
	Extension posturing	2
	Flaccidity	1

Speech

	Orientation	5
	Appropriate but disoriented speech	4
	Intelligible but inappropriate speech	3
	Unintelligible speech	2
	Absent vocalization	1

Eye Opening

	Spontaneous	4
	In response to verbal stimulation	3
	In response to painful stimulation	2
	No eye opening	1

practical issue in the use of the GCS is the timing of the assignment of the score. The GCS score can fluctuate for better or for worse from the moment of the injury to the initial evaluation and through the initial resuscitation. For lesser injuries the score is generally assigned at the time of the initial evaluation and for severe injuries at a specified time after the initial resuscitation, although protocols may vary. With due recognition of its limitations, the GCS is commonly condensed into 3 grades: mild TBI (score 13–15), moderate TBI (score 9–12), and severe TBI (score 3–8).

By this standard mild TBI still encompasses a significant range of severity. A patient who cannot recall the date, a lethargic patient who opens his eyes only with verbal encouragement, and a patient with completely normal responsiveness may all be categorized as "mild," but clearly they present distinct clinical circumstances. The term *minor* is sometimes applied to the mild end of the mild range, that is, to the patient with a GCS score of 15 and a normal neurologic examination. Implicit in this designation is the understanding that brain imaging is normal or has not yet been performed. A closely related concept is cerebral concussion. The strict definition of the term *concussion* is transient, traumatic disruption of continuing brain activity. Loss of consciousness, amnesia, and immediate traumatic convulsion are all evidence of concussion. Particularly among children, the presence or absence of such indisputable manifestations of disrupted brain activity cannot always be determined by history, and the term is stretched to include patients with persisting symptoms such as headache, dizziness, nausea, vomiting, or behavior changes.

This chapter addresses aspects of TBI of concern to physicians engaged in the primary care of children. Minor TBI and concussion are by far the most common problems in primary practice. Treatment is generally symptomatic and expectant, but informed judgments must be made to identify patients at substantial risk for life-threatening complications while minimizing the exposure of patients at very low risk to diagnostic radiation. Likewise, the salient issues in the management of TBI among athletes are not so much therapeutic as preventive: how to strike a judicious balance between participation in sports and avoidance of permanent cognitive disability from the cumulative effects of repeated injuries. The recognition of abusive injury is a fundamental task in pediatric office and emergency department practice. Primary practitioners may value some understanding of the management of severe TBI both for perspective and for counseling of families as well.

Minor Traumatic Brain Injury

There are 3 practical issues that arise in the care of the child who comes to medical attention after a minor head injury with a normal level of consciousness and a normal neurologic examination.

- Detection of evolving but not yet apparent injuries that will later become symptomatic or require neurosurgical intervention
- Management of symptoms
- Restriction of activities for avoidance of persisting neurocognitive disability from the cumulative effects of repeated injuries

This section will review guidelines and recent clinical research into the question of indications for brain imaging. It will also provide guidance for the emergency department and office management of acute and subacute symptoms. The question of restriction of activities will be taken up in the following section on TBI in athletics, which is the sector of child and adolescent life that harbors foreseeable risk of recurrent injury.

The risk of a latent, evolving, life-threatening intracranial process in the child with minor TBI is very small and very difficult to quantitate precisely, but it is not negligible. The prevalence of traumatic lesions on computed tomography (CT) scan among children with minor TBI has been reported between 0% and 7.6%. The clinical mandate, however, is not to identify abnormal CT scans but to rescue children who are destined for disability or death without timely treatment. To identify children who need neurosurgical intervention is a goal closer to the mandate, although not synonymous with it. The literature indicates that 20% to 60% of children with minor TBI and an abnormal CT scan will require neurosurgery, although these estimates seem very high to the writer. Between 0% and 5% of all children with minor TBI may require a neurosurgical procedure. With expansion of the denominator from "minor" to "mild" TBI (that is, GCS 13, 14, or 15), the prevalence of abnormal imaging and neurosurgical intervention increases substantially.

In 1999, in collaboration with the American Academy of Family Physicians, the American Academy of Pediatrics (AAP) attempted to provide some guidance for primary practitioners regarding diagnostic assessment and monitoring of children with minor TBI in the publication of a set of clinical guidelines. The scope of this document was very narrow.

- Children between 2 and 20 years of age
- With normal mental status and normal neurologic examination
- Without any physical findings suggestive of skull fracture
- Who have sustained an isolated head injury with witnessed loss of consciousness not exceeding 1 minute in duration
- Who have come to medical attention within 24 hours of the injury

Patients with preexisting neurologic conditions, coagulopathy, possible cervical spine injury, or possible abusive injury were excluded. For children without any loss of consciousness, observation by a competent adult was recommended, but brain imaging was not recommended. For children with brief loss of consciousness, the guidelines stated, "Cranial CT scanning may also be used, in addition to observation…." There was no comment on the duration or the technique of the recommended observation, matters which have not—before or since this publication—received any systematic study.

The unhelpfulness of the 1999 AAP statement illustrates the inadequacy of the evidence available at that time and highlights important subsequent work on the question of the indications for brain imaging. Curiously, the emphasis placed by the AAP statement on loss of consciousness has been undermined by subsequent investigations. In 2003 Palchuk et al reported an observational cohort study of 2,043 children with TBI of all degrees of severity. The presence of abnormal mental status, a history of vomiting, headache, scalp hematoma (among patients ≤2 years of age), or other signs of skull fracture identified all patients who required any acute intervention. The recursive partitioning process employed in this study rejected loss of consciousness as a significant predictor of need for intervention. A subsequent analysis confirmed that no child with *isolated* loss of consciousness or posttraumatic amnesia had an abnormal CT scan (95% CI: 0%–2.1%) or required acute intervention (95% CI: 0%–1.8%). The relatively simple decision rule based on the 5 factors mentioned above has not held up well, unfortunately, when applied to other comparable patient populations. The precise interpretation of the terms *headache* and *vomiting* seem to affect the sensitivity and specificity of the rule.

The search for guidelines has been taken up by large, multicenter, clinical research networks. The National Emergency X-ray Utilization Study—Phase II (NEXUS II) collected data prospectively on 13,728 patients of all ages who received CT scans for TBI at any of 21 participating North American institutions. Analysis of the entire cohort yielded a decision rule with a high sensitivity and a high negative predictive value for significant intracranial injury (Box 5-2). This rule was analyzed among the 1,666 children younger than 18 years enrolled in the study and among the 309 children younger than 3 years. Among the entire pediatric cohort, the sensitivity was 98.6% and the negative predictive value (NPV) was 99.1% (95% CI 96.9%–99.9%). Among the younger children, the rule performed even better with sensitivity and NPV both 100% (95% CI 78.2%–100%). A prospective validation of this rule is planned. Even though NEXUS II actually enrolled fewer children than some large single-institution studies, the results probably have better generalizability because interobserver misunderstandings about the meaning of the clinical and imaging criteria were resolved at an early stage in the coordination of the trial among the many centers.

The largest prospective, observational trial of this kind was reported by Dunning et al in 2006 from 10 hospital emergency departments in the northwest of England. Among the 22,772 children accrued, there were 281

Box 5-2. The NEXUS II Rule[a] (Presence of any of the following factors indicates a CT scan.)

Evidence of significant skull fracture

Altered level of alertness

Neurologic deficit

Persistent vomiting

Presence of scalp hematoma

Abnormal behavior

Coagulopathy

Age ≥65 years

Abbreviations: NEXUS II, National Emergency X-ray Utilization Study—Phase II; CT, computed tomography.
[a]Adapted from Dunning J, Daly JP, Lomas, JP, Lecky F, Batchelor J, Mackway-Jones K. Derivation of the children's head injury algorithm for the prediction of important clinical events decision rule for head injury in children. Arch Dis Child. 2006;91:885–891.

---

abnormal CT scans, 137 neurosurgical procedures, and 15 deaths. From this experience recursive partitioning was used to develop the children's head injury algorithm for the prediction of important clinical events (CHALICE) rule (Box 5-3). The CHALICE rule exhibited a sensitivity of 98% (95% CI 96%–100%) and a specificity of 87% (95% CI 86%–87%). It misclassified patients with clinically significant intracranial injury. The NPV was 0.9997 (95% CI 99.9%–100%), and although the interpretation of the NPV is sometimes clouded by its dependence on case mix, when it has been derived from such a large dataset from so many contributing institutions, such a high value inspires confidence. The weakness of the CHALICE rule, if any, is its complexity.

At the time of this writing, several other major multicenter efforts are underway in Canada and Europe to develop rules for indicating CT scans for children with minor TBI. Very likely all of these various rules will be validated by follow-up studies and investigated with respect to their adaptability in clinical practice and their implications for resource use. Eventually, practice guidelines will provide a foundation for evidence-based emergency department protocols. Depressed responsiveness, abnormal neurologic examination, repetitive vomiting, and physical signs of skull fracture are factors that have emerged as consistent indicators of brain imaging in the

---

Box 5-3. The CHALICE Rule[a] (Presence of any of the following factors indicates a CT scan.)

History

   Witnessed loss of consciousness of >5 min duration

   History of amnesia (either anterograde or retrograde) of >5 min duration

   Abnormal drowsiness (defined as drowsiness in excess of that expected by the examining doctor)

   >3 vomits after head injury (a vomit is defined as a single discrete episode of vomiting)

   Suspicion of NAI (defined as any suspicion of NAI by the examining doctor)

   Seizure after head injury in a patient who has no history of epilepsy

Examination

   GCS <14, or GCS <15 if <1 year old

   Suspicion of penetrating or depressed skull injury or tense fontanel

   Signs of a basal skull fracture (defined as evidence of blood or cerebrospinal fluid from ear or nose, panda eyes, Battle sign, hemotympanum, facial crepitus, or serious facial injury)

   Positive focal neurology (defined as any focal neurology, including motor, sensory, coordination, or reflex abnormality)

   Presence of bruise, swelling or laceration >5 cm if <1 year old

Mechanism

   High-speed road traffic accident either as pedestrian, cyclist, or occupant (defined as accident with speed >40 m/h)

   Fall of >3 m in height

   High-speed injury from a projectile or an object

Abbreviations: CHALICE, children's head injury algorithm for the prediction of important clinical events; CT, computed tomography; NAI, non-accidental injury; GCS, Glasgow Coma Scale.

[a]Adapted from Dunning J, Daly JP, Lomas, JP, Lecky F, Batchelor J, Mackway-Jones K. Derivation of the children's head injury algorithm for the prediction of important clinical events decision rule for head injury in children. Arch Dis Child. 2006;91:885–891.

rules that have been published to date, but the persistence and severity of headache, for instance, are factors that have exhibited variable significance and require further study. To attempt at this time to condense such a rapidly evolving body of knowledge into a succinct recommendation for the general physician would be intellectually unsupportable. Hopefully this brief review has served to emphasize the critical clinical issues in a fashion that informs clinical judgment.

Children who have been evaluated and released from an emergency department after a minor head injury not uncommonly reappear in the offices of their primary physicians the following week with continuing, non-specific symptoms such as headache, dizziness, anorexia, sleep disturbance, or other cognitive and behavioral changes. This scenario raises a practical question: When is repeat imaging indicated for the child who has had a negative initial evaluation? Davis et al reported the 1-month outcomes of 400 children younger than 18 years with mild TBI (GCS 13, 14, or 15) who had CT scans within 24 hours of injury showing no intracranial hemorrhage. Excluded from the study were out-of-state patients and patients who required surgery for depressed skull fractures. Included were patients with skull fractures, as long as there were no intracranial findings. Follow-up was conducted by review of hospital and clinic records and by searching a comprehensive statewide hospital discharge registry and a statewide death registry. Four of 400 patients were readmitted within 30 days for TBI complications. One patient had a seizure; one patient had post-concussive symptoms and otitis; one patient had a symptomatic hemorrhagic contusion; and one patient, who was chronically anticoagulated for congenital heart disease, had an acute subdural hematoma (ASDH) and required craniotomy. There were no deaths. Thus among patients not undergoing therapeutic anticoagulation, the cumulative rate of intracranial bleeding requiring neurosurgical intervention in the month following a normal CT scan, was 0% (95% CI 0%–0.7%). In the absence of extenuating circumstances, a normal CT scan after a mild TBI excludes the possibility of late surgical complications.

Persistence of symptoms for days or weeks after a minor head injury is referred to as the post-concussion syndrome. Typical symptoms include headache, dizziness, disturbed sleep, difficulty concentrating and other cognitive disturbances, irritability, and other behavioral changes. The post-concussion syndrome is quite common, depending on the criteria employed and the diligence with which it is sought, occurring in roughly 50% of adults. There are obvious obstacles to ascertainment of the prevalence of this condition in young children, but among school-aged children and adolescents it may approach the same prevalence as in adulthood. The prevalence, severity, and duration are enhanced by interest in litigation arising from the injury, but this factor is relatively uncommon in pediatric practice. Most patients with post-concussive symptoms recover within 12 weeks of the injury but, until they do recover, their symptoms can be very trouble-some and require management. Narcotics and habituating sedatives must be eschewed in the treatment of headaches. Acetaminophen and ibuprofen should be given in adequate doses early in the course of a headache, but continuing, periodic administration for days on end must be discouraged to avoid rebound. Some patients experience post-concussive headaches that seem qualitatively very similar to migraine and, if they do not get adequate relief from timely administration of non-narcotic analgesics, treatment with migraine-specific medications may be considered. In younger children prophylaxis with cyproheptadine may be helpful and, in older children and adolescents, this writer favors nortriptyline. Metoclopramide or ondansetron may be useful for patients with a fully developed migraine-like syndrome. Melatonin may be helpful in regulating disrupted sleep patterns, and nor-triptyline may likewise benefit sleep. The efficacy of these pharmacologic measures is difficult to judge, because the natural history of post-concussion syndrome is to resolve, and indeed reassurance may be the most effective intervention, particularly for cognitive and behavioral complaints. The rare patient whose symptoms do not remit in 12 weeks has a guarded prognosis and requires neurologic or psychiatric referral.

Traumatic Brain Injury Among Athletes

The management of mild TBI among athletes is a matter of practical inter-est for community-based practitioners who may be called on to evaluate affected patients on the sidelines as well as in the office, and it is also a topic of very active physiologic, clinical, and psychological research, a respectful review of which is far beyond the scope of this chapter.

What distinguishes the athletic context for mild TBI are the potential consequences of recurrent injury and the question of return to play. The sto-ries of world-class athletes who have suffered career-ending neurocognitive disabilities from repeated concussions have penetrated popular conscious-ness, but these anecdotes are merely the most visible examples of a signifi-cant public health problem endemic among less accomplished college and high school athletes, particularly among football players. The 1991 National Health Interview Survey estimated the incidence of sports-related concus-sion in the United States at 300,000 per year or 124 per 100,000 person years. Among college football players, the rate of concussion has been estimated at

0.81 per 1,000 athletic exposures (ie, games and contact practices). Players who have one concussion seem to be at greater risk for subsequent concussions during the same season.

The guiding principle in the care of the athlete with mild TBI is to forbid return to play until all post-concussive symptoms and signs have resolved. This principle has been inspired by the rare but catastrophic *second impact syndrome*. As the term suggests, the typical story features a young football player who suffers a blow to his head on the field. He may or may not lose consciousness, but he experiences headache, dizziness, and confusion, which he may conceal from his coach or minimize. He returns to play to be struck a second time, but now he does not get up. He becomes progressively less responsive. Within minutes his pupils are fixed and dilated. Emergency brain imaging shows diffuse swelling, and heroic neurosurgical efforts to control intracranial pressure (ICP) are unavailing. The physiological basis for such a calamity is unknown, but the initial "mild" injury is presumed to destabilize cerebrovascular autoregulation. The second impact is presumed to abolish vascular tone entirely, leading to sudden engorgement of the brain by intravascular blood, relentless brain swelling, and intracranial circulatory arrest. Reliable data do not exist, but the second impact syndrome is estimated to occur about once a year among American high school football players. Because of its rarity, the second impact syndrome has been impossible to study systematically, but the common thread among case reports is that victims have returned to play and have experienced a second injury before concussive symptoms from the first injury have resolved. The logical deduction from these infrequent observations is that forbidding return to play until all symptoms resolve prevents the second impact syndrome.

Study of the resolution of concussive symptoms has required development of instruments and scales for measurement of concussion severity. Early attempts to grade concussion were based on expert opinion. Perhaps the most widely recognized system was the practice parameter promulgated by the American Academy of Neurology (AAN). This document still provides helpful guidance in the sidelines assessment of the concussed athlete, emphasizing particularly the importance of enhancement of symptoms and signs by physical exertion. The AAN practice parameter, like contemporaneous proposals developed by the American College of Sports Medicine, the Colorado Medical Society in cooperation with the National Collegiate

Athletic Association, and by many other authorities, placed emphasis on the presence of absence of loss of consciousness. More recent efforts to develop an evidentiary basis for concussion grading have examined the correlation between an expanded set of concussive symptoms and the severity of the concussion syndrome, as measured by total number of symptoms, duration of symptoms, and persistence of cognitive disability. Close scrutiny has de-emphasized somewhat the importance of loss of consciousness. Self-report of memory difficulty at the first follow-up visit is a much stronger predictor of the subsequent course of the illness, for instance, than a history of loss of consciousness on the field.

With research instruments such as the Graded Symptom Checklist (GSC, Box 5-4), the Standardized Assessment of Concussion, and the Balance Error Scoring System, the question of the time course for concussion resolution has been addressed in a quantitative fashion. Among college football players, the GSC falls to half of its acute value within 24 to 48 hours of injury, and mean scores generally return to preinjury baseline levels by 7 days. Median duration of individual symptoms is 48 hours, and about 90% of athletes are completely symptom free by 7 days. Likewise, cognitive symptoms and balance disturbances generally resolve with a week of the injury. In view of what is known about the tempo of the resolution of the concussion syndrome, the National Athletic Trainers' Association has recommended that athletes who have experienced loss of consciousness or amnesia be forbidden to return to play on the same day, and that athletes who have experienced lesser insults be permitted to return only if they are free of symptoms and signs at rest and after exertion for more than 20 minutes after coming off the field. The disinclination of the National Football League (NFL) to conform to this conservative practice has been the object of critical attention in the clinical and the popular press.

The principle of return to play contingent on complete resolution of symptoms has been inspired by dread of the second impact syndrome, but it has entered clinical practice as a measure to prevent cumulative and permanent brain injury. Although anecdotes abound, cumulative cognitive disability from repetitive injury is difficult to study systematically in humans because of the long time frame for the accumulation of injuries. Retrospective recall of past concussions is subject to serious bias, and prospective, longitudinal studies are very expensive and difficult. Even the

Box 5-4. The Graded Symptom Checklist for Concussion[a]

- Blurred vision
- Dizziness
- Drowsiness
- Excess sleep
- Easily distracted
- Fatigue
- Feeling "in a fog"
- Feeling "slowed down"
- Headache
- Inappropriate emotions
- Irritability
- Loss of consciousness
- Loss of coordination
- Loss of orientation
- Memory problems
- Nausea
- Nervousness
- Personality change
- Poor balance/coordination
- Poor concentration
- Ringing in ears
- Sadness
- Seeing stars
- Sensitivity to light
- Sensitivity to noise
- Sleep disturbance
- Vacant stare/glassy eyes
- Vomiting

---

[a]*Symptoms may be noted to be absent or present, or they may be graded for severity using a Likert scale. The checklist can be used at the time of the initial injury and at follow-up visits. The proponents of the GSC recommend that no athlete who has suffered a concussion be allowed to return to play until all symptoms are absent, both at rest and after exertion. Rigid adherence to this rule is problematic, however, because athletes who have never suffered a concussion may be expected to endorse some of these symptoms. Baseline scores are not zero.*

prospective investigations lavishly funded by the NFL have been criticized because of bias in recruitment of subjects and limited duration of follow-up. Furthermore, preliminary data suggest important variation in individual susceptibility to the effects of repeated injury. In the absence of evidence-based guidelines, the resolution of symptoms rule strikes a compromise between the extremes of career termination after a single injury, which is unreasonable and unacceptable to athletes and families, and unrestricted return to play, which seems imprudent based on clinical experience and current pathophysiological concepts.

Abusive Traumatic Brain Injury

The role of the primary physician in the management of abusive TBI lies predominantly in recognition. The historical hallmark of abusive injury is discrepancy between the mechanism of injury described by the child's caretaker and the pattern of injury actually observed by the clinician. Recognition of such discrepancy is therefore dependent on an understanding of the expected pathological consequences of common childhood events. Although the judicial system may call, at times, for doctrinaire pronouncements, only general statements are possible, but generalizations nevertheless provide guidance in the decision whether to pursue further medical, social, and forensic investigations.

Falls are the most common cause of head injury in early childhood, and falls of 4 feet or less, that is, falls from adults' arms, falls off changing tables and beds, and ground-level falls among toddlers, are very common childhood experiences. Kravitz famously reported a 47% rate of acknowledgment of such falls by mothers of infants attending his pediatric clinics and office practices, and he estimated that there were 1.75 million such falls in homes in the United States in 1967. In another frequently cited publication, Helfer reviewed hospital incident reports for 85 infants who fell out of cribs and off examination tables. In this carefully observed study group, there was one skull fracture and not a single serious injury. An interpreter of the Helfer paper must bear in mind the implications of the Kravitz paper. None having been observed in 85 cases, the Helfer paper does not establish that falls off furniture never cause serious TBI; rather, it allows calculation of a 95% confidence interval of 0% to 3.5% for the rate of serious TBI among infants who fall off furniture. Furthermore, any mechanism of injury that causes an occasional skull fracture holds the potential to cause an occasional epidural hematoma (EDH), so the true rate of serious TBI is unlikely to be nil. The Kravitz paper, on the other hand, establishes that the denominator—the population of infants who experience such falls—is enormous. So a small-but-not-nil rate of serious TBI in an enormous population of falling infants must yield a rare life-threatening injury. The astute clinician should certainly be suspicious of serious TBI attributed to a short fall, but the honest expert witness must concede that such an event is not impossible but only very improbable.

Household falls are very common, and they can result in skull fractures. There are distinguishing features of the clinical or radiographic patterns of infant skull fracture that suggest mechanisms of injury other than an innocent household fall. Household falls typically cause single, linear, nondisplaced fractures. In infants such fractures usually extend from one suture to another. The parietal bone is by far the most common site. Cephalohematomas, that is, scalp hematomas between the bone and the periosteum delimited by the cranial sutures, are common and commonly expand slowly over 2 to 4 days. So for caretakers to bring an infant to medical attention because of scalp swelling several days after a household fall is not necessarily neglectful and is not by itself an indication to initiate a child abuse investigation. Fractures that fall outside these generalizations are more suspicious: multiple fractures, stellate fractures, fractures that cross sutures, and diastatic fractures. Diastatic fractures, that is, fractures with a gap between the fragments, are particularly notable because they are associated with laceration of the underlying dura and contusion of the underlying brain. This triad of injuries—diastatic fracture, dural laceration, and brain contusion—is the substrate for the spontaneous development over weeks to a few months of the so-called growing skull fracture or traumatic pseudomeningoencephalocele. Association of rib or extremity fractures with a skull fracture is seldom the result of a short, vertical, household fall and is a reasonable basis for suspicion of abuse.

The other common household fall is down stairs. Fortunately, falls down stairs very seldom cause serious TBI. Joffe and Ludwig reviewed 363 consecutive children evaluated in an emergency department after falls down stairs. Children who fell more than 4 steps did not suffer worse injuries than children who fell fewer. Skull fractures were seen, particularly in younger children, but there were no life-threatening injuries. No patient required intensive care. Children with serious TBI for whom the caretaker offers a history of a fall downs stairs should be evaluated for abuse. The exception to this generalization is the infant encumbered by a baby walker, who is clearly at risk for life-threatening TBI from a fall down stairs.

Caffey's historic descriptions of the injuries sustained by abused children featured ASDHs associated with humeral fractures. The combination of ASDH with humeral fractures or posterior rib fractures typifies shaken baby syndrome. The actual role of shaking in the infliction of such injuries has been the subject of unedifying debate, but there is no dispute about the specificity of ASDH among infants with severe TBI—in the absence of an insult such as a car crash that can be confirmed by disinterested observers—as an indicator of abuse. Likewise, bilateral retinal hemorrhages in the infant with TBI—in the absence of a medically plausible explanation—are fairly specific for abuse. Infant victims of high-speed car crashes, for instance, very seldom exhibit retinal hemorrhages even in the presence of severe TBI.

Other pathological patterns of TBI and other degrees of severity carry variably specific associations with abusive injury. Epidural hemorrhage is a particular concern. Epidural hemorrhage is not a brain injury, but a skull injury. It is analogous to cephalohematoma, only adjacent to the internal aspect of the skull, and it is not so common. Any traumatic insult that can cause a skull fracture can therefore cause an EDH, so EDH might be anticipated to be less powerfully associated with abusive injury than ASDH. Shugerman reviewed records of 93 children younger than 3 years with EDH or ASDH seen at a Harborview Medical Center and Children's Hospital Medical Center in Seattle. Of 59 cases of ASDH, 28 (47%) were abusive, but only 2 of 34 (6%) cases of EDH were abusive. There were 16 examples of EDH after short, vertical household falls and falls down stairs, reflecting referral to tertiary centers of uncommon complications of common injuries from a large population base.

Another problematic injury is chronic subdural hematoma (CSDH) in infancy. Chronic subdural hematoma arises as a complication of asymptomatic or unrecognized ASDH. The acute bleeding is believed to arise from the bridging veins that drain the cortical convexities, passing through the subarachnoid space to empty into the dural venous sinuses. The subdural space does not exist in the untraumatized state, but stretch or torsion of the bridging veins causes bleeding at their junction with the dural sinuses that dissects open the subdural space, where the blood subsequently collects. Subdural hemorrhage often liquefies and disappears without intervention, but for unknown reasons in a minority of instances the hematoma may become self-propagating. Expansion of the subdural space may stretch bridging veins and render them more susceptible to rupture. Another contributing factor may be fibrinolytic metabolites of coagulation proteins within the hematoma itself. The infant with CSDH commonly reaches medical attention ill, with irritability, anorexia, vomiting, failure to thrive, macrocephaly, bulging fontanel, and seizures. Computed tomography scan shows low-density fluid collections between the brain and the skull, but this modality cannot always distinguish between CSDH and prominence of the subarachnoid spaces (SAS), which is a common, transient, developmental phenomenon in infancy. Ultrasound can often identify CSDH, but magnetic resonance imaging (MRI) is the study of choice. Symptomatic CSDH in infancy is not pathognomonic of abusive injury, but it is certainly an indication for comprehensive medical investigation and for filing with appropriate child protection agencies.

Transient, developmental prominence of the SAS, commonly called *external hydrocephalus* (EH) or *benign extracerebral collections of infancy* and commonly misnamed *benign subdural effusions,* is a troublesome issue in the evaluation of infant TBI above and beyond the difficulties that it creates in the interpretation of CT scans. External hydrocephalus is by far the most common imaging diagnosis among infants with statistical macrocephaly (ie, head circumferences above the 95th percentile). Such infants are otherwise well: They thrive. They have flat anterior fontanels and apposed sutures. And aside from difficulties with head control on a purely mechanical basis early in infancy, they develop normally. They do not require neurosurgical treatment. Problems arise when MRI shows a small, asymptomatic CSDH in addition to prominence of the SAS (Figure 5-1). Development of CSDH in this setting is probably analogous to the development of CSDH among the elderly with brain atrophy. Because the brain does not fill the cranial cavity, it is subject to exaggerated rotational displacements after minor impacts. The bridging veins, which are elongated, are therefore subject to exaggerated tension and torsion. The prevalence of CSDH among infants with EH has not been documented credibly, but in this writer's experience, it is not negligible. Craniocerebral disproportion is also believed to be a factor in the development of subdural hemorrhage in glutaric aciduria type 1, a well-known mimic of abusive infant TBI. Most infants with ASDH in the setting of EH have small collections and are completely asymptomatic. Whether EH predisposes to symptomatic ASDH or CSDH is unknown. How frequently,

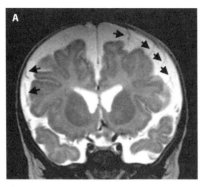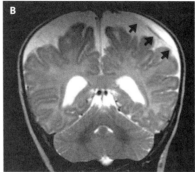

Figure 5-1.
External hydrocephalus with incidental chronic subdural hematoma. Coronal T2-weighted magnetic resonance imaging of an infant with marked macrocephaly shows very prominent subarachnoid spaces. Bridging veins pass from the cortical surface through the subarachnoid spaces to the dural venous sinuses (black arrow heads) (5-1A). An image from the same sequence farther posterior shows a subdural fluid collection of signal intensity different from cerebrospinal fluid, a chronic subdural hematoma (black arrow heads). This collection eventually disappeared without treatment (5-1B).

if ever, asymptomatic CSDH in the setting of EH is a reflection of abusive injury is unknown, and thus there is no consensus among pediatricians and pediatric neurosurgeons about what constitutes an appropriate medical investigation or social response to the identification of such lesions.

Physicians have professional, ethical, and legal obligations to report suspicious injuries to child protection agencies. What constitutes a suspicious injury is a matter of medical judgment based on familiarity with patterns, mechanisms, and temporal courses of common head injuries both abusive and otherwise. The primary objective is to protect the patient from additional physical injury, but sparing families the stress and potential disruption of misguided child protective service investigations based on misunderstandings of innocent childhood events is desirable as well. Cooperation between the primary physician and the neurosurgical consultant is critical in striking an informed balance.

Severe Traumatic Brain Injury

Competence in the detailed management of severe TBI is outside the scope of primary care practice, but in certain regions of the country, primary practitioners may have occasion to participate in the emergency department care of trauma victims. Some familiarity with the intensive care management of TBI may be a useful perspective in counseling and supporting affected families as well.

The first response to the acutely injured patient with severe TBI is subsumed under the principles that guide the care of any patient with life-threatening trauma: establishment of an airway, assurance of adequate ventilation, and support of circulation. Prompt and effective resuscitation in the trauma bay is probably the most potent medical therapy for severe TBI, and its importance may overshadow all the complex, technological interventions to which patients are subjected subsequently in the intensive care unit. While hypoxia and hypercarbia are certainly threatening to the already injured brain, analysis of prognostic factors in large datasets of patients with traumatic coma points to the especially malign effect of systemic hypotension. The adverse influence of hypotension has been documented amply among children as well as among adults. Restoration of intravascular volume and support of mean arterial pressure (MAP) are highest priorities in the initial care of the patient with severe TBI.

Assessment of the cervical spine is a critical issue in trauma care, but it is particularly salient in the evaluation of the patient with severe TBI, who cannot report neck pain or cooperate with neurologic examination. The prevalence of cervical fracture, dislocation, or spinal cord injury among comatose trauma victims is 8%, and despite protocolized trauma system care, roughly 4% of these injuries escape initial detection with potentially catastrophic results. What constitutes adequate imaging of the cervical spine in the setting of severe TBI is an unsettled question, most of all in young children. Helical CT scanning of the cervical spine with thin axial images and 2-dimensional coronal and sagittal reconstructions is an increasingly prevalent practice, because this study can be performed quickly and concurrently with scans of the head, chest, abdomen, and pelvis. It is very sensitive for fracture and dislocation, and at many institutions, a normal CT scan of the cervical spine of good quality is sufficient for clinical clearance and relaxation of precautions. There is a theoretical concern that CT scan may overlook destabilizing, purely ligamentous injuries that have undergone spontaneous reduction restoring normal vertebral alignment. Such injuries can only be detected by MRI, but MRI is time-consuming and requires specialized, non-ferromagnetic equipment for physiological monitoring and support. Fortunately, occult but significant injuries that elude detection by CT scanning are so infrequent that there is reasonable doubt whether they actually occur. Unfortunately, imaging criteria for cervical spine evaluation has received much less study among children than among adults. At this writer's children's hospital, clinical neurosurgical assessment and helical CT scanning are employed together in cervical spine clearance among comatose patients.

The thrust of the management of severe TBI is prevention of additional "secondary" brain injury from damaging pathophysiological processes set in motion at the instant of the original "primary" injury. After the critical phase of initial resuscitation in the emergency department, and after neurosurgical evacuation of intracranial hematomas, the effort to prevent secondary injury continues in the intensive care unit. The theoretical focus of this effort is to ensure delivery of adequate supplies of oxygen and other metabolic substrates to the brain. The operational focus is to maintain adequate cerebral perfusion by support of MAP and control of ICP. Therapies for reduction of ICP are undertaken in a graduated, step-wise fashion, exhausting the benefits of measures with lower complexity and risks of complications before moving to measures with greater risks (Box 5-5). Among the high-risk therapies, decompressive craniectomy is currently in the ascendance (Figure 5-2). Although it entails a moderately involved sequence of surgical

---

Box 5-5. Therapies for Control of Intracranial Pressure

Lower Risk

    Elevation of head of bed

    Analgesia

    Sedation

    Neuromuscular blockade

    Hypertonic saline/mannitol

    Cerebrospinal fluid drainage

Higher Risk

    Hyperventilation

    Barbiturate coma

    Decompressive craniectomy

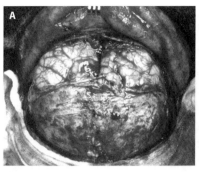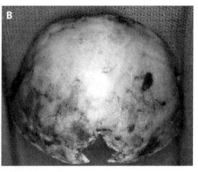

Figure 5-2.
Bifrontal decompressive craniectomy for abusive severe TBI in infancy. The retractor is applied to the reflected frontal scalp. A bifrontal craniectomy has been performed. The dura is open and the frontal lobes are exposed, a thin acute subdural hematoma having been removed (5-2A). The bifrontal craniectomy flap, including most of the anterior fontanel (5-2B).

procedures, it is extremely effective in controlling elevated ICP. It usually facilitates quick reduction in the intensity of other therapies, and there is preliminary evidence that it improves outcomes, specifically among children.

The therapies listed in Box 5-5 have been available for at least 30 years. Whatever progress has been made recently in the management of severe TBI has been in the organization of care—at the level of regional trauma systems and within the intensive care unit. Implementation of regional trauma systems has reduced overall mortality rates for children and, by inference, mortality rates for severe TBI. Hulka et al compared pediatric trauma outcomes in Oregon and Washington states before (1985–1987) and after (1991–1993) Oregon implemented a statewide trauma system. The incidence of serious injury (injury severity score >15) declined in both states between the 1985–1987 epoch and the 1991–1993 epoch. The incidence of trauma admissions to rural facilities declined in both states as well, demonstrating a trend toward more frequent transfer to referral centers apart from the implementation of an organized system. Nevertheless, risk-adjusted odds of death for seriously injured children were lower in Oregon in the second epoch. On a larger scale, Nathens et al compared injury death rates in states with and without regionalized trauma systems. Reduction in the risk of death in the 0- to 14-year age stratum was 17% for states with regionalized systems. Systematization of care seems to have improved outcomes on the level of intensive care as well. In 1995 the Brain Trauma Foundation published its landmark *Guidelines for the Management of Severe Head Injury,* a formal review of published evidence with grading of therapeutic recommendations. This effort was criticized at the time because of the weak foundation of the clinical data on which the superstructure of analysis had been erected, but it did serve to provoke awareness of practice variation and development of clinical protocols. Implementation of protocols based on the guidelines seems to have improved outcomes and reduced costs at several institutions. Subsequently published guidelines for management of severe TBI specifically in children rest on an even more limited evidentiary base, but hopefully they too will promote standardization of care and stimulate much needed clinical research.

The simple clinical emphasis on maintaining perfusion and oxygenation of the brain that is the current foundation for intensive care of severe TBI scarcely reflects the complexity of the experimental data developed in the last 3 decades to illuminate the physiology, biochemistry, and molecular biology of brain injury. Unfortunately, attempts to translate experimental insights into clinical advances have been very expensive, limited to adult patients, and without exception unsuccessful. There have been no clinical trials of novel pharmaceuticals for protection of the brain against secondary traumatic injury among children. On the horizon about to open at the time of this writing is a phase 3 trial of moderate therapeutic hypothermia. Phase 2 data have established the safety of hypothermia to 32°C to 33°C among children younger than 13 years admitted within 6 hours of injury, and although there was no clear benefit in mortality or ICP control in the pilot study, the preliminary evidence suggested improved cognitive outcomes at 6 months. These trials of hypothermia are the only clinical research in severe childhood TBI ever conducted with the support of federal funds. In the absence of a major new political commitment to translational research in trauma care, similar to the commitment to cancer research in the 1970s, there is little intermediate-term prospect for the appearance of new therapies for severe TBI. Improvements in outcome must come from more systematic and effective use of existing therapies.

Conclusion

Traumatic brain injury in childhood is difficult to manage. Treatment very seldom restores lost neurologic or cognitive functions, although medical interventions can sometimes prevent complications or secondary insults. It is much better to prevent the primary insult. Guidance for families in injury prevention is a core component of children's health care, as is advocacy with business and government for safety in the childhood environment. The AAP, through its Section and Committee on Injury, Violence, and Poison Prevention (www.aap.org/sections/ipp/default.htm), offers not only resources useful for patient care but also a platform for attacking the problem of childhood TBI in the arena of public health. Providers who wish to take a proactive approach to the well-being of children must practice both in the office and in the community.

Bibliography

General

Langlois JA, Rutland-Brown W, Thomas KE. Traumatic brain injury in the United States: emergency department visits, hospitalizations, and deaths. Atlanta, GA: Centers for Disease Control and Prevention, National Center for Injury Prevention and Control; 2004

Teasdale G, Jennett B. Assessment of coma and impaired consciousness. A practical scale. *Lancet.* 1974;2:81–84

Mild and Minor Traumatic Brain Injury

American Academy of Pediatrics Committee on Quality Improvement, American Academy of Family Physicians Commission on Clinical Policies and Research. The management of minor closed head injury in children. *Pediatrics.* 1999;104:1407–1415

Davis RL, Hughes M, Gubler KD, Waller PL, Rivara FP. The use of cranial CT scans in the triage of pediatric patients with mild head injury. *Pediatrics.* 1995;95:345-349

Dunning J, Daly JP, Lomas JP, Lecky F, Batchelor J, Mackway-Jones K. Derivation of the children's head injury algorithm for the prediction of important clinical events decision rule for head injury in children. *Arch Dis Child.* 2006;91:885–891

Mower WR, Hoffman JR, Herbert M, Wolfson AB, Pollack CV Jr, Zucker MI. Developing a clinical decision instrument to rule out intracranial injuries in patients with minor head trauma: methodology of the Nexus II investigation. *Ann Emerg Med.* 2002;40:505–514

Palchak MJ, Holmes JF, Vance CW, et al. A decision rule for identifying children at low risk for brain injuries after blunt head trauma. *Ann Emerg Med.* 2003;42:492–506

Palchak MJ, Holmes JF, Vance CW, et al. Does an isolated history of loss of consciousness or amnesia predict brain injuries in children after blunt head trauma? *Pediatrics.* 2004;113:e507–e513

Traumatic Brain Injury Among Athletes

American Academy of Neurology. Practice parameter: the management of concussion in sports (summary statement). Report of the Quality Standards Subcommittee. *Neurology.* 1997;48:581–585

Erlanger D, Kaushik T, Cantu R, et al. Symptom-based assessment of the severity of a concussion. *J Neurosurg.* 2003;98:477–484

Guskiewicz KM, Bruce SL, Cantu RC, et al. National Athletic Trainers' Association position statement: management of sport-related concussion. *J Athl Train.* 2004;39:280–297

Guskiewicz KM, McCrea M, Marshall SW, et al. Cumulative effects associated with recurrent concussion in collegiate football players: the NCAA Concussion Study. *JAMA.* 2003;290: 2549–2555

McCrea M, Guskiewicz KM, Marshall SW, et al. Acute effects and recovery time following concussion in collegiate football players: the NCAA Concussion Study. *JAMA.* 2003;290: 2556–2563

McCrea M, Kelly JP, Randolph C, et al. Standardized Assessment of Concussion (SAC): on-site mental status evaluation of the athlete. *J Head Trauma Rehabil.* 1998;13:27–35

Pellman EJ, Viano DC, Casson IR, Arfken C, Feuer H. Concussion in professional football: players returning to the same game—part 7. *Neurosurgery.* 2005;56:79–90

Quality Standards Subcommittee of the American Academy of Neurology. Management of concussion in sports: Centers for Disease Control and Prevention. http://www.cdc.gov/ncipc/pub-res/tbi_toolkit/physicians/concussion_sports.pdf. Accessed October 24, 2008

Saunders RL, Harbaugh RE. The second impact in catastrophic contact-sports head trauma. *JAMA.* 1984;252:538–539

Abusive Traumatic Brain Injury

Bechtel K, Stoessel K, Leventhal JM, et al. Characteristics that distinguish accidental from abusive injury in hospitalized young children with head trauma. *Pediatrics.* 2004;114:165–168

Caffey J. Multiple fractures in the long bones of infants suffering from subdural hematoma. *AJR Am J Roentgenol.* 1946;56:163–173

Chiaviello CT, Christoph RA, Bond GR. Infant walker-related injuries: a prospective study of severity and incidence. *Pediatrics.* 1994;93:974–976

Feldman KW, Bethel R, Shugerman RP, Grossman DC, Grady MS, Ellenbogen RG. The cause of infant and toddler subdural hemorrhage: a prospective study. *Pediatrics.* 2001;108:636–646

Helfer RE, Slovis TL, Black M. Injuries resulting when small children fall out of bed. *Pediatrics.* 1977;60:533–535

Joffe M, Ludwig S. Stairway injuries in children. *Pediatrics.* 1988;82:457-461

Johnson DL, Braun D, Friendly D. Accidental head trauma and retinal hemorrhage. *Neurosurgery.* 1993;33:231–234

Kravitz H, Driessen G, Gomberg R, Korach A. Accidental falls from elevated surfaces in infants from birth to one year of age. *Pediatrics.* 1969;44:869–876

Papasian NC, Frim DM. A theoretical model of benign external hydrocephalus that predicts a predisposition towards extra-axial hemorrhage after minor head trauma. *Pediatr Neurosurg.* 2000;33:188–193

Ravid S, Maytal J. External hydrocephalus: a probable cause for subdural hematoma in infancy. *Pediatr Neurol.* 2003;28:139–141

Shugerman RP, Paez A, Grossman DC, Feldman KW, Grady MS. Epidural hemorrhage: is it abuse? *Pediatrics.* 1996;97:664–668

Strauss KA, Puffenberger EG, Robinson DL, Morton DH. Type I glutaric aciduria, part 1: natural history of 77 patients. *Am J Med Genet C Semin Med Genet.* 2003;121:38–52

Tarantino CA, Dowd MD, Murdock TC. Short vertical falls in infants. *Pediatr Emerg Care.* 1999;15:5–8

Severe Traumatic Brain Injury

Adelson PD, Bratton SL, Carney NA, et al. Guidelines for the acute medical management of severe traumatic brain injury in infants, children, and adolescents. *Pediatr Crit Care Med.* 2003;4:S2–S75

Adelson PD, Ragheb J, Kanev P, et al. Phase II clinical trial of moderate hypothermia after severe traumatic brain injury in children. *Neurosurgery.* 2005;56:740–754

Bullock R, Chesnut RM, Clifton GL, et al. Guidelines for the management of severe head injury: Brain Trauma Foundation; 3rd ed. 1995

Cho DY, Wang YC, Chi CS. Decompressive craniotomy for acute shaken/impact baby syndrome. *Pediatr Neurosurg.* 1995;23:192–198

Fakhry SM, Trask AL, Waller MA, Watts DD, IRTC Neurotrauma Task Force. Management of brain-injured patients by an evidence-based medicine protocol improves outcomes and decreases hospital charges. *J Trauma.* 2004;56:492–499

Hulka F, Mullins RJ, Mann NC, et al. Influence of a statewide trauma system on pediatric hospitalization and outcome. *J Trauma.* 1997;42:514–519

Kokoska ER, Smith GS, Pittman T, Weber TR. Early hypotension worsens neurological outcome in pediatric patients with moderately severe head trauma. *J Pediatr Surg.* 1998;33:333–338

Nathens AB, Jurkovich GJ, Rivara FP, Maier RV. Effectiveness of state trauma systems in reducing injury-related mortality: a national evaluation. *J Trauma.* 2000;48:25–30

Palmer S, Bader MK, Qureshi A, et al. The impact on outcomes in a community hospital setting of using the AANS traumatic brain injury guidelines. Americans Association of Neurological Surgeons. *J Trauma.* 2001;50:657–664

Piatt JH Jr. Detected and overlooked cervical spine injury in comatose victims of trauma: report from the Pennsylvania Trauma Outcomes Study. *J Neurosurg Spine.* 2006;5:210–216

Ruf B, Heckmann M, Schroth I, et al. Early decompressive craniectomy and duraplasty for refractory intracranial hypertension in children: results of a pilot study. *Crit Care.* 2003;7:R133–R138

Taylor A, Butt W, Rosenfeld J, et al. A randomized trial of very early decompressive craniectomy in children with traumatic brain injury and sustained intracranial hypertension. *Childs Nerv Syst.* 2001;17:154–162

Cerebrovascular Disorders in Children

Christos D. Katsetos, MD, PhD, FRCPath
Edward R. Smith, MD
R. Michael Scott, MD

Introduction

Although stroke is less common in children compared with adults, it represents an important cause of mortality and morbidity in the pediatric population. Incidence rates vary widely around the world, ranging from 1.3 to 13 per 100,000 children. In the United States, the incidence of childhood stroke is estimated to be between 2 and 8 per 100,000. However, these figures might have previously underestimated the increased risk of cerebrovascular disease among newborns, the latter accounting for nearly 25% of strokes in children. Ischemic stroke is the pathologic correlate in up to 14% of patients presenting with neonatal seizures. It is estimated that more than half of children with stroke will develop permanent cognitive or motor disability, and approximately one-third will develop a recurrent stroke.

The World Health Organization defines stroke as "rapidly developing clinical signs of focal (or global) disturbance of cerebral function, with symptoms lasting 24 hours or longer or leading to death with no apparent cause other than of vascular origin." The definition includes ischemic and hemorrhagic cerebral infarction and intracerebral and subarachnoid hemorrhage. Clinical presentation is variable and includes acute or recurrent neurologic manifestations, as well as evolving neurologic deficits.

Stroke in children and adolescents is divided into *ischemic* and *hemorrhagic*. The former is further subdivided into *arteriopathic* and *non-arteriopathic*.

Although an excess of 100 risk factors have been reported in the literature, no definitive underlying cause is identified in about one-third of childhood stroke cases, which are designated as *cryptogenic*.

The principal causes for ischemic stroke are underlying developmental cardiac abnormalities and coagulation defects, whereas vasculopathies/

arteriopathies of divergent origins remain important underpinning factors or correlates of pathogenesis. In children, vascular malformations of the central nervous system (CNS) account for most hemorrhagic strokes.

Risk factors for pediatric stroke are diverse and fall into the following general categories:

A) Faulty development of vascular structures, such as in arteriovenous malformations (AVMs); vein of Galen malformations (VOGMs); arteriovenous fistulas (AVFs); and cavernous malformations (CMs), formation of new vessels (neovascularization) in the context of brain tumors or structural changes in preexisting blood vessels (aneurysms or arterial dissections)

B) Progressive arteriopathies/vasculopathies (moyamoya syndrome or heritable arteriopathies)

C) Systemic, infective/post-infective vascular lesions (varicella vasculo-pathy) and immune-mediated vascular diseases (vasculitis-vasculopathy sequence)

D) Hematologic disorders (sickle cell disease) and acquired or congenital abnormalities of hemostasis predisposing to thrombosis (thrombophilias and immune-mediated prothrombotic states

E) Congenital and acquired heart disease (infective endocarditis)

F) Venous thrombosis and thrombophlebitis

G) Metabolic diseases such as mitochondrial myopathy, encephalopathy, lactic acidosis, and stroke-like episodes, and hyperhomocysteinemia/homocystinuria

H) Traumatic or spontaneous arterial dissection

Unfortunately, many of these conditions are difficult to identify prior to the onset of symptoms. However, once diagnosed, prompt referral to an appropriate specialist or specialized interdisciplinary hospital setting devoted to the diagnosis and treatment of childhood cerebrovascular diseases is critical to achieve the best possible outcome.

General Principles in the Diagnosis and Evaluation of Cerebrovascular Disease in Children

Identification and diagnosis of children with cerebrovascular disease can be difficult. Particularly challenging in this regard is the early and accurate diagnosis of ischemic stroke as well as the identification of its cause. Both are critically important because they will dictate the choice of treatment and the prediction of outcome. The clinical presentation of stroke in children varies according to age and the anatomical location of the ischemic or hemorrhagic lesion as well as the mode of onset. Frequently, a stroke may go unrecognized in a child. This is especially true in neonates, some of whom may initially appear normal and develop neurologic deficits months later. A number of cases will present acutely to the emergency department, a circumstance that calls for full awareness of the clinical spectrum of stroke in children on the part of emergency department physicians. Similarly, the correct elucidation of the stroke's etiology often takes time, causing delays in diagnosis and, potentially, change of management.

It is often impossible to determine, on clinical grounds, whether an ischemic stroke (cerebral infarction) is the consequence of embolism or thrombosis. As a rule, a sudden onset points to cerebral embolism but there are no reliable clinical correlates to predict etiology/pathogenesis, especially in infants and toddlers. The determination of arterial versus venous origin of cerebral infarction is also important. A venous infarct, occurring in the setting of venous sinus thrombosis or thrombophlebitis is more likely to have a hemorrhagic nature.

Symptoms and signs depend largely on the location and size of the infarct. The most common presenting symptoms and signs are headache, alteration of consciousness, hemiparesis, vomiting, and seizures (Box 6-1). Typical cortical signs attributable to internal carotid artery (ICA) and/or middle cerebral artery occlusion include hemiparesis, hemianesthesia, and aphasia, whereas hemichorea has been described with basal ganglionic infarcts. As alluded previously, stroke-associated seizures are more common in children compared with adults, being the second most common symptom after weakness in the young. Acute ataxia and other cerebellar and brain stem signs, vertigo, vomiting, dysarthria, seizures, and visual field defects (hemianopsia) are present in patients with posterior circulation infarcts.

Box 6-1. Clinical Features of Headache Suggestive of an Intracranial Lesion

Sleep-related headache

Absence of family history of migraine

Vomiting

Absence of visual symptoms (migraine scotoma)

Headache of less than 6 months duration

Confusion

Abnormal neurologic examination findings

There are some important general screening tools that may help to identify patients at risk for cerebrovascular disease.

Family History

Family history may be important in the process of screening patients for the presence of cerebrovascular disease. A small number of genetic conditions associated with vasculopathies or structural anomalies of blood vessels are known to have an increased risk of cerebrovascular disease (Box 6-2) or with hematologic disorders and prothrombotic states (thrombophilias) (Box 6-3). In particular, a family history of strokes, intracranial bleeding, connective tissue disorders, or myocardial infarction at a young age should be a cause for concern.

Review of Systems

A careful review of systems may provide clues suggestive of the presence of cerebrovascular disease in children. Headaches, seizures, focal neurologic deficits (weakness, numbness, visual field problems), or cognitive decline may be present. Symptoms suggestive of previous transient ischemic attacks (TIAs) or strokes may be indicative of underlying cerebrovascular disease. Evidence of syndromes known to be associated with intracranial vascular disease should be addressed in the patient interview. In addition to the genetic syndromes discussed previously, one should be attuned to the possibility of systemic lupus erythematosus, cardiac disease (especially infectious endocarditis with the risk of mycotic aneurysms or high-output cardiac failure in infants suggestive of VOGMs) or high-risk drug use, such as cocaine.

Box 6-2. Genetic Conditions Associated With Vasculopathies or Structural Anomalies of Blood Vessels

Vasculopathies
- Moyamoya syndrome
- Hereditary hemorrhagic telangectasia
- Ehlers-Danlos syndrome
- Fabry disease
- Homocystinuria
- α1 antitrypsin deficiency
- Marfan syndrome
- Autosomal dominant polycystic kidney disease

Structural anomalies of blood vessels
- Sturge-Weber syndrome
- Fibromuscular dysplasia
- Hereditary hemorrhagic telangectasia
- Neurofibromatosis type I
- Multiple familial cavernous malformations
- Multiple familial intracranial aneurysms

Examination

Obvious neurologic deficits should cue the examiner to the potential of cerebrovascular disease: focal weakness or numbness in a cortical distribution, visual field deficits, or disturbances or speech or language. The presence of a systolic bruit over the eye, head, or neck may suggest the presence of an AVM or carotid disease, and any focal neurologic signs will help to localize it. A bruit may be found in between 15% and 40% of patients with AVMs. It is best heard over the ipsilateral eye or mastoid region. Arteriovenous shunts of large volume may also be associated with tachycardia, cardiomegaly, or even cardiac failure, especially in infants and children, and particularly when the vein of Galen is involved. However, other than potential neurologic deficits, the typical patient with a cerebrovascular lesion will not have any obvious findings on general physical examination to suggest an underlying problem.

Although rare, there are a number of findings on physical examination that merit urgent evaluation with imaging. These findings, listed in Box 6-4, are often associated with neurologic emergencies and should prompt immediate referral to a tertiary care center with experienced neurologists and neurosurgeons available to provide treatment if necessary.

Box 6-3. Genetic and Immune-mediated Prothrombotic States (Thrombophilias)[a]

Antithrombin III deficiency

Factor V Leiden

Protein C deficiency

Protein S deficiency

Activated protein C resistance

Hyperhomocysteinemia/homocystinuria[b]

   (total plasma homocysteine >95th percentile)

Thrombophilic mutations recommended as part of routine screening of pediatric stroke patients

Factor V 1691 GA

Prothrombin 20210GA

Methylenetetrahydrofolate reductase C677T

Immune-mediated prothrombotic states

Lupus anticoagulant

Anti-phospholipid antibodies

Anti-cardiolipin antibodies[c]

---

[a]*Factors found to be more common in children with first-time arterial ischemic stroke. This association was especially significant for protein C deficiency and the (Methylenetetrahydrofolate reductase) C677T mutation. (From Haywood S, Liesner R, Pindora S, Ganesan V. Thrombophilia and first arterial ischaemic stroke: a systematic review. Arch Dis Child. 2005;90:402–405.)*

[b]*Heterozygous and/or homozygous gene mutations of enzymes involved in homocysteine metabolism may be associated with an increased risk for thrombosis and stroke by giving rise to hyperhomocysteinemia. FV 1691 A and PT 20210 A mutations must be part of routine screening of pediatric stroke patients. (From Akar N, Akar E, Ozel D, Deda G, Sipahi T. Common mutations at the homocysteine metabolism pathway and pediatric stroke. Thromb Res. 2001;102:115–120.)*

[c]*Increased anticardiolipin antibody IgG titers do not predict recurrent stroke or transient ischemic attacks in children. (Lanthier S, Kirkham FJ, Mitchell LG, et al. Increased anticardiolipin antibody IgG titers do not predict recurrent stroke or TIA in children. Neurology. 2004;62:194–200.)*

Initial Clinical and Laboratory Evaluation

A thorough evaluation of underlying cardiac abnormalities in the context of congenital or acquired heart disease is mandatory, because these disorders, particularly those associated with complex cardiac anomalies, constitute collectively the most common causes of cerebral infarction in children. In view of the high frequency of underlying cardiac abnormalities in patients with arterial ischemic stroke (AIS), the consultation of a pediatric cardiologist is

---

Box 6-4. Red Flags on Examination

Bradycardia, hypertension, decreased respirations (Cushing response)

Dilated pupil, hemiparesis (uncal herniation)

Fixed downward gaze (Parinaud syndrome)

Lethargy, tense open anterior fontanel

Ataxia with nausea and vomiting

Sudden onset of a third nerve palsy, including dilatation of the pupil

Sudden onset of the "worst headache of my life"

---

often sought. Electrocardiography and chest x-ray are standard and may be complemented by ambulatory cardiac rhythm monitoring and echocardiography as clinically dictated. Overall, the diagnostic yield of echocardiography is low if cardiac examination and prior studies have been normal.

From the standpoint of AIS, complete blood count will provide important clues for hemoglobinopathies, polycythemia rubra vera, thrombocytopenic purpura, and infections. Amongst hemoglobinopathies, sickle cell disease (SCD) is by far the most important nosologic correlate to childhood stroke, although other hemoglobinopathies may also be associated with cerebrovascular complications. A significant percentage of ischemic stroke patients have prothrombotic disorders, often associated with other stroke-related risk factors. These disorders are summarized in Box 6-3. From the standpoint of a hemorrhagic stroke, laboratory evaluation for thrombocytopenia, bleeding disorders (hemophilias, acquired coagulation defects/vitamin K deficiency), and hematopoietic malignancies (leukemia) are indicated.

Lumbar puncture and cerebrospinal fluid (CSF) examination are indicated in patients with unexplained fever and/or acute focal deficits, provided that there is no concomitant brain swelling and significant mass effect, to rule out infective causes such as herpes simplex encephalitis mimicking stroke. Stroke may be one of the presentations of early tuberculous meningitis, meningovascular syphilis, and HIV-associated CNS disease. Serologic studies for syphilis may be considered in adolescent stroke patients. Although fulminant bacterial meningitis can potentially give rise to ischemic infarcts, stroke is not the typical presentation in this clinical setting.

Neuroimaging Evaluation

In general, the diagnosis of cerebrovascular disease is made with an imaging study. A variety of modalities are available, each with relative advantages and shortcomings. The evaluation of children suspected of harboring cerebrovascular disease varies depending on the particular entity being considered in the differential diagnosis.

Computed tomography (CT) is an excellent initial study for hemorrhage, delayed stroke, or larger vascular lesions. One of the obvious shortcomings of CT is failure to identify small cerebral infarcts, particularly of recent onset. The use of CT angiography (CTA) can markedly increase the sensitivity of detection of cerebrovascular lesions, including dissection and aneurysms. However, CT studies expose children to radiation, and the use of contrast is associated with a small but real risk of allergic reaction. The presence of braces or other metal objects, such as piercings, may produce artifact and should be removed if possible. In the setting of an emergency, an axial CT of the brain is the most common screening modality.

Magnetic resonance imaging (MRI), MR angiography (MRA), and MR venography (MRV) have revolutionized the diagnosis of cerebrovascular disease in children. Magnetic resonance imaging is superior to CT for the evaluation of cerebral infarction. There is little risk other than the very rare reaction to gadolinium, the need for sedation/general anesthesia (to reduce motion artifact in children unable to tolerate the confines of the scanner) and, in infants, the potential for hypothermia in the cooled MRI suite. Magnetic resonance imaging/MRA can provide exquisitely detailed images of the brain, abnormalities of larger cerebral vessels, and excellent reconstructions of vascular lesions in 3 planes, and can also provide evidence of recent infarction with diffusion weighted images. Magnetic resonance angiography is indicated in patients who are deemed at risk from conventional angiography (such as in patients with SCD in whom angiography could exacerbate sickling) or in patients who have a high index of suspicion for a presumptive vascular lesion. Magnetic resonance venography is strongly indicated if there is a high index of clinical suspicion for dural venous sinus thrombosis. Magnetic resonance imaging/MRA is generally used as the initial study in a non-emergent setting.

There are specific clinical situations in which standard angiography is diagnostically superior to MRA. The former is strongly indicated in patients with subarachnoid and/or intracerebral hemorrhage, where the risk of re-bleeding as a result of a missed AVM or aneurysm far exceeds the risk associated with angiography per se. Digital subtraction catheter angiography (DSA) is the gold standard for imaging of most vascular lesions. Digital subtraction angiography provides the greatest detail of intracranial and extracranial vessels, including rates of flow and the capacity for selective study of individual segments of specific vessels. In addition, DSA, which is performed by an interventional radiologist, allows for diagnostic and therapeutic procedures to be performed in the same clinical setting. However, DSA carries a greater risk for complications compared with the other procedures described previously and should only be performed by experienced interventional radiologists.

Disease Categories and Specific Disease Entities

Structural Anomalies of Blood Vessels

Intracranial Aneurysms

Aneurysms of the CNS are extremely rare in the pediatric population. While the etiology of CNS aneurysms in adults is frequently related to chronic conditions or acquired factors, such as hypertension and smoking, the pathogenesis of pediatric aneurysms is often quite different, including trauma, infection, and predisposing genetic disorders (Box 6-5). There are further differences between adult and pediatric aneurysms with regard to location, size, and presentation. Given the rarity of these lesions and the differences from their more common adult counterparts, it is important for the clinician caring for children with aneurysms to both recognize the disease and be able to distinguish appropriate differences in treatment between the 2 age groups.

An aneurysm should be considered whenever symptoms suggestive of a subarachnoid hemorrhage (SAH) are present; namely, the acute onset of the "worst headache of my life," often associated with neck stiffness, photophobia, and/or altered consciousness. Although AVMs are far more common in children, these findings should prompt an urgent head CT, with a subsequent CTA if a hemorrhage is found. Rapid transfer to a tertiary care center with neurosurgical staffing should be undertaken.

Box 6-5. Conditions Associated With Pediatric Intracranial Aneurysms

Genetic

Polycystic renal disease

Tuberous sclerosis

Fibromuscular dysplasia

Ehlers-Danlos syndrome

Pseudoxanthoma elasticum

Familial intracranial aneurysms

Thalassemia minor

Sickle cell disease

Glucose-6-phosphatase deficiency

Congenital

Persistent fetal patterns of cerebral vasculature

Coarctation of the aorta

Moyamoya syndrome

Acquired

Infectious aneurysms (mycotic)

Syphilis

Human immunodeficiency virus

Concurrent tumors (intracranial tumors, cardiac myxoma)

Trauma

Screening for aneurysms is limited to a very select group of patients. Currently, children with a history of autosomal dominant polycystic kidney disease (PCKD) (1%–9% of children with PCKD may have aneurysms), Ehlers-Danlos syndrome type IV, and α1-antitrypsin deficiency should be considered for screening. In addition, patients with a family history of 2 or more first-degree relatives with documented aneurysmal SAH should be considered for screening (about 1.2%–8% of children meeting this criteria will have an aneurysm). There does not seem to be an increased risk with only one affected relative.

Screening should consist of a MRI/MRA or, if not available, a CTA. There are no clear guidelines on whether follow-up is needed if a study reveals no aneurysms. It has been the practice at Children's Hospital Boston to obtain the initial study then, if negative, to repeat it at 21 years of age prior to transitioning to an adult practitioner (assuming that no new symptoms develop in the interval period).

Treatment is centered on removing the aneurysm from circulation while maintaining normal brain perfusion. This can be achieved surgically, commonly with clip ligation, or endovascularly, with intraluminal obliteration of the aneurysm by coils or stenting. In rare cases, the artery may be sacrificed when collateral circulation exists to supply the brain. Not all aneurysms will require intervention, and decisions regarding treatment should be made at an experienced center by a multidisciplinary team of neurointerventionalists, intensivists, and neurosurgeons.

Arteriovenous Malformations (Including Hereditary Hemorrhagic Telangiectasia)

Arteriovenous malformations consist of direct arterial-to-venous connections without intervening capillaries. They can occur in the cerebral hemispheres, brain stem, and spinal cord. Functional neural tissue does not reside within the lesion.

It is generally believed that arteriovenous connections develop early in embryogenesis from a localized failure of vascular channels to differentiate into normal arteries, capillaries, and veins. Arteriovenous malformations can increase in size over time. This growth has been attributed to both "mechanical" expansion of the lesion, resulting from dilation of existing vessels "stretched" by high flow and also by recruitment of new collateral arterial feeders. Ischemia and surrounding micro-hemorrhages with resultant gliosis may promote enlargement of the AVM by destruction of the surrounding parenchyma.

Arteriovenous malformations may be diagnosed after evaluation for seizures, headache, or focal neurologic deficits. However, up to 80% to 85% of children are diagnosed with an AVM after a hemorrhage. Similar to aneurysms, AVMs can cause neurologic injury by hemorrhage, presumably caused by high-pressure arterial blood breaching the weakened dilated vessels. In contrast to the SAH associated with ruptured aneurysms, AVM typically gives rise to intracerebral hemorrhage because of the location of the AVM within the brain. A non-traumatic intracerebral hemorrhage in a child should raise concerns for the presence of an AVM (or tumor). Arteriovenous malformations can also produce deficits through mass effect or from cerebral ischemia that is due to diversion of blood to the AVM from the normal cerebral circulation ("steal").

If a child hemorrhages, re-bleeding rates are approximately 6% for the first 6 months, then 3% per year afterward. Hemorrhagic events from an AVM in children have been associated with a 25% mortality rate. These statistics have 2 important clinical implications. First, because the early rate of re-bleeding is relatively low, definitive treatment of AVMs is conducted on an elective basis after the patient has stabilized following the initial hemorrhage. Second, even though the annual hemorrhage rate is low, the cumulative lifetime risk is high. Assuming a 3% per year hemorrhage rate, the risk over 20 years, for instance, is 46%. Thus treatment of cerebral AVMs in children is always indicated whenever it is feasible.

Comprehensive evaluation of a patient with an AVM includes a detailed history, clinical examination, and radiographic studies to delineate the anatomy of the lesion. Most patients presenting with a new-onset neurologic deficit, an unusually severe headache ("worst headache of my life"), or seizures are often initially evaluated by CT scan. Computed tomography angiography has increasingly been employed as a method to better delineate AVM anatomy, particularly in the setting of an acute hemorrhage, as an initial study on presentation to the emergency department due to its speed, availability, and ease of use. In addition, the index of suspicion for an AVM is high when an intracerebral hemorrhage is found in a child or young adult without an antecedent history of trauma. If a child presents with an intracerebral hemorrhage without a clear cause, AVM should be considered, and repeat imaging in 4 to 6 weeks should be performed to evaluate the hemorrhage cavity after the clot has cleared.

Magnetic resonance imaging is of significant value to the diagnosis and to the understanding of the anatomy of AVMs. Even if there is a high suspicion of AVM based on the CT findings, and an angiogram is planned, an MRI will commonly be performed to better localize parenchymal structures relative to the AVM. Susceptibility imaging will sometimes disclose evidence of previous hemorrhage as a dark "bloom" around a nidus. Chronic ischemia, presumably a result of "steal" phenomena, may be identified on MRI as bright signal of the surrounding brain on FLAIR (fluid attenuation inversion recovery) or T2 images.

Traditional DSA continues as the definitive investigation to evaluate intracerebral AVMs, because it permits the nature and extent of the lesion to be established and its blood supply and venous drainage to be determined. Occasionally, angiography can fail to demonstrate an AVM despite suggestive imaging findings on CT or MRI usually because of partial or complete thrombotic occlusion of feeding vessels. Other suggested causes of an angiographically occult vascular malformation include small size, compression by adjacent clot, and destruction at the time of hemorrhage. In the setting of intracranial hemorrhage without a clearly proximate cause, reimaging with MRI at 6 weeks post-hemorrhage is often recommended to screen for an occult lesion. Even with patients who present with a hemorrhage resulting from an obvious AVM, re-imaging with angiography and MRI at 6 weeks postictus should be performed.

In approximately 7% to 25% of cases of cerebral AVM, there is an associated arterial aneurysm, whereas 1.4% of patients with intracranial aneurysms have coexistent AVMs. Aneurysms may arise from hemodynamic stresses resulting from the presence of the AVMs. Many times, these flow-related aneurysms will spontaneously regress following the reduction in blood flow after treatment of the AVM.

The goal of treatment of AVMs is to remove the risk of bleeding or growth. This is best accomplished with surgical excision, if possible. Radiation therapy (including radiosurgery) has also had excellent success in treating these lesions. Embolization is often a significant aid in the treatment of AVMs, making lesions smaller and more amenable to surgery and/or radiation. However, it rarely has any use as a stand-alone therapy, as embolized vessels will often recanalize over time.

All patients with AVMs need to be followed, even if the AVM has been treated. There are rare cases of regrowth of AVMs in growing children, and lesions may be incompletely treated, with recurrences found at later dates. Follow-up varies by institution, but often involves annual angiograms or MRA studies for several years posttreatment. Non-treated AVMs also need to be followed. Even if an individual AVM cannot be resected or radiated, changes in parts of the AVM (such as development of flow-related aneurysms) may be treatable.

Arteriovenous Fistulas/Vein of Galen Malformations

Arteriovenous fistulas (AVFs) and vein of Galen malformations (VOGMs) are grouped together as they are similar entities in many ways. Both are direct connections between cerebral arteries and existing veins. Unlike AVMs, they do not usually have a nidus and, in some cases of AVFs, may exist as a single pathologic connection between an artery and vein. In VOGMs, multiple small arterial vessels directly drain into the vein of Galen (Figure 6-1). The result of this type of direct connection is markedly increased venous pressure, leading to increased intracranial pressure and potential hemorrhage. In some VOGMs the connections have such rapid flow rates that children can present with high-output cardiac failure.

Vein of Galen malformations are congenital lesions and are not known to have a genetic predisposition. Arteriovenous fistulas may be congenital or acquired; they may occur after trauma or in settings of venous stasis, as is seen in transverse sinus thrombosis after severe mastoiditis, presumably by rupture of the thin-walled dural arteries traversing the dural sinus. The one genetic condition associated with multifocal AVFs that has been described in children is hereditary hemorrhagic telangiectasia (HHT). The same screening study, MRI/MRA, done for AVMs in patients with HHT, can also be useful in evaluating for AVFs.

Symptoms from AVFs and VOGMs result from venous hypertension and high flow. Symptoms are dependent on location and, historically, these lesions have been divided into 2 regions: anterior-inferior and posterior-superior. Involvement of the cavernous sinus in the anterior-inferior distribution can produce vision loss, proptosis, chemosis, ophthalmoplegia, and pain. Posterior-inferior lesions can present with tinnitus, headache, hydrocephalus, hemorrhage, and seizure. Any location can present with headache, hemorrhage, and a bruit.

Angiography remains the gold standard for evaluation of these lesions. Because of the morbidity associated with conventional angiography in neonates, diagnostic angiography for VOGMs is generally deferred until the time of endovascular treatment. Features that are important in determining the optimal therapeutic approach include the number of feeding arteries, the status of the venous outflow of the shunt and of the brain, and the severity of arterial "steal" from the cerebral circulation.

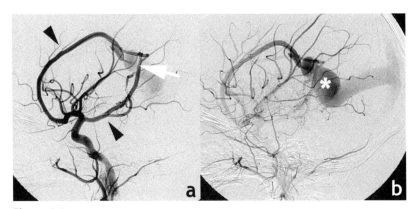

Figure 6-1.
Cerebral arteriogram performed in an infant with a loud cephalic bruit and high output cardiac failure. Early in the arterial phase there is a jet of contrast (white arrow) entering a large venous varix through an arteriovenous fistula (Figure 6-1A). Two large arterial feeders are visible (black arrowheads). Slightly later, but still in the arterial phase, contrast fills the varix (white asterisk) and an anomalous vein that passes from the varix to the superior sagittal sinus (Figure 6-1B). The diagnosis is vein of Galen malformation. (Courtesy of Dr Joseph E. Piatt, Chief of Neurosurgery, St Christopher's Hospital for Children, Philadelphia, PA.)

Pediatric AVFs and VOGMs should be considered for treatment. Minimally symptomatic lesions without reflux into cortical veins may be observed, as a number of them will close spontaneously. However, the findings of vision loss, severe exophthalmos, progressive ophthalmoplegia, and progressive dural sinus thrombosis with cortical venous drainage should prompt urgent treatment. High-flow VOGMs should be treated, often endovascularly. These children commonly present with concomitant hydrocephalus, believed to be secondary to increased venous pressure. Treatment of the VOGM will frequently result in resolution of the hydrocephalus without need for a shunt.

Treatment is generally via endovascular occlusion of the lesion, either via transarterial embolization or transvenous occlusion of the draining dural sinus. Surgery or radiosurgery, with or without adjunctive endovascular therapy, has been used less frequently, and outcomes for non-endovascular treatment of AVFs are generally less satisfactory than with endovascular occlusion.

Cavernous Malformations

Cavernous malformations are also referred to as *cavernomas, cavernous angiomas,* and *cavernous hemangiomas.* They are composed of a compact mass of sinusoidal-type vessels with low flow that are immediately contiguous with one another and have no intervening normal parenchyma. Cavernous malformations are often undetectable on angiogram, and are therefore grouped with the heterogenous entity of angiographically occult vascular malformations. Cavernous malformations are often well-circumscribed, unencapsulated masses identified grossly as having a purple lobulated "mulberry" appearance and are further identified by neuroimaging by a characteristic rim of hemosiderin seen on susceptibility images on MRI (Figure 6-2).

Cavernous malformations may never give rise to symptoms, being discovered incidentally at autopsy, or may be responsible for a variety of neurologic complaints. Cavernous malformations can develop anywhere in the CNS and, if symptomatic, most commonly present with headache, seizure, or focal neurologic deficit. Intracranial CMs cause symptoms by (relatively) low-pressure hemorrhages that exert mass effect on surrounding brain tissue. The extravasation of blood into brain parenchyma creates a hemosiderin ring that predisposes susceptible tissue to seizures.

Cavernous malformations are relatively common lesions, with an estimated prevalence of 0.5% in autopsy and MRI studies. Fifty percent to 80% of all lesions are sporadic. Single CMs are found in 75% of sporadic cases and 8% to 19% of familial cases. The presence of multiple lesions often indicates either a familial form of CMs or radiation-induced CMs. Familial CMs are rare, but if there is a history of other first-degree relatives with intracranial CMs, screening may be indicated. In particular, patients with relatives with multiple intracranial CMs are more likely to have CMs themselves. Guidelines for screening include first-degree relatives with multiple CMs or a family history of hereditary hemorrhagic telangiectasia. Screening should consist of an MRI with susceptibility images to identify previous hemorrhage.

Many patients who present with deficit from hemorrhage of CMs often have poor long-term resolution of symptoms and can be at risk of temporal clustering of hemorrhages in a short period. These lesions can progress in a relentless fashion, causing stepwise development of neurologic deficits.

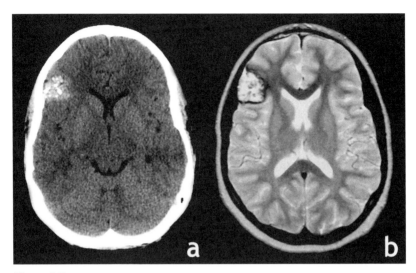

Figure 6-2.
A computed tomography scan of the head without contrast (Figure 6-2A) shows a slightly radiodense lesion in the right frontal cortex with punctate calcifications. An axial T2-weighted magnetic resonance scan (Figure 6-2B) shows that the high signal intensity core of this lesion is surrounded by a ring of low signal intensity hemosiderin. These imaging features are diagnostic of cavernous malformation, cavernous hemangioma or "cavernoma." (Courtesy of Dr Joseph H. Piatt, Chief of Neurosurgery, St Christopher's Hospital for Children, Philadelphia, PA.)

Given this natural history, several authors have advocated early treatment of CMs in children, as the long life span anticipated in the pediatric patient may favor a more aggressive approach. Indications for treatment generally include symptomatic lesions or lesions with demonstrated growth on serial imaging studies. If the CM is in an unfavorable location, such as the brain stem or thalamus, treatment may focus on supportive measures. In general, there is no role for chemotherapy or embolization for CMs and the use of radiation therapy is highly controversial. Outcomes for surgical therapy have been remarkably good, although lesion location has been noted to affect prognosis.

Follow-up is indicated in these patients, as lesions can recur if not completely excised, and generation of new lesions has been documented, particularly in the setting of radiation-induced CMs. In most patients, a postoperative MRI is the imaging modality of choice, often obtained at 6 weeks to 6 months postoperatively. There is sparse literature on the usefulness of long-term follow-up imaging. It is the practice at the authors' institution to obtain follow-up imaging at 1-year intervals for up to 2 years postoperatively.

Patients with multiple CMs should have periodic imaging to ascertain progression of any lesions. In the pediatric population, the lifelong risk of a lesion, which demonstrates repeated hemorrhage or growth, is significant and merits consideration of resection. With this in mind, annual imaging is obtained in this population.

Vasculopathies/Arteriopathies

Moyamoya Syndrome

Moyamoya syndrome is a vasculopathy characterized by chronic progressive stenosis to occlusion at the apices of the intracranial ICAs, including the proximal anterior cerebral arteries and middle cerebral arteries. It has been associated with approximately 6% of childhood strokes. As progressive stenosis occurs, there is simultaneous development of characteristic arterial collateral vessels at the base of the brain. These collateral vessels, when visualized on angiography, have been likened to the appearance of "a puff of smoke"—*moyamoya* in Japanese.

Some authors have distinguished between moyamoya disease, the idiopathic form of moyamoya, and moyamoya syndrome, defined as the vasculopathy found in association with another condition, such as neurofibromatosis, SCD, or Down syndrome. The precise etiology of this vasculopathy remains unclear, but its progressive course, coupled with a good response to surgical therapy, has resulted in study of this entity in far greater detail than might be expected from its relative rarity.

Overall, most children present with recurrent TIAs, stroke, seizures, or headaches; only about 3% of pediatric patients in the Children's Hospital Boston series had an intracerebral hemorrhage as their first symptom, a presentation far more common in adults with moyamoya.

There are a number of clinical conditions associated with moyamoya. These include prior radiotherapy to the head or neck for optic gliomas, craniopharyngiomas, and pituitary tumors; genetic disorders, such as Down syndrome, neurofibromatosis type 1 (with or without hypothalamic-optic pathway tumors), large facial hemangiomas, sickle cell anemia, and other hemoglobinopathies; autoimmune disorders such as Graves disease, congenital cardiac disease, renal artery stenosis, meningeal infections, including tuberculous meningitis, among others.

Moyamoya syndrome should be considered in any child who presents with symptoms of cerebral ischemia, especially if the symptoms are precipitated by physical exertion, hyperventilation, or crying. In addition to signs of recent or remote cerebral infarction, MRI reveals the characteristic peppering of the basal ganglia by flow voids representing the moyamoya collaterals (Figure 6-3). To confirm the diagnosis of moyamoya syndrome and to visualize the anatomy of the vessels involved and the patterns of flow through the hemispheres, conventional cerebral arteriogram is typically required (Figure 6-4).

The prognosis of moyamoya syndrome is difficult to predict because the natural history of this disorder is not well known. The progression of disease can be slow, with rare, intermittent events, or can be fulminant, with rapid neurologic decline. However, regardless of the course, it seems clear that moyamoya syndrome, both in terms of arteriopathy and clinical symptoms,

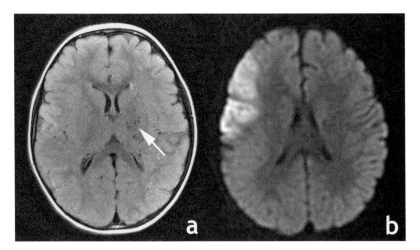

Figure 6-3.
Axial magnetic resonance images of the brain show an acute cerebral infarct in the right frontal region. The infarct is essentially undetectable on the FLAIR (fluid attenuation inversion recovery) sequence (Figure 6-3A), but it is demarcated vividly by high signal intensity changes on the diffusion-weighted image (Figure 6-3B). The cluster of punctate signal voids in the left putamen (white arrow) reflects tiny collateral arteries in this patient with moyamoya disease. (Courtesy of Dr Joseph H. Piatt, Chief of Neurosurgery, St Christopher's Hospital for Children, Philadelphia, PA.)

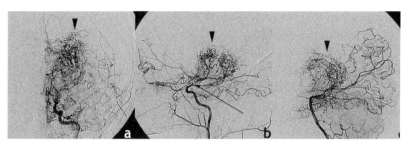

Figure 6-4.

Anteroposterior (Figure 6-4A) and lateral (Figure 4B) views of a left common carotid arteriogram and a lateral view (Figure 6-4C) of a vertebral arteriogram in a child with moyamoya disease illustrate the "puff of smoke" appearance (black arrowheads) of tiny collateral arteries conveying blood flow from the uninvolved posterior circulation to the ischemic brain in the distribution of the occluded internal carotid artery (long black arrow in 4B). (Courtesy of Dr Joseph H. Piatt, Chief of Neurosurgery, St Christopher's Hospital for Children, Philadelphia, PA.)

inevitably progresses in untreated patients. It has been estimated that 50% to 66% of patients with moyamoya have symptomatic progression of the disease with poor outcomes if left untreated. This number contrasts strikingly to an estimated rate of only 2.6% of symptomatic disease progression in surgically treated pediatric patients. In general, neurologic status at time of treatment, more so than age of the patient, predicts long-term outcome.

Treatment includes medical measures to improve blood flow to the brain, avoidance of dehydration, use of anti-thrombotic agents such as aspirin, and maintenance of normotension and normocarbia. Patients diagnosed with moyamoya syndrome should be started on aspirin therapy (barring other medical contraindications), and parents should be instructed to keep affected children well hydrated and to try to discourage crying, which causes cerebral vasoconstriction through lowering carbon dioxide partial pressure.

However, these maneuvers will ultimately fail without surgical revascularization of the ischemic brain. Revascularization can be accomplished directly, by bypass grafting to one of the major branches of the middle cerebral artery, or indirectly by encouragement of development of collateral vessels. Many surgical techniques for indirect revascularization have been described. A popular technique is pial synangiosis, in which a segment of the superficial temporal artery is mobilized with proximal and distal continuity and laid on the surface of the brain. The underlying ischemia of the brain evokes a rapid and luxuriant growth of collateral vessels from the transposed superficial temporal artery. In general, indirect procedures such as pial synangiosis are more suitable for children because small arterial caliber makes bypass grafting problematic.

Importantly, if surgical revascularization is performed prior to disabling infarction in moyamoya syndrome, even if severe angiographic changes are present, the prognosis tends to be excellent. Even in asymptomatic patients, surgical revascularization has been reported to protect against infarction. However, if left untreated, both the angiographic process and the clinical syndrome invariably progress, producing clinical deterioration with potentially irreversible neurologic deficits over time.

Careful follow-up of patients with moyamoya is warranted. The experience of Children's Hospital Boston suggests that at least 14% of unilateral patients will progress to requiring surgery on the second side within an average of 2.2 years. Of those patients who were treated operatively (for either bilateral or unilateral disease), the need for additional revascularization procedures ranges from 1.8% to 18%. These data suggest that periodic clinical and radiographic examinations of patients with moyamoya disease, even if treated, should be performed on a regular basis.

Other Arteriopathies Associated With Cerebrovascular Disease
There are a number of other arteriopathies that are associated with cerebrovascular disease in children. While many conditions are listed in the section on aneurysms, several deserve special note. In particular, fibromuscular dysplasia, Marfan syndrome, and Ehlers-Danlos syndrome type IV merit particular attention.

Fibromuscular dysplasia, identified by bead-like arteriopathic changes in affected arteries, has been associated with carotid dissection and intracranial aneurysms. Fibromuscular dysplasia is rare, present in approximately 0.02% of the US population, and is more commonly found in females. Patients may present with neck pain or TIAs. Evaluation requires MRI/MRA, including the proximal carotid arteries. Management of this disease is controversial, but many favor medical treatment with antiplatelet agents. Rarely, surgery or endovascular therapy may be used to bypass or dilate affected vessel segments.

Marfan syndrome is a genetic connective tissue disorder caused by defects in the fibrillin gene. Marfan affects approximately 1 per 10,000 individuals in the United States, with variable expression of symptoms, some of which do not manifest until adulthood. Patients are often unusually tall, thin, and have hypermobile joints. They are at risk for dissections of cerebral vessels (and the aorta) and aneurysms. Workup includes a MRI/MRA and referral to a tertiary care center for neurosurgical and cardiac evaluation.

Ehlers-Danlos syndrome is actually a family of connective tissue disorders sharing a variety of errors in the metabolism of collagen. Similar to the other arteriopathies discussed, these patients may present with hypermobile joints, delayed healing, and easy bruising. Of particular importance is one subtype of Ehlers-Danlos, type IV. Patients with this "vascular" variant of Ehlers-Danlos are prone to acute rupture of intracranial and intra-abdominal arteries with severe morbidity and shortened life expectancies. Patients with Ehlers-Danlos type IV should be considered for MRI/MRA screening for intracranial aneurysms, but it should be noted that they have notoriously fragile blood vessels, and the reported mortality rate for any type of vascular surgical procedure is high.

Congenital and Acquired Heart Disease

Heart disease, whether congenital or acquired, is the most common cause of ischemic stroke in children, accounting approximately for 25% of all arterial stroke and 20% and 17% of cases following cardiac surgery and catheterization respectively. Any structural lesion of the heart can potentially lead to stroke, although complex anomalies within the nosological context of congenital heart disease (CHD), particularly those associated with cyanotic heart disease and polycythemia, are the most serious predisposing lesions by virtue of increasing the likelihood for both thrombosis and embolism. Common CHD examples associated with stroke include tetralogy of Fallot, membranous ventricular septal defects, patent ductus arteriosus, and anomalous pulmonary venous drainage. Right-to-left cardiac shunts may give rise to a paradoxical (venous) embolus. In the clinical setting of tetralogy of Fallot, emboli may be septic and evolve into cerebral abscesses. There is a strong relationship between CHD, Down syndrome, and stroke.

Cerebral embolism has also been described in children with cardiac rhabdomyomas in the context of tuberous sclerosis, and atrial and anterior mitral valve myxomas, as well as primary tumors of the heart.

Although many patients have a known history of CHD before the onset of cerebral ischemia, a significant percentage of cases have a previously unknown or unsuspected structural defect of the heart. It has been shown that, in patients with cryptogenic stroke, the prevalence of a patent foramen ovale is almost twice as high relative to the general healthy population. This has lead to speculation about a potential role of intracardiac right-to-left shunts as an underlying causal factor in AIS in children. To date, percutaneous catheter (transcatheter) closure of the patent foramen ovale is the most common interventional procedure performed in adult congenital heart disease units. However, even though the prevalence of patent foramen ovale is similar in children, this procedure is performed much less commonly in the pediatric age group despite a similar susceptibility of defect-related morbidity for cerebrovascular disease and stroke. Currently, the only strong indication for the performance of percutaneous closure of the foramen ovale in children is evidence of recurrent paradoxical embolism in patients with an aneurysmal atrial septum and a patent foramen ovale. Percutaneous closure of the patent foramen ovale would seem to be a safe and effective intervention to prevent recurrent stroke in children. Moreover, it is envisioned that as the complication rate for device implantation abates, percutaneous closure may become more widely used in the pediatric interventional cardiology setting.

Infective endocarditis is considered an important cause of cardiogenic AIS in children, with an incidence of approximately one-third of that of adults (0.6 per 100,000/year) but a high mortality rate of 11% to 20%. Predisposing factors are different in children compared with adults with congenital heart disease, accounting for most cases (50%–75%) followed by rheumatic heart disease (12%). In a significant percentage of patients there are no overt cardiac abnormalities (14%–40%).

It is well established that 20% to 40% of adult patients with infective endocarditis will go on to develop neurologic complications, principally cerebral infarction, bacterial meningitis, intracerebral hemorrhage, and mycotic aneurysms. Even though neurologic complications are less well elucidated in the pediatric setting, up to 60% of children suffering a stroke as a result of infective endocarditis will potentially develop permanent neurologic deficits, with an added risk of recurrent stroke in up to 50% of them.

A recently published retrospective study of a cohort of pediatric patients conducted at Children's Memorial Hospital of Chicago revealed that 7 of 115 pediatric patients with endocarditis, 4 of whom had congenital heart disease, went on to develop cerebral infarcts. Most of them involved the territorial distribution of the middle cerebral artery, with focal weakness being the most common presenting sign. Three patients manifested mycotic aneurysms, all of which were successfully surgically repaired. Two patients received aspirin therapy without adverse effects. While all patients survived, neurologic sequelae were variable. The most severe neurologic deficits were seen in the 2 youngest patients (aged 3 and 14 weeks), both of whom required prolonged hospital stays. Even though children may have better outcomes than adults, routine surveillance to rule out mycotic aneurysms in patients with new neurologic deficits coupled with aspirin prophylaxis should be considered in the medical management of infective endocarditis-associated cerebrovascular disease.

Venous Thrombosis and Thrombophlebitis

Venous thrombosis is a less common cause of stroke than AIS. Yet, venous stroke has a proclivity for younger patients, including children and newborns, thus calling for heightened awareness in this regard among pediatricians and child neurologists. Dural or cerebral venous sinus (sinovenous) thrombosis and cortical vein thrombosis in children are not always amenable to early recognition because their clinical manifestations are often less overt or specific compared with arterial ischemic infarcts. Early and accurate diagnosis requires a high level of experience and prompt intervention, taking advantage of recent advances in neuroimaging and management for these disorders.

A common clinical setting for intracranial venous thrombosis is dehydration, particularly among infants. Clinical presentations include symptoms secondary to increased intracranial pressure such as lethargy, anorexia, headache, vomiting, and coma (associated with dural sinus thrombosis), as well as focal or generalized seizures and focal signs (associated with cortical vein thrombosis). As a rule, there is evidence of cerebral sinus venous thrombosis on neuroimaging, especially using MRV.

Predisposition to intracranial venous thrombosis is, in part, genetically determined, with several inherited thrombophilias accounting for about one-quarter of all cases (see below).

The treatment of intracranial venous thrombosis begins with rehydration and continuing support of intravascular volume. In cases in which dehydration is the precipitating clinical event, no additional treatment may be indicated. In other instances, anticoagulation may be considered. Low molecular weight heparin is often used acutely because of its simplicity and relative safety. Recommendations regarding long-term anticoagulation depend on laboratory findings from the obligatory investigation of clotting. Disruption or dissolution of large thrombi in the major dural sinuses by endovascular techniques is technically feasible and may be appropriate for carefully selected, unstable patients.

Infective, Postinfective, and Immune-Mediated Vascular Diseases (Vasculitis)

Vasculopathies Associated With Infections

Central nervous system infections are frequently involved in the pathogenesis of cerebral vasculopathy and constitute a major etiologic category for stroke in children. Inflammation of cerebral blood vessels associated with infection (infective vasculitis) results in acute, subacute, or delayed vascular damage (vasculopathy) and cerebral infarction, principally in the form of arterial or venous ischemic strokes. By comparison, intra- or extra-axial hemorrhages, which are directly attributed to an infective process of the CNS, are less common. Stroke may occur in the setting of fulminant or inadequately treated bacterial, tuberculous, or luetic meningitis; Lyme disease; *Mycoplasma pneumoniae* infection; vasoinvasive fungal infections (aspergillosis, mucormycosis); or viral disease. To this end, herpes zoster virus (HZV), HIV, and Japanese encephalitis are the most significant viral agents implicated in childhood cerebrovascular disease and stroke.

While hemorrhagic stroke is less frequent than ischemic stroke in children in the clinical setting of CNS infection, it can still lead to potentially devastating neurologic deficits. It is usually due to ruptured intracranial mycotic aneurysms secondary to bacterial or angioinvasive fungal infections. In addition, aneurysms arising in the background of viral infections (ie, HZV vasculopathy, HIV vasculopathy, or noninfective immune-mediated vasculitides, such as primary angiitis of the central nervous system) can potentially undergo spontaneous rupture, causing massive SAH or intracerebral hemorrhages.

Among viral-induced CNS vasculopathies associated with stroke, HZV CNS vasculopathy and HIV CNS vasculopathy are particularly important in the pediatric population.

Herpes Zoster Virus-Associated Cerebrovascular Disease and Stroke

Herpes zoster virus (varicella-zoster virus or chickenpox) infection constitutes a major risk factor for ischemic stroke in children, estimated in 1 in 15,000.

The neurologic manifestations of HZV-associated cerebrovascular disease may be variable, with a typical onset months following clinically apparent disease; in some cases it can occur without any prior history of skin rash. Central nervous system vasculitis and resultant obliterative vasculopathy can occur after primary varicella infection or HZV reactivation, either spontaneously in immunologically competent children or in patients with history of risk factors for immunologic compromise.

The most typical presentation of HZV-associated cerebrovascular disease is occlusive ischemic stroke involving large cerebral arteries. That said, ischemic lesions secondary to occlusive disease of small-sized cerebral vessels can also occur either singly, giving rise to a multifocal leukoencephalopathy, or in combination with large vessels. Large-vessel disease seems to be more common among immunologically competent children, whereas small-vessel disease is more common among immunocompromised patients.

The diagnostic approach in suspected cases includes MRI, cerebral angiography, and CSF examination with molecular virology testing. For the diagnosis of HZV-associated CNS vasculopathy, 3 criteria must be met: (1) HZV infection within the preceding 12 months; (2) evidence of unilateral, proximal large-vessel stenosis; and (3) detection of HZV DNA by polymerase chain reaction (PCR) or detection of HZV IgG in the CSF.

In immunologically compromised patients, especially in children with HIV/AIDS, the presumptive mode of spread is direct infection of the blood vessel walls by HZV. In the setting of HZV and HIV coinfection, there may be combined large- and small-vessel involvement, accounting for an overlapping pattern of cerebral infarcts and multifocal leukoencephalopathy.

The prognosis of HZV-associated cerebrovascular disease is unpredictable and may range from rapid resolution and an overall favorable neurologic outcome to a fatal outcome. The rate of recurrent strokes associated with HZV is significant (approximately 45%), while residual neurologic deficits are present in a high percentage of patients (approximately 70%).

At the present time, the management of children is based on the principles of therapy used for adult patients. In this regard, the standard treatment protocol comprises anticoagulation (low-dose aspirin with or without low-molecular-weight heparin), acyclovir for 7 to 10 days, and a short course of oral corticosteroids for 3 to 5 days. The rationale for treatment with acyclovir and/or other antiviral agents is to prevent or abate the progression of the vasculitic changes owing to a continuous or recurrent virus-triggered vascular injury. Persistence of HZV infection in the cerebral vessels has been confirmed by detectable HZV DNA sequences by PCR in the cerebrospinal fluid several months following the onset of neurologic manifestations. Along these lines, it has been observed that when HZV-associated vasculopathy develops months after varicella infection, antiviral treatment is often effective.

In recent years, the International Herpes Management Forum has proposed guidelines regarding diagnosis and management of CNS syndromes associated with HZV, with special attention to HZV-associated vasculopathy (Box 6-6).

Box 6-6. International Herpes Management Forum Guidelines[a]

1. Children with focal vasculopathy due to HZV should undergo treatment with intravenous acyclovir (500 mg/m^2 body surface area) for 7 days.

2. Immunologically compromised patients may require longer treatment, but antiviral therapy should be discontinued if CSF HZV DNA and anti-HZV antibody are negative (966).

3. Corticosteroids (prednisone 60–80 mg/d for 3–5 days) should be considered as they may contribute to the abatement of HZV-associated CNS vasculitis.

Abbreviations: HZV, herpes zoster virus; CSF, cerebrospinal fluid; CNS, central nervous system.
[a]Gilden D. Varicella zoster virus and central nervous system syndromes. Herpes. 2004;11(suppl 2):89A–94A.

Cerebrovascular Disease and Stroke in Pediatric HIV/AIDS

An increased incidence of ischemic and hemorrhagic stroke and aneurysmal arteriopathy is encountered in the setting of pediatric HIV/AIDS. Most cases are transmitted either vertically or are acquired perinatally. In a study of 426 HIV-infected pediatric patients who were evaluated at the National Cancer Institute from 1986 to June 2001 for participation in approved therapeutic research trials, only 11 (2.6%) were found to have focal neurologic signs coupled by definable cerebrovascular lesions by neuroimaging. Most patients had advanced HIV disease and had received antiretroviral treatment. The incidence of HIV-associated cerebrovascular disease in children is unclear and potentially underappreciated.

Central nervous system vasculitis/vasculopathy in children with HIV/AIDS may be associated with aberrant immune cell responses triggered by HIV infection of the CNS or be the consequence of coinfection, particularly with HZV. Angiocentric mononuclear inflammatory cell infiltrates with evidence of lymphocytic vasculitis (comprised of cytotoxic CD3+/CD8+ T cells) and multifocal cerebral infarcts have been described in infants and young children with HIV infection without evidence of concomitant viral or other opportunistic infection. Collectively, HIV-associated vasculitis, together with other viral co-infections exhibiting a tropism for blood vessels such as HZV, as well as thromboembolism of cardiac origin and autoimmune thrombocytopenia, may contribute to aneurysmal vasculopathy, cerebral infarction, and hemorrhage, all of which are recognized cerebrovascular complications in children with HIV/AIDS. Moreover, small-vessel CNS vasculitis may be responsible for the calcific vasculopathy underlying CNS perfusion deficits and the mineralizations of the basal ganglia and thalami, which are common neuroimaging findings in children with HIV/AIDS. It is postulated that CNS vasculitis may potentially result in calcific vasculopathy, fibrointimal fibroplasia, and aneurysmal arteriopathy. In the brain parenchyma, a vasculitis-vasculopathy sequence may disrupt the blood-brain barrier and cause endothelial cell injury, prothrombotic phenomena, and vascular occlusion leading to perfusion deficits and stroke in children with HIV/AIDS.

As most HIV-infected children are for the most part asymptomatic during the early stages of the disease, screening of high-risk children, preferably by MRI, is recommended for the early detection of cerebrovascular abnormalities. However, at this time the role of antiretroviral drugs for prophylaxis against cerebral vasculopathy or stroke is unclear and awaits further investigation.

Less common secondary systemic vasculitides likely to involve the CNS and cause cerebrovascular disease in children include polyarteritis nodosa and Churg-Strauss syndrome (allergic granulomatosis), the muco-cutaneous lymph node syndrome (Kawasaki disease), and certain collagen vascular diseases.

Kawasaki disease may exhibit CNS involvement principally in the form of aseptic meningitis and encephalopathy. Stroke, seizures, cranial nerve palsies, retinal lesions, and neuromuscular manifestations are less frequent. Focal neurologic findings and MRI lesions are attributed to CNS ischemia resulting from vasculitis; however, angiography or brain biopsy confirm-ing vasculitis is only seldom reported. In these patients, high-dose aspirin (80–100 mg/kg/d) for 14 days in conjunction with immune globulin intrave-nous administration in a single dose of 2 g/kg seems to be highly effective in ameliorating the arteritis and myocardial complications.

Hematologic Disorders: Sickle Cell Disease and Prothrombotic Disorders (Thrombophilias)

Sickle Cell Disease and Stroke

Within the nosological spectrum of hemoglobinopathies, it is the homozy-gous SCD that accounts for most stroke cases. Other hemoglobinopathies, such as thalassemia, may present with stroke, as part of an increased procliv-ity for thromboembolic complications mostly in the form of silent strokes, or occasionally in association with concomitant thrombophilias (also see section on prothrombotic disorders).

Children with SCD are at a high risk for strokes. The cumulative risk increases according with age, ranging from 11% at age 20 years to up to 24% by age 45 years. Recurrence is a major issue: The occurrence of an initial stroke carries with it a greater than 50% risk of subsequent strokes.

Most SCD-associated childhood strokes are in the form of arterial infarction (Figure 6-5). Parenchymal and subarachnoid hemorrhages may also occur but are less common in children.

While AIS may occur during a thrombotic crisis, most patients show no clinically apparent premonitory symptoms or signs. In fact, nearly

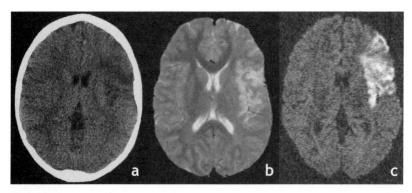

Figure 6-5.
Sickle cell disease. An axial non-contrast computed tomography (CT) scan demonstrates a low-density area in the distribution of the left middle cerebral artery consistent with an infarct (Figure 6-5A). Axial non-contrast T2-weighted magnetic resonance imaging (MRI) demonstrates a hyperintense area (Figure 6-5B). Axial diffusion weighted MRI demonstrates an area of hyperintensity corresponding to the lesion demonstrated on both CT and MRI, consistent with cytotoxic edema in acute infarction (Figure 6-5C). (Courtesy of Dr Eric N. Faerber, Director of Radiology, St Christopher's Hospital for Children, Philadelphia, PA.)

three-quarters of children with homozygous SCD experience subclinical, commonly referred to as *silent* (or covert), cerebral infarcts, which lack overt neurologic manifestations and are detected only by neuroimaging.

The pathophysiologic basis of SCD-related stroke relates to blood vessel occlusion and intravascular hemolytic anemia. Small-vessel occlusion, which is of the same kind that gives rise to painful somatic episodes, is the main underlying cause for microcirculatory hemodynamic derangements in the CNS. That being said, both small and large cerebral blood vessels may be involved. On clinical grounds, large artery infarction is most commonly recognized, most often involving the distal internal carotid arteries and proximal middle cerebral arteries, leading to diminished perfusion of the corresponding arterial territories of supply or, especially at the level of the circle of Willis, through artery-to-artery embolization.

Effective stroke prevention in children with SCD can be achieved nowadays by transcranial Doppler ultrasonography (TCD), which can greatly facilitate early and timely detection and prompt therapeutic intervention by means of prophylactic blood transfusion. Transcranial Doppler ultrasonography measures blood flow velocity in the large arteries of the circle of Willis. As a rule, severe anemia causes velocity increases, which subsequently attain a focal distribution when vascular occlusion ensues, resulting in compromise of the diameter of the arterial lumens. Healthy children and adults without evidence of anemia have velocities of approximately 90 cm/s and 60 cm/s respectively, whereas, in patients with SCD, the mean velocity is approximately 130 cm/s.

Currently the risk for stroke in all children with SCD is directly related to increase in TCD velocity. This has been convincingly shown in 2 independent studies.

The first of the 2 studies was designated Stroke Prevention Trial in Sickle Cell Anemia (STOP) (1995–2000). It included children who had 2 TCD studies with velocities of 200 cm/s or higher. In this high-risk pediatric population, it was found that patients who did not receive transfusions exhibited a stroke risk of 10% per year, which was dramatically decreased to less than 1% per year with regular blood transfusions. STOP was halted ahead of time when it became evident that regular blood transfusions in this group of SCD patients led to a sharp (90%) decline in the onset of first stroke. Since then, regular blood transfusions are recommended for SCD patients who meet the TCD criteria of STOP.

A sequel randomized controlled study known as STOP II was carried out, which aimed at identifying a subset of children in whom withdrawal of transfusion could be attempted without increasing the risk for stroke. Children with initially abnormal TCD velocities (characterized either by ≥200 cm/s) treated with regular blood transfusions for 30 months or more, which resulted in reduction of the TCD to less than 170 cm/s, were eligible for participation in the randomized STOP II trial. Half of the patients who were entered in the STOP II trial continued to undergo transfusion, while there was discontinuation of transfusions in the other half. However, STOP II had to be halted early on safety grounds as many patients in whom transfusions were discontinued reverted back to the high-risk group with TCD velocity measurements exceeding or equal to 200 cm/s. There were also 2 instances of stroke among these patients.

At the present time there are no evidence-based guidelines for the discontinuation of transfusion once these children have been classified as high risk for stroke on the basis of TCD criteria. Thus long-term chronic transfusion therapy to maintain hemoglobin S levels below 30% is indicated in children with SCD and intracranial large vessel stenosis. The benefits of such an indefinite transfusion are 2-fold and include: (1) prevention of recurrence in most patients with a prior stroke and (2) prevention of a first stroke in those children exhibiting high TCD velocities. Unfortunately, these patients remain at risk for the undesirable long-term sequela of transfusion, including effects on growth and iron overload. The latter has recently become easier to manage with the use of oral iron chelator compounds.

As many patients with SCD and cerebral ischemia have chronic, progressive stenosis of the internal carotid artery and its major branches, the underlying physiological disturbance is similar to moyamoya disease. Such patients are sometimes characterized as having moyamoya syndrome. Favorable experiences with surgical revascularization for symptomatic cerebral ischemia in the setting of SCD have been reported from a number of institutions. In the context of recent advances in transfusion therapy, however, no consensus has yet formed around the role of revascularization in SCD.

Inherited or Acquired Prothrombotic Disorders (Thrombophilias)

As alluded previously, the etiology of stroke in children is unknown in more than one-third of the patients. However, the true incidence of stroke linked etiologically to various prothrombotic disorders (thrombophilias) is unknown and, to some extent, controversial. In a retrospective study performed in a cohort of 212 pediatric patients with stroke at the University College London, Ganesan and colleagues reported that genetically determined or acquired conditions causing thrombophilia are rare. On the other hand, other studies have found prothrombotic abnormalities in as many as half of children with stroke, most of whom may harbor more than one risk factor, mainly vasculopathies, hemoglobinopathies, and coagulation defects such as elevation of lipoprotein-associated phospholipase A(2) and C677T mutation of the methylenetetrahydrofolate reductase gene.

That being said, the view that prothrombotic abnormalities in stroke, especially in recurrent stroke, are less common in children compared with adults remains entrenched. Although an evaluation of certain prothrombotic conditions is routinely performed in adults with stroke, the same is not the case in the pediatric setting. Traditionally, the coagulation battery of tests included protein C, protein S, antithrombin III, lupus anticoagulants, and anticardiolipin antibodies. More tests have been added to include homocystine level, factor VIII level, mutations for factor V Leiden and prothrombin G20210A, and lipoprotein-associated phospholipase A(2) level. As such, the extended battery of laboratory diagnosis testing for prothrombotic disorders has recently disclosed additional risk factors in the clinical setting of pediatric stroke, thus calling for a thorough evaluation of newly emerging prothrombotic abnormalities in these patients.

Inherited thrombophilias, either alone or in concert with other prothrombotic risk factors, such as antiphospholipid antibodies and hyperhomocysteinemia (Box 6-3), account for an expanding spectrum of AIS and cerebral venous thrombosis cases. Factor V Leiden is the most common genetic risk factor in this regard and is followed by the prothrombin gene mutation G20210A and deficiencies of protein S, protein C, and antithrombin III, all of which are known to cause venous infarcts in the neonatal setting. In the latter scenario, rigorous thrombophilia screening is indicated for both the mother and the newborn. Importantly, the co-inheritance of 2 or more known mutations markedly increases patient susceptibility to cerebral venous thrombosis.

At present, there are no evidence-based guidelines for stroke prevention and/or management in children with inherited or acquired thrombophilic disorders. However, it is recommended that all children with stroke undergo a thrombophilia workup regardless of family history.

Stroke Associated With Leukemia and Disseminated Intravascular Coagulopathy

Cerebrovascular disease is a serious, potentially fatal complication of acute leukemia. There are at least 3 recognizable clinicopathological patterns of predominantly hemorrhagic stroke. These include (a) hemorrhagic infarction developing in the clinical setting of severe neutropenia (agranulocytosis) due to hematogenously disseminated vasoinvasive aspergillosis or mucormycosis, (b) massive cerebral hemorrhage associated with coagulation defects including disseminated intravascular coagulopathy (DIC), and (c) multiple cerebral hemorrhages due to leukemic cell infiltration into the brain associated with marked leukocytosis and intravascular leukostasis. Disseminated intravascular coagulopathy–related lobar hemorrhages are especially common in the setting of acute myelogenous leukemia. The detection of multiple lobar hemorrhages by neuroimaging (often conforming to a cortical-white matter junctional distribution) is a strong diagnostic indicator in favor of intravascular leukostasis and "blast crisis" and are thus tantamount to metastatic leukemic deposits.

Cerebral arterial or venous thrombosis and hemorrhage may be associated with exposure to chemotherapeutic agents such as L-asparaginase, which is typically used in rescue chemotherapy regimens for acute lympho-blastic leukemia.

Disseminated intravascular coagulopathy-associated cerebral hemor-rhages may be fulminant and potentially fatal. They are usually parenchy-mal or subdural, rarely exhibiting a subarachnoid pattern of distribution. The finding of systemic thrombotic or hemorrhagic complications should heighten suspicion for DIC. The diagnosis of DIC can be established by examination of the peripheral smear, platelet count (patients with platelet counts falling below 20,000 mm^3 are at imminent risk of spontaneous cere-bral hemorrhage), and tests of coagulation function. The management of acute DIC is controversial and should be individualized in accordance with the clinical setting.

Cerebrovascular Disease and Metabolic Disorders

Several hereditary metabolic disorders are known culprits of cerebrovascular disease and stroke.

Mitochondrial myopathy, encephalopathy, lactic acidosis, and stroke-like episodes is a maternally inherited mitochondrial disorder that pro-duces stroke-like events in young adults but also in children. These patients may manifest with epilepsia partialis continua and recurrent cortical and subcortical infarctions. Segmental vascular stenosis has been documented by MRA during the acute phase of first stroke-like episodes with subse-quent improvement.

Fabry disease is an X-linked lysosomal storage disease caused by defi-ciency of the enzyme α-galactosidase A, which results in the accumulation of the neutral glycosphingolipid globotriaosylceramide in the walls of small blood vessels, potentially resulting in stroke in adults.

Diabetic Ketoacidosis, Cerebral Edema, and Stroke

Approximately 16% of children with new-onset diabetes present with *diabetic ketoacidosis* (DKA) at the time of diagnosis. In the pediatric set-ting, cerebral edema is a rare but important and serious complication incurred during DKA episodes, which is associated with significant mor-bidity and mortality.

Heralding symptoms of subclinical cerebral edema include headache, vomiting, and lethargy, while rapid neurologic deterioration may ensue concomitant with overt diffuse cerebral edema. A study by Edge and colleagues analyzing all cases of DKA-associated cerebral edema in England, Scotland, and Wales, reported through the British Paediatric Surveillance Unit during a 2-year period (1996–1998), identified a total of 34 cases of cerebral edema out of 2,940 episodes of DKA. The calculated risk of developing cerebral edema was 6.8 per 1,000 episodes of DKA, which was higher in new (11.9 per 1,000 episodes) as opposed to established (3.8 per 1,000) cases of juvenile diabetes. Cerebral edema was associated with a significant mortality (24%) and morbidity (35% of survivors).

As a rule, cerebral edema in the setting of DKA responds to mannitol administration, with usual recovery expected within hours. However, there are instances with fatal outcome attributed to brain herniation as a result of fulminant or inadequately treated DKA-associated brain swelling.

Stroke in the setting of DKA should be suspected when focal neurologic deficits are apparent. It should be noted that children with new onset type I diabetes mellitus, exhibiting hyperglycemia and DKA, are prone to thrombosis. These may include venous sinus thrombosis with venous infarcts as well as arterial infarcts. Also, there are rare instances of cerebral hemorrhage described in this clinical setting.

Hyperhomocysteinemia/Homocystinuria and Stroke

Homocystinuria is an autosomal recessive syndrome, which gives rise to premature atherosclerosis and venous thrombosis and has been directly implicated in pediatric stroke. Hyperhomocysteinemia without a full-blown homocystinuria phenotype has been described in connection with cystathionine beta-synthase deficiency. The link between hyperhomocysteinemia with prothrombotic disorders and stroke is especially relevant and noteworthy in this regard.

Pathologic mechanisms of stroke in hyperhomocysteinemia/homocystinuria include carotid intraluminal thrombosis, arterial dissection, and possible artery-to-artery or cardiac embolisms. Some stroke cases associated with hyperhomocysteinemia have no known diagnosis of homocystinuria. Thus there is good rationale for screening for hyperhomocysteinemia in young stroke patients who lack an overt phenotype of classic homocystinuria. Family screening is also advisable as it may reveal additional members with clinically silent homocystinuria and hypercystinuria.

Arterial Dissection and Stroke in Children

An arterial dissection is a tear in one or more layers of the arterial wall. Once the integrity of the vessel wall is disrupted, blood collects within the vessel wall, and this hematoma typically compromises or obliterates the lumen of the vessel. Hemodynamic compromise from encroachment on the lumen can cause cerebral ischemia. Artery-to-artery embolism from thrombus accumulating at the site of the intimal injury is another potential mechanism of cerebral ischemia. A dissection that breaches the adventitia causes subarachnoid hemorrhage.

Unfortunately, arterial dissections in children usually present with TIA or cerebral infarction; detection of arterial dissection before the onset of neurologic symptoms requires an exceptionally high level of suspicion. There are diverse causes of arterial dissection. Arterial dissections may be seen in the setting of major, complex craniofacial trauma, or the precipitating injury may seem minor and inconsequential. Oral penetrating trauma is a classical cause of internal carotid artery injury in the tonsillar fossa, and carotid dissection can be seen similarly as a complication of tonsillectomy and adenoidectomy. Also, carotid artery dissection must be considered as a cause of stroke in children who have suffered head and neck burns, even on a delayed basis during the recovery phase of burn injury. Among the less well-recognized causes of arterial dissection and stroke are traumatic injuries as a result of child abuse, as a consequence of roller coaster rides, or in association with musculoskeletal abnormalities such as Klippel-Feil syndrome or tethering of the vertebral artery in the congenital arcuate foramen of the atlas vertebra.

In a large meta-analysis based on MEDLINE and other relevant bibliographic searches (1966 to 2000) of the English-language literature, Fullerton and colleagues at the University of California at San Francisco critically appraised the clinical characteristics of anterior circulation arterial dissections (ACAD) and posterior circulation arterial dissections (PCAD) in patients younger than 18 years. Three-quarters of patients with ACAD and almost 9 in 10 patients with PCAD were male. This marked male preponderance was not explained solely on the basis of trauma. All patients had evidence of cerebral ischemia at the time of diagnosis. Headache was reported in approximately half of patients. Unlike in adults, ACAD in children are most commonly intracranial. Spontaneous ACAD (without preceding trauma) tends to be intracranial, while posttraumatic ACAD is more often extracranial. The vertebral artery at the level of the C1-C2 vertebral bodies was found to be the most common location for PCAD, accounting for roughly half of all cases reported. Overall, neither recurrent cerebral ischemia nor recurrent dissections were frequent occurrences. The former was seen in approximately 15% of PCAD and 5% of ACAD cases, while the latter were encountered in 10% of the ACAD group and in no cases of the PCAD group.

In a subsequent retrospective study conducted by 2 Canadian pediatric ischemic stroke registry centers, arterial dissection was identified as the principal cause of stroke in 16 out of 213 AIS patients (8%). In this cohort, 38% of patients had prior warning symptoms while 50% had an unequivocal history of head or neck trauma. The clinical presentation included, in a descending order of frequency, focal deficits (88%), headache (44%), altered consciousness (25%), and seizures (13%). Extracranial vessel dissection was found in three-quarters of cases, while involvement of the anterior circulation was found in just over a half of the patients. Full neurologic recovery was attained in 43% of the children, whereas the rest of the patients had mild to moderate deficits (44%) or severe deficits (13%). Fourteen out of 16 children (88%) received antithrombotic treatment. Resolution of abnormalities was evidenced in 60% of vessels as determined by follow-up angiography. There was a statistically significant relationship between total occlusion and failure of ultimate recanalization.

Occasionally, patients may present with delayed neurologic symptoms and multiple or multifocal cerebral infarcts secondary to bilateral extracranial traumatic carotid artery dissection.

The use of newer, noninvasive neuroimaging modalities, including MRI, MRA, and dynamic CT, may facilitate early diagnosis of arterial dissection when patients have ill-defined premonitory symptoms or TIAs. The diagnosis of vertebral artery dissection requires MRA or conventional vertebral angiography (Figure 6-6).

Treatment is dependent on the anatomical site of the lesion. Dissections of the extracranial carotid and vertebral arteries are managed generally by anticoagulation or antiplatelet therapy. Data demonstrating superior efficacy of one or the other of these alternatives do not exist, but antiplatelet therapy is much simpler to administer. Surgical reconstruction,

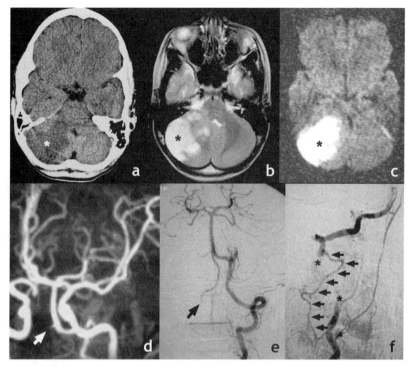

Figure 6-6.

Vertebral artery dissection in an 11-year-old male with altered mental status following wrestling injury. Axial non-contrast computed tomography (Figure 6-6A) demonstrates a low density in the right cerebellar hemisphere consistent with an infarct (white asterisk). Axial non-contrast T2-weighted magnetic resonance imaging (MRI) (Figure 6-6B) demonstrates a hyperintense area in the right cerebellar hemisphere consistent with an infarct (black asterisk). Axial diffusion weighted MRI (Figure 6-6C) demonstrates a hyperintense area in the right cerebellar hemisphere consistent with cytotoxic edema in acute infarction (black asterisk). Time-of-flight magnetic resonance angiography (Figure 6-6D) demonstrates occlusion of the distal right vertebral artery. A small stump is present (white arrowhead). Selective left vertebral angiogram (Figure 6-6E) demonstrates normal left vertebral artery and non-visualization of the right vertebral artery (black arrowhead). Selective right vertebral angiogram (Figure 6-6F) demonstrates the stumps of the occluded right vertebral artery (black asterisks) with collateral circulation (black arrowheads). (Courtesy of Dr Eric N. Faerber, Director of Radiology, St Christopher's Hospital for Children, Philadelphia, PA.)

endovascular stenting, and vessel ligation can be considered in the setting of recurrent embolic stroke or enlargement of an associated pseudoaneurysm, but such measures seem seldom to be necessary among children. Treatment of intracranial dissections is highly individualized and may involve endovascular stenting, extracranial-intracranial bypass grafts, and other arterial reconstructions with or without ligation or trapping of the involved vessel.

Web Sites

Children's Hemiplegia and Stroke Association: www.chasa.org

American Stroke Association: www.strokeassociation.org

National Stroke Association: www.stroke.org

The Brain Attack Coalition: www.stroke-site.org

The National Institute of Health/National Institute of Neurological Disorders and Stroke: www.stroke.ninds.nih.gov

Bibliography

General

Bernard TJ, Goldenberg NA, Armstrong-Wells J, Amlie-Lefond C, Fullerton HJ. Treatment of childhood arterial ischemic stroke. *Ann Neurol.* 2008;63:679–696

Braun KP, Kappelle LJ, Kirkham FJ, DeVeber G. Diagnostic pitfalls in paediatric ischaemic stroke. *Dev Med Child Neurol.* 2006;48:985–990

Braun KP, Rafay MF, Uiterwaal CS, Pontigon AM, DeVeber G. Mode of onset predicts etiological diagnosis of arterial ischemic stroke in children. *Stroke.* 2007;38:298–302

Brobeck BR, Grant PE. Pediatric stroke: the child is not merely a small adult. *Neuroimaging Clin N Am.* 2005;15:589–607, xi

deVeber G. Arterial ischemic strokes in infants and children: an overview of current approaches. *Semin Thromb Hemost.* 2003;29:567–573

deVeber G. In pursuit of evidence-based treatments for paediatric stroke: the UK and chest guidelines. *Lancet Neurol.* 2005;4:432–436

deVeber G. Stroke and the child's brain: an overview of epidemiology, syndromes and risk factors. *Curr Opin Neurol.* 2002;15:133–138

Ganesan V, Prengler M, Wade A, Kirkham FJ. Clinical and radiological recurrence after childhood arterial ischemic stroke. *Circulation.* 2006;114:2170–2177

Jordan LC, Hillis AE. Hemorrhagic stroke in children. *Pediatr Neurol.* 2007;36:73–80

Kirton A, deVeber G. Ischemic stroke complicating pediatric cardiovascular disease. *Nat Clin Pract Cardiovasc Med.* 2007;4:163–166

Lynch JK, Han CJ. Pediatric stroke: what do we know and what do we need to know? *Semin Neurol.* 2005;25:410–423

Lynch JK, Pavlakis S, deVeber G. Treatment and prevention of cerebrovascular disorders in children. *Curr Treat Options Neurol.* 2005;7:469–480

Molofsky WJ. Managing stroke in children. *Pediatr Ann.* 2006;35:379–384

Roach ES. Etiology of stroke in children. *Semin Pediatr Neurol.* 2000;7:244–260

Santos CC, Sarnat HB, Rouch ES. Cerebrovascular disorders. In: Menkes JH, Sarnat HB, Maria BL, eds. *Child Neurology.* Philadelphia, PA: Lippincott Williams & Wilkins; 2006:829–856

Seidman C, Kirkham F, Pavlakis S. Pediatric stroke: current developments. *Curr Opin Pediatr.* 2007;19:657–662

Thorvaldsen P, Asplund K, Kuulasmaa K, Rajakangas AM, Schroll M. Stroke incidence, case fatality, and mortality in the WHO MONICA project. World Health Organization Monitoring Trends and Determinants in Cardiovascular Disease. *Stroke.* 1995;26:361–367

Structural Anomalies of Blood Vessels

Aiba T, Tanaka R, Koike T, Kameyama S, Takeda N, Komata T. Natural history of intracranial cavernous malformations. *J Neurosurg.* 1995;83:56–59

Barker FG II, Amin-Hanjani S, Butler WE, et al. Temporal clustering of hemorrhages from untreated cavernous malformations of the central nervous system. *Neurosurgery.* 2001;49:15–24

Baumgartner JE, Ater JL, Ha CS, et al. Pathologically proven cavernous angiomas of the brain following radiation therapy for pediatric brain tumors. *Pediatr Neurosurg.* 2003;39:201–207

Brown RD Jr, Wiebers DO, Torner JC, O'Fallon WM. Incidence and prevalence of intracranial vascular malformations in Olmsted County, Minnesota, 1965 to 1992. *Neurology.* 1996;46: 949–952

Burger IM, Murphy KJ, Jordan LC, Tamargo RJ, Gailloud P. Safety of cerebral digital subtraction angiography in children: complication rate analysis in 241 consecutive diagnostic angiograms. *Stroke.* 2006;37:2535–2539

Frim DM, Scott RM. Management of cavernous malformations in the pediatric population. *Neurosurg Clin N Am.* 1999;10:513–518

Gault J, Sarin H, Awadallah NA, Shenkar R, Awad IA. Pathobiology of human cerebrovascular malformations: basic mechanisms and clinical relevance. *Neurosurgery.* 2004;55:1–17

Haitjema T, Disch F, Overtoom TT, Westermann CJ, Lammers JW. Screening family members of patients with hereditary hemorrhagic telangiectasia. *Am J Med.* 1995;99:519–524

Kim EJ, Halim AX, Dowd CF, et al. The relationship of coexisting extranidal aneurysms to intracranial hemorrhage in patients harboring brain arteriovenous malformations. *Neurosurgery.* 2004;54:1349–1358

Malek AM, Halbach VV, Dowd CF, Higashida RT. Diagnosis and treatment of dural arteriovenous fistulas. *Neuroimaging Clin N Am.* 1998;8:445–468

Malek AM, Halbach VV, Higashida RT, Phatouros CC, Meyers PM, Dowd CF. Treatment of dural arteriovenous malformations and fistulas. *Neurosurg Clin N Am.* 2000;11:147–166, ix

Ogilvy CS, Stieg PE, Awad I, et al. AHA scientific statement: recommendations for the management of intracranial arteriovenous malformations: a statement for healthcare professionals from a special writing group of the Stroke Council, American Stroke Association. *Stroke.* 2001;32:1458–1471

Porter PJ, Willinsky RA, Harper W, Wallace MC. Cerebral cavernous malformations: natural history and prognosis after clinical deterioration with or without hemorrhage. *J Neurosurg.* 1997;87:190–197

Raaymakers TW, Rinkel GJ, Ramos LM. Initial and follow-up screening for aneurysms in families with familial subarachnoid hemorrhage. *Neurology.* 1998;51:1125–1130

Satomi J, van Dijk JM, Terbrugge KG, Willinsky RA, Wallace MC. Benign cranial dural arteriovenous fistulas: outcome of conservative management based on the natural history of the lesion. *J Neurosurg.* 2002;97:767–770

Willemse RB, Mager JJ, Westermann CJ, Overtoom TT, Mauser H, Wolbers JG. Bleeding risk of cerebrovascular malformations in hereditary hemorrhagic telangiectasia. *J Neurosurg.* 2000;92:779–784

Willinsky RA, Fitzgerald M, TerBrugge K, Montanera W, Wallace M. Delayed angiography in the investigation of intracerebral hematomas caused by small arteriovenous malformations. *Neuroradiology.* 1993;35:307–311

Vasculopathies

Danchaivijitr N, Cox TC, Saunders DE, Ganesan V. Evolution of cerebral arteriopathies in childhood arterial ischemic stroke. *Ann Neurol.* 2006;59:620–626

Fung LW, Thompson D, Ganesan V. Revascularisation surgery for paediatric moyamoya: a review of the literature. *Childs Nerv Syst.* 2005;21:358–364

Ikezaki K. Rational approach to treatment of moyamoya disease in childhood. *J Child Neurol.* 2000;15:350–356

Imaizumi T, Hayashi K, Saito K, Osawa M, Fukuyama Y. Long-term outcomes of pediatric moyamoya disease monitored to adulthood. *Pediatr Neurol.* 1998;18:321–325

Jea A, Smith ER, Robertson R, Scott RM, Research Committee on moyamoya disease in Japan. Moyamoya syndrome associated with Down syndrome: outcome after surgical revascularization. *Pediatrics.* 2005;116:e694–e701

Kuroda S, Hashimoto N, Yoshimoto T, Iwasaki Y. Radiological findings, clinical course, and outcome in asymptomatic moyamoya disease. Results of multicenter survey in Japan. *Stroke.* 2007;38:1430–1435

Rosser TL, Vezina G, Packer RJ. Cerebrovascular abnormalities in a population of children with neurofibromatosis type 1. *Neurology.* 2005;64:553–555

Schievink WI, Link MJ, Piepgras DG, Spetzler RF. Intracranial aneurysm surgery in Ehlers-Danlos syndrome Type IV. *Neurosurgery.* 2002;51:607–611

Scott RM, Smith JL, Robertson RL, Madsen JR, Soriano SG, Rockoff MA. Long-term outcome in children with moyamoya syndrome after cranial revascularization by pial synangiosis. *J Neurosurg Spine.* 2004;100(2 suppl *Pediatrics*):142–149

Uchino K, Johnston SC, Becker KJ, Tirschwell DL. Moyamoya disease in Washington State and California. *Neurology.* 2005;65:956–958

Ullrich NJ, Robertson R, Kinnamon DD, et al. Moyamoya following cranial irradiation for primary brain tumors in children. *Neurology.* 2007;68:932–938

Congenital and Acquired Heart Disease

Ballerini L, Cifarelli A, Ammirati A, Gimigliano F. Patent foramen ovale and cryptogenic stroke. A critical review. *J Cardiovasc Med* (Hagerstown). 2007;8:34–38

Coward K, Tucker N, Darville T. Infective endocarditis in Arkansas children from 1990 through 2002. *Pediatr Infect Dis J.* 2003;22:1048–1052

Kenny D, Turner M, Martin R. When to close a patent foramen ovale. *Arch Dis Child.* 2008;93:255–259

Lewena S. Infective endocarditis: experience of a pediatric emergency department. *J Paediatr Child Health.* 2005;41:269–272

Omeroglu RE, Olgar S, Nisli K, Elmaci T. Recurrent hemiparesis due to anterior mitral leaflet myxomas. *Pediatr Neurol.* 2006;34:490–494

Venkatesan C, Wainwright MS. Pediatric endocarditis and stroke: a single-center retrospective review of seven cases. *Pediatr Neurol.* 2008;38:243–247

Venous Sinus Thrombosis and Thrombophlebitis

Sébire G, Tabarki B, Saunders DE, et al. Cerebral venous sinus thrombosis in children: risk factors, presentation, diagnosis and outcome. *Brain.* 2005;128(pt 3):477–489

Infective, Postinfective, and Immune-Mediated Vascular Diseases (Vasculitis)

Askalan R, Laughlin S, Mayank S, et al. Chickenpox and stroke in childhood: a study of frequency and causation. *Stroke.* 2001;32:1257–1262

Benseler S, Schneider R. Central nervous system vasculitis in children. *Curr Opin Rheumatol.* 2004;16:43–50

Dubrovsky T, Curless R, Scott G, et al. Cerebral aneurysmal arteriopathy in childhood AIDS. *Neurology.* 1998;51:560–565

Frank Y, Lu D, Pavlakis S, Black K, LaRussa P, Hyman RA. Childhood AIDS, varicella zoster, and cerebral vasculopathy. *J Child Neurol.* 1997;12:464–466

Gilden DH, Mahalingam R, Cohrs RJ, Kleinschmidt-DeMasters BK, Forghani B. The protean manifestations of varicella-zoster virus vasculopathy. *J Neurovirol.* 2002;8(suppl 2):75–79

Hoffmann M, Berger JR, Nath A, Rayens M. Cerebrovascular disease in young, HIV-infected, black Africans in the KwaZulu Natal province of South Africa. *J Neurovirol.* 2000;6:229–236

Katsetos CD, Fincke JE, Legido A, et al. Angiocentric CD3(+) T-cell infiltrates in human immunodeficiency virus type 1-associated central nervous system disease in children. *Clin Diagn Lab Immunol.* 1999;6:105–114

Kleinschmidt-DeMasters BK, Gilden DH. Varicella-zoster virus infections of the nervous system: clinical and pathologic correlates. *Arch Pathol Lab Med.* 2001;125:770–780

Mazzoni P, Chiriboga CA, Millar WS, Rogers A. Intracerebral aneurysms in human immunodeficiency virus infection: case report and literature review. *Pediatr Neurol.* 2000;23:252–255

Moriuchi H, Rodriguez W. Role of varicella-zoster virus in stroke syndromes. *Pediatr Infect Dis J.* 2000;19:648–653

Patsalides AD, Wood LV, Atac GK, Sandifer E, Butman JA, Patronas NJ. Cerebrovascular disease in HIV infected pediatric patients: neuroimaging findings. *AJR Am J Roentgenol.* 2002;179:999–1003

Takeoka M, Takahashi T. Infectious and inflammatory disorders of the circulatory system and stroke in childhood. *Curr Opin Neurol.* 2002;15:159–164

Hematologic Diseases: Sickle Cell Disease and Prothrombotic Disorders (Thrombophilias)

Abboud MR, Cure J, Granger S, et al. Magnetic resonance angiography in children with sickle cell disease and abnormal transcranial Doppler ultrasonography findings enrolled in the STOP study. *Blood.* 2004;103:2822–2826

Adams RJ, Brambilla D, Optimizing Primary Stroke Prevention in Sickle Cell Anemia (STOP 2) Trial Investigators. Discontinuing prophylactic transfusions used to prevent stroke in sickle cell disease. *N Engl J Med.* 2005;353:2769–2778

Files B, Brambilla D, Kutlar A, et al. Longitudinal changes in ferritin during chronic transfusion: a report from the Stroke Prevention Trial in Sickle Cell Anemia (STOP). *J Pediatr Hematol Oncol.* 2002;24:284–290

Ganesan V, Prengler M, McShane MA, Wade AM, Kirkham FJ. Investigation of risk factors in children with arterial ischemic stroke. *Ann Neurol.* 2003;53:167–173

Gökben S, Tosun A, Bayram N, et al. Arterial ischemic stroke in childhood: risk factors and outcome in old versus new era. *J Child Neurol.* 2007;22:1204–1208

Grabowski EF, Buonanno FS, Krishnamoorthy K. Prothrombotic risk factors in the evaluation and management of perinatal stroke. *Semin Perinatol.* 2007;31:243–249

Johal SC, Garg BP, Heiny ME, et al. Family history is a poor screen for prothrombotic genes in children with stroke. *J Pediatr.* 2006;148:68–71

Kawanami T, Kurita K, Yamakawa M, Omoto E, Kato T. Cerebrovascular disease in acute leukemia: a clinicopathological study of 14 patients. *Intern Med.* 2002;41:1130–1134

Kirkham FJ. Therapy insight: stroke risk and its management in patients with sickle cell disease. *Nat Clin Pract Neurol.* 2007;3:264–278

Lee MT, Piomelli S, Granger S, et al. Stroke Prevention Trial in Sickle Cell Anemia (STOP): extended follow-up and final results. *Blood.* 2006;108:847–852

Nelson KB. Thrombophilias, perinatal stroke, and cerebral palsy. *Clin Obstet Gynecol.* 2006;49:875–884

Pegelow CH, Wang W, Granger S, et al. Silent infarcts in children with sickle cell anemia and abnormal cerebral artery velocity. *Arch Neurol.* 2001;58:2017–2021

Simma B, Martin G, Müller T, Huemer M. Risk factors for pediatric stroke: consequences for therapy and quality of life. *Pediatr Neurol.* 2007;37:121–126

Skardoutsou A, Voudris KA, Mastroyianni S, Vagiakou E, Magoufis G, Koukoutsakis P. Moyamoya syndrome in a child with pyruvate kinase deficiency and combined prothrombotic factors. *J Child Neurol.* 2007;22:474–478

Wang WC, Morales KH, Scher CD, et al. Effect of long-term transfusion on growth in children with sickle cell anemia: results of the STOP trial. *J Pediatr.* 2005;147:244–247

Wu YW, Lynch JK, Nelson KB. Perinatal arterial stroke: understanding mechanisms and outcomes. *Semin Neurol.* 2005;25:424–434

Zafeiriou DI, Prengler M, Gombakis N, et al. Central nervous system abnormalities in asymptomatic young patients with S beta-thalassemia. *Ann Neurol.* 2004;55:835–839

Cerebrovascular Disease and Metabolic Disorders

Akar N, Akar E, Ozel D, Deda G, Sipahi T. Common mutations at the homocysteine metabolism pathway and pediatric stroke. *Thromb Res.* 2001;102:115–120

Chou HF, Liang WC, Zhang Q, Goto Y, Jong YJ. Clinical and genetic features in a MELAS child with a 3271T>C mutation. *Pediatr Neurol.* 2008;38:143–146

Clarke JT. Narrative review: Fabry disease. *Ann Intern Med.* 2007;146:425–433

Edge JA, Hawkins MM, Winter DL, Dunger DB. The risk and outcome of cerebral oedema developing during diabetic ketoacidosis. *Arch Dis Child.* 2001;85:16–22

Hanas R, Lindgren F, Lindblad B. Diabetic ketoacidosis and cerebral oedema in Sweden—a 2-year paediatric population study. *Diabet Med.* 2007;24:1080–1085

Kelly PJ, Furie KL, Kistler JP, et al. Stroke in young patients with hyperhomocysteinemia due to cystathionine beta-synthase deficiency. *Neurology.* 2003;60:275–279

Noguchi A, Shoji Y, Matsumori M, Komatsu K, Takada G Stroke-like episode involving a cerebral artery in a patient with MELAS. *Pediatr Neurol.* 2005;33:70–71

Silliman S. Mendelian and mitochondrial disorders associated with stroke. *J Stroke Cerebrovasc Dis.* 2002;11:252–264

Arterial Dissection and Stroke in Children

Bacigaluppi S, Rusconi R, Rampini P, et al. Vertebral artery dissection in a child. Is "spontaneous" still an appropriate definition? *Neurol Sci.* 2006;27:364–368

Bernard TJ, deVeber GA, Benke TA. Athletic participation after acute ischemic childhood stroke: a survey of pediatric stroke experts. *J Child Neurol.* 2007;22:1050–1053

Carvalho KS, Edwards-Brown M, Golomb MR. Carotid dissection and stroke after tonsillectomy and adenoidectomy. *Pediatr Neurol.* 2007;37:127–129

Chamoun RB, Mawad ME, Whitehead WE, Luerssen TG, Jea A. Extracranial traumatic carotid artery dissections in children: a review of current diagnosis and treatment options. *J Neurosurg Pediatrics.* 2008;2:101–108

Cushing KE, Ramesh V, Gardner-Medwin D, et al. Tethering of the vertebral artery in the congenital arcuate foramen of the atlas vertebra: a possible cause of vertebral artery dissection in children. *Dev Med Child Neurol.* 2001;43:491–496

Fullerton HJ, Johnston SC, Smith WS. Arterial dissection and stroke in children. *Neurology.* 2001;57:1155–1160

Ganesan V, Chong WK, Cox TC, Chawda SJ, Prengler M, Kirkham FJ. Posterior circulation stroke in childhood: risk factors and recurrence. *Neurology.* 2002;59:1552–1556

Hasan I, Wapnick S, Kutscher ML, Couldwell WT. Vertebral arterial dissection associated with Klippel-Feil syndrome in a child. *Childs Nerv Syst.* 2002;18:67–70

Lee YH, Chen CL, Pan SC. Acute stroke in the burn patient. *J Burn Care Res.* 2007;28:351–354

Lin JJ, Chou ML, Lin KL, Wong MC, Wang HS. Cerebral infarct secondary to traumatic carotid artery dissection. *Pediatr Emerg Care.* 2007;23:166–168

Lotze TE, Paolicchi J. Vertebral artery dissection and migraine headaches in children. *J Child Neurol.* 2000;15:694–696

Rafay MF, Armstrong D, Deveber G, Domi T, Chan A, MacGregor DL. Craniocervical arterial dissection in children: clinical and radiographic presentation and outcome. *J Child Neurol.* 2006;21:8–16

Chapter 7

Neurocutaneous Disorders

H. Huntley Hardison, MD
Ignacio Valencia, MD
Agustín Legido, MD, PhD, MBA

Introduction

Neurocutaneous disorders or phakomatoses are a group of conditions that affect both the nervous system and the skin. Van der Hoeve first coined the term in 1932 because of the lens-like retinal tumors (phakomata) seen in several of these disorders. Others, citing the Greek root *phakos,* meaning "mother spot" or birthmark, apply the term to disorders of abnormal tissue growth or tumor formation

Embryologically, both the skin and the nervous system are derived from the ectoderm. The phakomatoses give rise to malformations and abnormal growth in the form of tumors in the nervous system and abnormalities of the skin and its appendages. However, cutaneous features are not present in all phakomatoses (ie, von Hippel-Lindau syndrome), and may include others outside the skin and nervous system, so the term can be misleading. Box 7-1 lists disorders associated with specific cutaneous findings.

Neurofibromatosis Type 1

Epidemiology and Genetics

Neurofibromatosis type 1 (NF1) is the most common of the neurocutaneous disorders occurring in 1 per 2,500 to 3,000 persons. The prevalence is similar in both genders and all ethnic groups.

The disease is linked to a defect in the gene *NF1,* which is located on the long arm of chromosome 17 in the region q11.2. The gene encodes the protein neurofibromin, which undergoes post-translational modification (farnesylation or attachment of an isoprenoid to the C-terminal cysteine residue) in the cytoplasm, and then it attaches to the inner cell membrane. The functions of neurofibromin are to suppress tumor growth and regulate

---

Box 7-1. Neurocutaneous Disorders: Specific Cutaneous Abnormalities and Associated Disorders[a]

Hyperpigmented Lesions

Neurofibromatosis

Epidermal nevus syndrome

Neurocutaneous melanosis

Incontinentia pigmenti

Hypopigmented Lesions

Tuberous sclerosis complex

Incontinentia pigmenti achromians

Hypomelanosis of Ito

Vascular Lesions

Sturge-Weber syndrome

Ataxia-telangiectasia

Maffuci syndrome

Osler-Weber-Rendu syndrome

Hemiatrophy/Hemihypertrophy

Klippel-Trénaunay-Weber syndrome

Retinal Involvement

Von Hippel-Lindau disease

Wyburn-Mason syndrome

---

[a]*Modified from Thiele EA, Korf BR. Phakomatoses and allied conditions. In: Swaiman KF, Ashwal S, Ferriero DM, eds. Pediatric Neurology. Principles & Practice. Philadelphia, PA: Mosby Elsevier; 2006:771, with permission from Elsevier.*

---

ras-mediated cell proliferation; its N-terminus is associated with microtubule assembly.

Neurofibromatosis type 1 may be inherited as an autosomal dominant trait. However, half of affected persons have the disease due to spontaneous mutations; and there is variable penetrance among persons with the defective gene. Offspring of patients with NF1 have a 50% risk of inheriting the disease.

Clinical Characteristics

Neurofibromatosis type 1 may present with a variety of clinical manifestations, including disorders of the
skin, bone, and nervous system. The
most common skin finding is an oval-
shaped area of homogeneous hyperpigmentation, which usually has a
smooth border. The areas of increased
pigment have the color of coffee with
milk. Hence, they are called café-au-
lait spots (CALS; Figure 7-1).

Neurofibromatosis type 1 usually
presents with multiple CALS. Occasionally, however, it may manifest
as bone dysplasia or nervous system
tumor. Bone dysplasias include bowing of the long bones and pseudo-

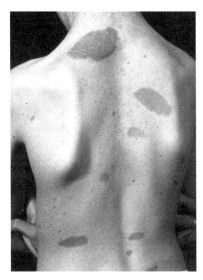

Figure 7-1.
Café au-lait-spots of neurofibromatosis
type 1.

arthrosis, either in infancy or later in life. Nervous system tumors that are
common in children with NF1 include glioma of the optic pathway, which
may cause optic disc pallor or visual difficulty, and neurofibroma of spinal
roots, which may present with focal weakness or pain.

Physical Examination

It is important to think about NF1 whenever the examination shows any of
its clinical manifestations. The purpose of the examination is to confirm the
diagnosis of NF1 and to monitor the child for signs of progressive disease.
On the other hand, a few CALS may be seen in otherwise normal children.

In addition to CALS, other skin manifestations of NF1 include freckles
and neurofibromas. Freckles are small pigmented macules, and in NF1 they
tend to occur in areas of skin folds (axilla, groin). Hypopigmented macules
may also be seen. Juvenile xanthogranulomas are orange-colored papules
that appear transiently on the head and trunk. There is an increased risk of
chronic myeloid leukemia in children with NF1 and xanthogranulomas.

Lisch nodules are asymptomatic pigmented iris hamartomas that are pathognomonic for NF1. Rarely, children with NF1 have retinal hamartomas, which usually also remain asymptomatic.

Neurofibromas are benign peripheral nerve sheath tumors, which can be cutaneous, subcutaneous, and plexiform. Cutaneous neurofibromas are pedunculated skin tumors, which may catch on clothing or cause transient itching. Subcutaneous neurofibromas are recognized by palpation, and they may be either tender or cause tingling in the distribution of the affected peripheral nerve. Plexiform neurofibromas consist of a mixture of defective Schwann cells and other supporting cells that grow around nerve fibers and along peripheral nerves. The overlying skin may have a large area of irregular hyperpigmentation. Subcutaneous and plexiform neurofibromas may evolve into malignant peripheral nerve sheath tumors, which are difficult to detect and metastasize widely. Signs of malignant transformation of a neurofibroma include the following: persistent pain that either lasts for longer than 1 month or disturbs sleep, new or unexplained neurologic deficit or sphincter disturbance, alteration in the texture from soft to hard, and rapid increase in size.

Bone abnormalities may be present at birth or they may develop later in patients with NF1. Bowing of the long bones may be associated with fracture, and there can be delayed healing with formation of a false joint (pseudoarthrosis). Scoliosis usually affects the lower cervical and upper thoracic spine. It can involve as many as 6 segments, causing rapidly progressive distortion of the vertebral bodies and the ribs.

Dysplasia of the renal or carotid arteries occurs in a few patients with NF1. Hypertension in patients with NF1 may be due to renal artery stenosis or to pheochromocytoma in adults. Cerebral artery dysplasia may cause moyamoya disease and stroke.

Cognitive problems are, however, the most common neurologic complication of NF1. It has been estimated that more than 50% of patients with NF1 have neurobehavioral impairments, such as attention-deficit/hyperactivity disorder, visual/spatial learning disabilities, pervasive developmental disorder, and other cognitive developmental problems. Several mechanisms by which NF1 gene mutations cause these cognitive problems have been suggested, including excessive Ras signaling, increased γ-aminobutyric acid–mediated inhibition, and interaction of neurofibromin through filamin proteins with a dopamine receptor (Drd3). This information may provide new ideas about the pathogenesis of cognitive defects in NF1 and may facilitate the development of novel targeted therapeutic interventions.

Psychiatric dysfunction is noted in one-third of patients, with dysthymia most prevalent. There is an increased rate of depression, anxiety, and personality disorders. The cosmetic and medical aspects of this disease have a significant impact in the patients' quality of life.

Developmental assessment and follow-up are important to recognize early signs of learning disability and behavior problems. Repeated neurologic evaluation is also important for the recognition of progressive disease. Screening for symptoms of psychiatric conditions is also warranted.

The pediatrician should look for acute or progressive sensory deficit, motor deficit, incoordination, or sphincter dysfunction that may indicate intracranial or spinal lesions. Increased intracranial pressure is an emergency that may be associated with headache on waking, morning vomiting, and altered consciousness. Pulsating exophthalmos is due to herniation of the temporal lobe through a defect in the wing of the sphenoid bone. Scoliosis may deform the spine and be associated with cord compression and respiratory compromise.

Diagnosis

The National Institutes of Health (NIH) Consensus Development Conference formulated diagnostic criteria for NF1. The diagnosis of NF1 is a clinical decision, and the diagnostic criteria are sensitive enough to recognize children who are at risk for progressive disease and specific enough to recognize children who may be otherwise normal (Box 7-2).

The differential diagnoses of NF1 include other forms of neurofibromatosis, conditions with café-au-lait patches, or with pigment changes confused with café-au-lait patches. Also, tumors or localized body overgrowth can be mistaken for neurofibromas.

Children with mosaic NF1 may fulfill the criteria because they have 6 or more CALS and either skin-fold freckling or neurofibromas. However, the skin manifestations are limited to one segment of the body. The risk for progressive disease and having an affected child is low because this condition is caused by a somatic mutation of gene *NF1*. Children with multiple

Box 7-2. Diagnostic Criteria for Neurofibromatosis Type 1 (NF1)[a]

Two or more of the following:

Six or more cutaneous macules (café-au-lait spots) that are in diameter
>0.5 cm in children
>1.5 cm in adults

Neurofibromas
Two or more cutaneous or subcutaneous neurofibromas
One plexiform neurofibroma

Axillary or inguinal freckling

Optic pathway glioma

Two or more Lisch nodules (iris hamartomas)

Bony dysplasia, including
Sphenoid wing dysplasia
Bowing of the long bones with or without pseudoarthrosis

First degree relative with NF1

[a]*From Neurofibromatosis.* Natl Inst Health Consensus Dev Conf Consens Statement. *1987;6(12):1–17.*

CALS with no other criteria and no family history of the disease should be followed as if they have NF1, because 95% may develop NF1. Watson syndrome is the combination of pulmonary stenosis, cognitive impairment, and CALS. There are few, if any, cutaneous neurofibromas. Other forms of neurofibromatosis include neurofibromatosis 2 and schwannomatosis.

McCune-Albright syndrome is associated with CALS, but affected children have delayed sexual maturation and large, irregular areas of increased pigment that tend not to cross the midline. Conditions that are confused with NF1 because of pigmented cutaneous macules include LEOPARD (lentigines [multiple], electrocardiographic conduction abnormalities, ocular hypertelorism, pulmonary stenosis, abnormalities of genitalia, retardation of growth, deafness) syndrome, neurocutaneous melanosis, Peutz-Jeghers syndrome, and piebaldism (congenital poliosis and leukoderma). Localized overgrowth syndromes include Klippel-Trénaunay-Weber syndrome and Proteus syndrome. Conditions causing tumors that are confused with NF1 include lipomatosis, Bannayan-Riley-Ruvalcaba syndrome, fibromatoses, and multiple endocrine neoplasia type 2B.

The defective gene responsible for NF1 was identified more than 25 years ago. Since that time, the rate of positive molecular genetic testing among children who meet the NIH consensus criteria for NF1 has risen from under 20% to 95% using a combination of molecular techniques. The cost is expensive, and it may take several weeks for results to be available. Genetic testing is not necessary unless the results are helpful in managing the child with signs of NF1.

Magnetic resonance imaging (MRI) of the brain or spine is indicated if there are signs of increased intracranial pressure or neurologic deficit. Follow-up of optic gliomas also requires MRI. A significant percentage of patients with NF1 have one or more increased signal lesions on T2-weighted images in the basal ganglia, thalamus, brain stem, and cerebellum. The significance of these findings is unclear.

Treatment

The patient with NF1 should be followed in a multidisciplinary neurofibromatosis clinic or a specialist with experience in the evaluation and management of the disease. The role of the clinic is to diagnose difficult cases, manage and monitor complex disease, and educate and support the patient and family. At the present time, treatment options are symptomatic.

Clinical trials have shown mixed results for agents such as thalidomide and pirfenidone, an antifibrotic agent, in patients with plexiform neurofibromas. If the patient is concerned about the cosmetic effect of CALS, one may recommend sunscreen and skin moisturizers. If a neurofibroma is disfiguring or causes loss of function, the patient should be referred to a surgeon who is experienced in the removal of this type of tumor. Chemotherapy of orbital optic nerve gliomas is reserved for the older child who experiences loss of vision. If surgical removal of a malignant peripheral nerve sheath tumor is incomplete, the patient may benefit from radiation or chemotherapy. Bone disorders may present a difficult situation for the orthopedic surgeon because of impaired healing.

Natural History and Prognosis

Forty-one children with multiple CALS were followed in the neurofibromatosis clinic at Children's Hospital in Boston, where each child underwent annual physical and ophthalmologic examinations. Twenty-four (58%) were diagnosed with NF1 following the appearance of skin-fold freckling (16), Lisch nodules (4), neurofibromas (2), or the combination of skin-fold freckling and either Lisch nodule or neurofibromas (2). Nine children (22%) were diagnosed with segmental neurofibromatosis (6), Bannayan-Riley-Ruvalcaba syndrome (1), multiple lentigines syndrome (1), and polyostotic fibrous dysplasia (1). A diagnosis was not established in 8 (19%) children, but 5 of them were seen only 2 times 1 year apart. The diagnosis was usually established within 3 years of initial evaluation and by 5 years of age.

The clinical outcome of NF1 is variable. Tumors of the spine or optic nerves are most likely to have an adverse effect on the patient's quality of life. The risk of malignant peripheral nerve sheath tumors is about 10%, and the tumors tend to occur among young adults.

In summary, the diagnostic outcome among children with multiple CALS is that three-fifths develop diagnostic signs of NF1, one-fifth have segmental neurofibromatosis or other neurocutaneous disorders, and one-fifth have no definitive diagnosis. Not establishing a diagnosis may be related to shortened time of follow-up. Annual physical examinations and appropriate specialist consultations help in establishing the diagnosis, early detection of complications, and management of progressive disease. Genetic counseling is important for patients and their families. Molecular testing and imaging studies are indicated if they may help in making management decisions.

Neurofibromatosis Type 2

Epidemiology and Genetics

Neurofibromatosis type 2 (NF2) is an autosomal dominant neurocutaneous disorder that is clinically and genetically distinct from NF1 and occurs in approximately 1 in 25,000 to 50,000 individuals.

Neurofibromatosis type 2 is caused by inactivating mutations on chromosome 22q11.2. The NF2 protein product, known as *merlin* or *schwannomin,* also suppresses tumor formation, and its dysfunction accounts for the common occurrence of central nervous system (CNS) tumors, typically bilateral vestibuloacoustic nerve schwannomas (so-called acoustic neuromas), although other types of tumors may develop, such as meningiomas, gliomas, and ependymomas.

Clinical Characteristics

The most common presentation is bilateral hearing loss. There are other symptoms associated with compression of other structures in the cerebello-pontine angle by the acoustic neuroma. Therefore, patients can also present with symptoms of facial palsy, ataxia, or compression of the trigeminal nerve with altered sensation in the face. Spinal cord compression may be another presenting symptom if there are spinal cord tumors. In patients with other types of tumors, the associated clinical symptoms and signs may be present.

Neurofibromatosis type 2–associated skin tumors can overlap in appearance with those in NF1, including NF2 plaques (discreet, slightly raised, well-circumscribed patches of roughened skin that are usually <2 cm in diameter and may be hyperpigmented and/or hairy), nodular schwannomas (mobile, subcutaneous, well-circumscribed lesions that have similar appearance to NF1 lesions but are schwannomas rather than neurofibromas by pathology), and dermal neurofibromas (intradermal papillary violoceous skin tumors similar to those in NF1 but occurring in far fewer numbers).

Physical Examination

A thorough examination of the cranial nerves and cerebellum should be performed. Most commonly, patients will show bilateral hearing loss that can be detected with a tuning fork. Skin needs to be carefully examined for typical lesions.

Diagnosis

The presence of bilateral acoustic neuromas is diagnostic of NF2. Other patients can be diagnosed with NF2 if they have a first-degree relative with NF2 and a unilateral acoustic neuroma, or 2 other of the common findings (meningioma, glioma, schwannoma, or juvenile cortical cataract) (Box 7-3).

The differential diagnosis should include other causes of hearing loss, such as Meniere disease, acoustic trauma, vascular malformations of the posterior fossa, and rare genetic causes.

Magnetic resonance imaging with gadolinium is the diagnostic test of choice, which typically will show bilateral enhancing lesions in the cerebello-pontine angles. Acoustic neuromas usually arise from the internal auditory canal extending into the cerebello-pontine angle. They typically

Box 7-3. Diagnostic Criteria for Neurofibromatosis Type 2 (NF2)[a]

Confirmed NF2
Bilateral vestibular schwannomas

OR

In a first-degree relative: NF2 and unilateral vestibular schwannoma

Before age 30 years or any 2 of the following: meningioma, schwannoma, gliomas, juvenile lens opacity

Presumptive NF2
Unilateral vestibular schwannoma before age 30 years and at least

One of the following: meningioma, schwannoma, gliomas, juvenile lens opacity

OR

Two or more meningiomas and unilateral vestibular schwannoma

Before age 30 years or at least one of the following: meningioma, schwannoma, gliomas, juvenile lens opacity

[a]*From Gutmann DH, Aylsworth A, Carey JC, et al. The diagnostic evaluation and multidisciplinary management of neurofibromatosis 1 and neurofibromatosis 2. JAMA. 1997;278:51–57. Reprinted with permission from the American Medical Association.*

are isointense or hypointense on T1-weighted images and hyperintense on T2-weighted images. There is usually enhancement with contrast.

Magnetic resonance imaging of the brain should be ordered at the onset of the complaint of bilateral hearing loss, or if there are any signs of compression in the cerebello-pontine angle or posterior fossa. In other instances, the MRI is performed in asymptomatic children with positive family history as a screening tool.

The evaluation of brain stem auditory evoked potentials is another available test, but they are less sensitive and specific.

Referral to clinical genetics and neurosurgery should be performed at the time of diagnosis or suspicion of NF2. The frequency of follow-up will be determined by the activity of the disease.

Treatment

Treatment options for patients with bilateral acoustic neuromas include observation, surgery, stereotactic radiosurgery, stereotactic radiotherapy, and proton beam therapy.

Natural History and Prognosis

The evolution of NF2 varies from patient to patient. Most individuals experience first symptoms between the second and third decades of life. Because tumors grow slowly, delayed diagnosis is common. Other brain tumors can increase the morbidity in this group of patients.

Tuberous Sclerosis Complex

Epidemiology and Genetics

Tuberous sclerosis complex (TSC) is an autosomal dominant neurocutaneous disorder with a variable prevalence from 1 per 25,000 persons in Northern Ireland to 1 per 3,000 in Hong Kong.

Tuberous sclerosis complex is caused by mutations in 1 of 2 genes: *TSC1*, which is located in chromosome region 9q34.1 and encodes the protein hamartin, or *TSC2*, which is located in chromosome region 16p13.3 and encodes the protein tuberin. In normal cells, hamartin and tuberin form heterodimers that participate in the mammalian target of rapamycin signaling pathway, inhibiting cell growth and proliferation. Abnormalities in this interaction between hamartin and tuberin explain the similarities of clinical features among patients with mutations in either *TSC1* or *TSC2*. Mutations can be identified in 96% of patients with TSC, 26% of them are in *TSC1*, and 74% in *TSC2*. Mutations of *TSC2* are associated with more severe forms of the disease.

Clinical Characteristics

The most common presenting symptoms of infants and children with TSC are neurologic or cutaneous manifestations.

Epilepsy is the most common neurologic manifestation and occurs in 93% of children with TSC. The types of seizures include infantile spasms, focal, multifocal, and generalized, and may be difficult to control. However, in our experience, most children with TSC can achieve good seizure control; the sleep electroencephalogram (EEG) is helpful in predicting eventual seizure control. Neuropathological correlation of seizures are cortical hamartomas (tubers), heterotopic gray matter, subependymal nodules, and subependymal giant cell astrocytomas (SEGAs). The mechanism of epileptogenesis in TSC is unclear. In our laboratory, we have demonstrated that immunohistochemical analysis of surgically excised cortical tubers from children with TSC showed an absence of calcium-binding proteins in giant or ballooned cells, indicating the presence of dysfunctional circuits that are poorly protected from excitatory injury. The activation of inflammatory pathways in cortical tubers and SEGAs may be the consequence of the epilepsy or may play a pathogenic in its pathogenesis.

A common neurologic manifestation of TSC is cognitive impairment. The prevalence of mental retardation in TSC is estimated to be between 44% and 60%, and seems to be related to having seizures in infancy. Learning disabilities, attention-deficit disorder or attention-deficit/hyperactivity disorder (ADHD), behavioral difficulties, and autistic spectrum disorders are also frequently seen in patients with TSC and represent the area of greatest concern to parents and caregivers. The evolving neurocognitive literature suggests that frontal brain systems might be most consistently disrupted by TSC-related neuropathology, thus leading to abnormalities in regulatory and goal-directed behaviors.

The earliest cutaneous finding is a rounded spot of hypopigmentation that resembles the shape of a leaf from a mountain ash tree; hence it has been called an *ash leaf spot.* Now called *hypomelanotic macules,* the spots are found on the trunk or the extremities in 80% of patients (Figure 7-2). When illuminated in a dark room using a Wood light, visualization of hypomelanotic macules is enhanced because they reflect more ultraviolet light than the surrounding skin.

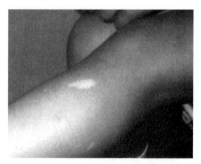

Figure 7-2.
Hypomelanotic macule (ash leaf spot) of tuberous sclerosis complex.

After early infancy and into adulthood, 70% of patients with TSC develop facial angiofibromas, which are small, firm nodules located on the face. They resemble acne but have a different distribution and tend to become more prominent with age. Periungual fibromas appear in 25% of adolescents and adults with TSC. They are firm nodules located around the fingernails.

Shagreen patches resemble the underside of untanned leather and are located on the trunk. They increase in prevalence from 20% of children with TSC to 80% of adults with the disease.

During infancy and childhood ophthalmologic examination may show retinal astrocytomas (mulberry lesions), hamartomas, or retinal achromatic patches.

Cardiac rhabdomyomas occur in about two-thirds of patients with TSC. They form during embryogenesis; therefore, they may be seen on imaging studies in utero or during early infancy. The cardiac tumors tend to regress with age, but they can grow or appear during puberty. They most frequently present during the neonatal period with unexplained heart failure; they may also cause cardiac arrhythmias or be asymptomatic.

Renal angiomyolipomas, typically multiple and bilateral, occur in about three-fourths of patients with TSC. Pulmonary lymphangiomyomatosis occurs in 1% to 2% of patients with TSC, and may manifest as spontaneous pneumothorax, dyspnea, cough, or hemoptysis.

Physical Examination

Physical examination should be directed to the demonstration of the physical findings described previously. As indicated before, the use of Wood light may be necessary. The skin and the nails should be examined carefully. Auscultation of the heart should be performed to rule out the presence of murmurs. Ophthalmologic evaluation should be detailed and, if necessary, consultation to an ophthalmologist should be requested.

Diagnosis

The diagnostic criteria for TSC were defined in a consensus conference, and they are listed in Box 7-4. A thorough evaluation, as indicated previously, should be performed to consider the major and minor features of the disease and to monitor for long-term complications. Computed tomography (CT) scan or MRI of the brain should be performed whenever the diagnosis is suspected. The neuroradiologic hallmark of TSC is the calcified subependymal nodule, best seen on CT (Figure 7-3). Cerebral malformations are best visualized with T2-weighted and fluid attenuated inversion recovery MRI images.

Box 7-4. Diagnostic Criteria for Tuberous Sclerosis Complex[a]

Definite Diagnosis
Two major features

OR

One major feature and 2 minor features

Probable Diagnosis
One major feature and one minor feature

Possible Diagnosis
One major feature

OR

Two minor features

Major Features	Minor Features
Facial angiofibroma	Multiple pits in dental enamel
Ungual fibroma	Hamartomatous rectal polyps
Shagreen patch	Bone cysts
Hypomelanotic macule	Cerebral white matter radial migration lines
Cortical tuber	Gingival fibromas
Subependymal nodule	Retinal achromatic patch
Subependymal giant cell tumor	"Confetti" skin lesions (groups of small,
Retinal hamartoma	lightly pigmented spots)
Cardiac rhabdomyoma	Multiple renal cysts
Renal angiomyolipoma	
Lymphangiomatosis	

[a]From Roach ES, Smith M, Huttenlocher P, Bhat M, Alcorn D, Hawley L. Diagnostic criteria: tuberous sclerosis complex. Report of the Diagnostic Criteria Committee of the National Tuberous Sclerosis Association. J Child Neurol. 1992;7: 221–224. Reprinted by permission of Sage Publications.

Serial ultrasound images of the heart help monitor the progress of cardiac rhabdomyomas. Ultrasound images of the kidneys detect renal hamartomas, angiomyolipomas, or cysts. They are useful in the evaluation of asymptomatic parents of children with TSC for manifestations of the disease to determine whether the patient has either inherited disease or a spontaneous mutation. Patients with TSC should undergo serial ultrasound images of the kidneys at least every 5 years to monitor for the development of renal abnormalities. If the patient has renal lesions, imaging studies should be done more frequently to monitor for progressive renal disease or development of polycystic kidney disease or renal cell carcinoma.

Chest CT scan may be needed in patients with symptoms or signs suggestive of lymphangiomyomatosis.

Tuberous sclerosis complex affects multiple organ systems, and it should be considered in the differential diagnosis of children with epilepsy (especially infantile spasms), developmental delay, and autism. Although many of the cutaneous manifestations of TSC are relatively unique to the disease, the diagnosis is confirmed by the coexistence of other findings suggestive of TSC. For example, an otherwise normal infant with one

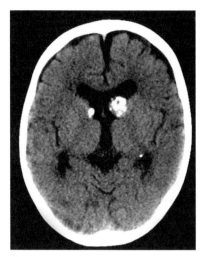

Figure 7-3.
Head computed tomography scan showing periventricular calcifications in tuberous sclerosis complex. (Courtesy of Dr Eric N. Faerber, Chief Department of Radiology, St Christopher's Hospital for Children, Philadelphia, PA.)

hypomelanotic macule may have a transient aberration of cutaneous pigmentation and not develop other manifestations of TSC.

Testing for *TSC1* and *TSC2* mutations has been available since 2002. Confirmatory testing for TSC is helpful in individuals who fail to meet the criteria for definite TSC and to improve genetic counseling. Also, confirmatory testing in an individual who already fulfills the diagnostic criteria for definite disease can help identify a mutation that can be sought in other family members. Prenatal genetic testing for TSC is possible when there is a defined mutation in a specific family.

Treatment

Treatment of children with TSC includes the management of epilepsy, intracranial hypertension, and learning disabilities. The choice of anticonvulsant medication depends on the type of epilepsy. Patients with medically refractory epilepsy may benefit from epilepsy surgery. Subependymal giant cell astrocytomas may obstruct the drainage of the lateral ventricles and cause hydrocephalus. These tumors can be excised.

Hydrocephalus may require shunt treatment. The manifestations of learning disability in children with TSC are variable; therefore, the child's education program should be individualized to address the needs of the patient in the least restrictive environment.

Cardiac rhabdomyomas may need surgical treatment. Renal angiomyolipomas have abnormal blood vessels that may cause acute life-threatening hemorrhage, especially if the diameter is greater than 3 cm. These large lesions may be treated successfully with embolization.

Natural History and Prognosis

The natural course of TSC varies from mild to severe, regardless of the severity of its presentation. Children with infantile spasms and difficult to control epilepsy are more likely to have intellectual problems. Life-threatening complications include respiratory failure due to pulmonary lymphangiomatosis, hemorrhage from renal angiomyolipoma, increased intracranial pressure from acute hydrocephalus, and malignant spread of renal cell carcinoma.

Sturge-Weber syndrome

Sturge-Weber syndrome (SWS) is a phakomatosis that affects the face and the pial-arachnoid surface of the brain. On the face, the hallmark of the disease is the port-wine stain (facial angioma or nevus flammeus) (Figure 7-4). Sturge-Weber syndrome also produces growing angiomas in the pia-arachnoid (leptomeningeal angiomatosis), leading to chronic brain ischemia with calcifications and progressive brain hemiatrophy.

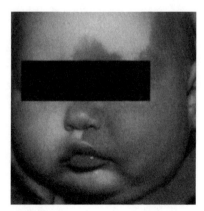

The typical angioma of SWS may result from the failure of the primitive cephalic venous plexus to regress and properly mature in the first trimester of development. The mechanisms underlying the pathobiology of these vascular lesions are unknown, but recent research findings has provided some possible explanations. Thus it

Figure 7-4.
Facial angioma (port-wine stain or nevus flammeus) in Sturge-Weber syndrome.

has been found that fibronectin expression is decreased in SWS meningeal vessels and increased in the parenchymal vessels. Fibronectin is a protein that has potent effects on angiogenesis, vessel remodeling, and vessel innervation density. Its altered expression could contribute to abnormal vascular structure and function in this disorder. It has also been suggested that the chronic hypoxia-ischemia induced by the SWS vascular lesions could activate key angiogenic factors. Recent studies have demonstrated that hypoxia-inducible factor-1 alpha (HIF1-alpha) and HIF2-alpha, which induce the angiogenic vascular endothelial growth factor and neuropilin, are elevated in SWS vessels, whereas the endothelial cell (EC) turnover is also enhanced, as evidenced by increased EC proliferation and apoptosis. Endothelial cell–specific HIF activation provides a setting that supports and sustains angiogenesis. A better understanding of these mechanisms could potentially help to develop therapeutic strategies to treat the so far incurable SWS vascular lesions.

Epidemiology and Genetics

Sturge-Weber syndrome occurs almost entirely sporadically and with equal frequency in the sexes. The incidence of port-wine stain is about 3 in 1,000 newborns, with 25% of them having SWS when the stain involves the first branch of the trigeminal nerve.

A variety of chromosomal abnormalities has been reported in association with SWS; however, somatic mutations have recently been cited as the probable cause of SWS. A report of one monozygotic twin with typical bilateral SWS reinforces the concept that if it has a genetic basis, it is likely to be a somatic mutation. Chromosomal abnormalities have also been found in fibroblast cultures derived from affected regions in 2 patients with SWS (dilated leptomeningeal blood vessels in one case and port-wine–derived skin tissue in another). These findings also suggest the presence of a somatic mutation in selected patients with SWS or chromosomal instability in the affected tissue.

Clinical Characteristics

The most common presenting symptom is a port-wine stain noted over the first division of the trigeminal nerve in the newborn period. This angioma may be difficult to detect in infants with darker skin. The risk of SWS is

higher with more extensive unilateral angioma involving the other trigeminal divisions or with bilateral trigeminal involvement. Some patients with
SWS will have associated vascular malformations in other body regions that
may be accompanied by overgrowth.

Ophthalmologic findings include glaucoma, which can occur in up to
70% of patients at any age. The risk of developing glaucoma is highest in the
first decade, but young adults occasionally develop glaucoma as well. Congenital glaucoma can present as buphthalmos and amblyopia at birth, due to
an anomalous chamber angle. Almost all patients with unilateral or bilateral
upper eyelid angioma present ipsilateral, unilateral, or bilateral choroid-
retinal angiomas. Other ophthalmologic complications include retinal
detachment, strabismus, hemianopsia, or cortical blindness.

The typical neurologic involvement is the leptomeningeal angiomatosis,
which usually occurs ipsilateral to the facial angioma in the occipitopari-
etal region. Sometimes it may be bilateral (20%). There is no relationship
between the size of the facial angioma and the severity of intracranial lesion.
It is hypothesized that impaired venous drainage in SWS interacting with
the overlying angioma produces thrombosis and stasis, resulting in hypoxia-
ischemia of the underlying cerebral tissue. This is responsible for the development of cortical atrophy, sclerosis, and calcification.

The most frequent correlate of the neuropathological lesions of SWS is
seizures, present in 55% to 90% of patients, more frequently manifesting
in the first 2 years of life, although they can present in adulthood. Epilepsy
is usually partial, or partial with secondary generalization; however, some
children may develop infantile spasms. The occurrence of seizures in the
setting of impaired perfusion may play a significant role in the brain injury
in SWS. A prolonged period of weakness on the contralateral side lasting
days or even weeks can follow a prolonged seizure. When the seizures are
recurrent and severe, developmental delay, permanent hemiparesis, and
cognitive deficits are frequent. Hemiparesis may also be the manifestation
of chronic hypoxia per se or acute stroke. The degree of cognitive impairment varies and ranges from normal to severe mental retardation; the
severity of intracranial lesion and epilepsy is directly related to the severity
of cognitive deficit.

Behavioral and emotional problems are also present in a significant percentage of patients, even in those who do not have epilepsy. About 20% of SWS patients have ADHD and 40% to 60% develop migraine headaches.

Physical Examination

The facial angioma must be defined carefully, and other possible associated skin lesions must be noted. The ophthalmologic examination should be detailed and, if necessary, it should be performed by a pediatric ophthalmologist. The neurologic evaluation should focus in demonstrating subtle signs of motor asymmetry (mild weakness or hyperreflexia) or visual field defects.

Diagnosis

The basis of the diagnosis of SWS is a thorough physical and neurologic examination. Typical facial angioma should be distinguished from the isolated port-wine stain and other skin lesions without neurologic manifestations.

Plain skull radiographs can show the gyral calcifications of the leptomeninges, termed *trolley track*. Computed tomography scan of the head can demonstrate the calcifications earlier. Magnetic resonance imaging with gadolinium is the neuroimaging modality of choice to demonstrate the abnormal intracranial vessels. It can be complemented with magnetic resonance angiography. Brain volumetrics can be performed with MRI, permitting early discovery of brain atrophy. Single-proton emission CT and positron emission tomography scans show regions of abnormal cerebral blood flow or glucose metabolism larger than the corresponding leptomeningeal angiomata seen on CT or MRI.

Electroencephalography is only necessary for the evaluation of epilepsy, but routine studies are not indicated if the patient does not have seizures.

Treatment

Antiepileptic drugs should be used to control seizures. In patients with intractable epilepsy, progressive brain atrophy, and hemiparesis, surgical procedures, including hemispherectomy (functional or anatomical), may be the treatment of choice.

Antithrombotic agents may diminish damage caused by thrombotic events precipitated by sluggish blood flow. Attention-deficit/hyperactivity disorder and migraine are treated symptomatically.

Patients should be monitored closely by an ophthalmologist for glaucoma with examination every 3 months for the first 2 years of life and yearly thereafter.

The cosmetic aspects of the facial angioma should be promptly addressed with families. With age, it often darkens and can become nodular. Pulsed dye laser treatments may be successful at fading the lesions. Results are best when started before 7 years of age, and treatment is safe in the first few weeks of life.

Children's educational needs need to be evaluated and fulfilled. Because the effects of SWS on individual patients and families are difficult to predict, support and education tailored to each family's specific needs are key.

Natural History and Prognosis

There is a spectrum of disease with some patients exhibiting almost no progression and some with very fast brain atrophy and intractable epilepsy. The neurologic outcome ranges from normal intellect and no seizures to intractable seizures with mental retardation. Although patients with widespread hemispheric or bihemispheric disease are at greater risk for neurologic complications, many function virtually normally. On the other hand, a subgroup of patients with limited CNS involvement as defined by neuroimaging studies may have a particularly malignant course with intractable epilepsy, headache, stroke-like episodes, and cognitive deterioration.

The severity of the epilepsy is related to the extent of the intracranial lesion and maybe to earlier seizure onset. In particular, the presence of seizures before 1 year of age with hypsarrhythmia on the EEG and status epilepticus is correlated with an unfavorable outcome. About half of the patients will be controlled on antiepileptic medications, whereas others will continue to develop refractory epilepsy, particularly those who have mental retardation. The clinical condition eventually stabilizes, leaving a patient who has residual hemiparesis, hemianopsia, mental retardation, and epilepsy, but without further deterioration.

Ataxia-Telangiectasia

Ataxia-telangiectasia (AT) is a rare, multisystem degenerative disorder affecting the skin, eye, CNS, and the immune response with increased infections, extreme sensitivity to radiation, and risk for malignancies.

Epidemiology and Genetics

Ataxia-telangiectasia is a monogenic autosomal recessive disorder with an incidence between 1 in 40,000 and 1 in 100,000. Carrier frequency is thought to be 1 in 100 to 200.

The disease is caused by mutations in the *ATM* gene located in 11q22-23. As a consequence, there is total loss of the ataxia-telangiectasia mutated (ATM) protein, which normally recognizes DNA damage and activates the DNA repair machinery and the cell cycle checkpoints to minimize the risk of genetic damage. More than 400 distinct AT mutations have been described in every part of the gene, and most of the patients are com-pounded heterozygotes inheriting distinct AT mutations from each parent. About 85% are null mutations, resulting in premature protein truncation, causing complete inactivation of the gene and absence of a protein product. Less than 15% are missense mutation or short-in-frame deletions or inser-tions. De novo mutations are rare. Almost all recurring mutations are found on unique haplotypes that represent founder effects and ancestral relation-ships between patients. There seems to be a phenotype-genotype relation-ship: truncating mutations are responsible for the most severe cases, whereas the mutations that allow the transcription of the protein cause a less severe clinical picture. Fifty percent of residual ATM protein activity, as is typical among heterozygotes, protects from the disease.

Clinical Characteristics

The condition usually presents with repetitive chronic bacterial sinopulmo-nary infections in infancy. Then children can manifest delayed psychomotor development and cerebellar ataxia during the first decade of life, usually at about 2 years, with other signs of cerebellar involvement (hypotonia, tremor, dysmetria, and incoordination). Signs of progression of neurologic degen-eration include extrapyramidal syndrome, peripheral neuropathy, nystag-mus, and eye movement abnormalities. Telangiectasias are chronic dilation of capillaries leading to the appearance of dark red blotches on the skin or the eyes. They present after the ataxia, usually at 3 to 6 years of age, as "small spider veins" in the bulbar conjunctiva (Figure 7-5), ears, cheeks, and the flexor surfaces in the antecubital fossa and the popliteal fossa. Café-au-lait spots, vitiligo, and seborrheic dermatitis may also be seen. Other clinical features include growth retardation, hypogonadism, and premature aging.

The immunodeficiency phenotype in AT is variable and usually manifests as decreased or absent IgA, IgE, and IgG2. There is also deficit of T-cell–mediated immunity, involving CD4 and CD8, with a negative tuberculin skin test and negative T-cell proliferation to mitogens. About 20% of patients develop a malignancy, usually acute lymphocytic leukemia or

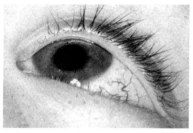

Figure 7-5.
Conjunctival telangiectasia in ataxia-telangiectasia.

lymphoma. Breast cancer is significantly increased in heterozygote women.

Some atypical patients with minimal signs and symptoms, such as very mild or very late-onset ataxia, or late-onset spinal muscular atrophy, can now be included in the diagnosis of AT because they either lack ATM protein or ATM kinase activity, or have mutations in the *ATM* gene.

Physical Examination

A detailed examination of the skin and the conjunctiva should demonstrate the typical telangiectasias. Neurologic evaluation should demonstrate the cerebellar type of ataxia and the accompanying neurologic findings described previously.

Diagnosis

The diagnosis is commonly based on the clinical triad of cerebellar ataxia, telangiectasia, and immunodeficiency causing repeated sinopulmonary infections. Brain MRI may show significant thinning of the molecular layer of the cerebellum and cerebellar atrophy.

Elevated levels of alpha fetoprotein are detected in 95% of patients with AT. Humoral and cellular immunity tests are abnormal, as indicated previously.

Cytogenetic investigation reveals chromosome instability, accelerated telomere shortening, radiosensitivity, and sensitivity to other DNA-damaging agents. Chromosome analysis of peripheral blood lymphocyte cultures reveals an increased incidence of translocations in the loci of immunoglobulin and T-cell receptor genes on chromosomes 7 and 14. The specific *ATM* gene mutations can be tested.

Differential diagnoses include other disorders that are due to mutations in genes other than AT. For example, mutations in the *MRE11* gene lead to the development of AT-like disorder, a less severe form of AT, and in *NBS1* gene to Nijmegen syndrome, phenotypically similar to AT but with a characteristic facial appearance and microcephaly.

The diagnosis of ataxia needs to consider other entities in the differential, like spinocerebellar ataxias; Friedrich ataxia; and Gaucher, Hartnup, Niemann-Pick, or Refsum disease.

Treatment

There is no specific treatment for AT. Sino-pulmonary infections require symptomatic treatment with antibiotics; gammaglobulin may also be helpful. Malignancies require specific therapies. Some neurologic symptoms (tremor) may improve with symptomatic treatment.

Natural History and Prognosis

Affected children are normal at birth, but by the age of 2 to 3 years they lose muscle coordination; by the age of 10 years they are usually confined to a wheelchair. Ataxia-telangiectasia is usually a slowly progressive disease, and most children die in the second or third decade of life.

Death is usually due to pneumonia, or chronic lung disease resulting from immunodeficiency, or from defects in chewing and swallowing due to progressive neurologic degeneration. The increased risk for malignancies also accounts for the lethality of AT.

Incontinentia Pigmenti

Incontinentia pigmenti (IP), also known as *IP type 2* or *Bloch-Sulzberger syndrome,* is a rare genodermatosis that affects mostly females (49:1) and is usually lethal for males in utero, although several cases of affected males have been reported. It is a multisystem disorder, primarily of ectodermal origin, characterized by skin, dental, ocular, and CNS abnormalities.

Epidemiology and Genetics

The perinatal incidence of IP is estimated to be about 1 in 50,000 births, but it is probably higher because the complex phenotype is difficult to diagnose. Most cases have been described in white persons, but the disorder may affect persons of other races as well. In a 1976 review of 653 patients, 55.4% had a definitive family history of IP.

The disorder is inherited as an X-linked dominant trait and is due to the mutation of the gene *NEMO,* located on Xq28, which encodes the regulatory subunit of the IkB kinase complex required for nuclear factor-*k*B activation. *NEMO* is an important signaling molecule and has a vital function in the transmission of information from the nucleus about the status of genotoxic damage. Loss of function mutation of *NEMO* accounts for 80% of cases. Hypomorphic mutations of *NEMO* result in IP in heterozygous females and in hypohidrotic ectodermal dysplasia associated with severe immunodeficiency (EDI) in surviving hemizygous males.

Occasional survival of affected males is attributed to the presence of an extra X chromosome (Klinefelter syndrome), postzygotic mutations, or hypomorphic alleles with less deleterious mutations and presentations along a continuum from IP to EDI.

Clinical Characteristics

The skin lesions may occur in 4 classically successive diagnostic stages.

- Stage 1. Linear inflammatory erythema, then vesicles and pustules that appear at birth or during the first 2 months of life and may last from weeks to months. Lesions are filled with eosinophils, and the inflammatory response is thought to represent a selection against the functionally defective cell clone.
- Stage 2. The inflammatory response is replaced by linear, hyperkeratotic warty or verrucous plaques. These lesions usually disappear within several months, but may last until 1 year of age.
- Stage 3. As the warty lesions resolve, the child is left with persistent linear hyperpigmentation. A linear hyperpigmentation that follows the dermatome lines (Blaschko lines) is very characteristic of IP (Figure 7-6).
- Stage 4. The presence of hypopigmented or depigmented linear macules on the lower extremities and trunk (pallor and scarring) is the final phase that appears during adulthood.

  Stages, however, may overlap or not occur at all in a same patient.

  Tooth abnormalities include anodontia of deciduous or permanent teeth, conical teeth, microdontia, and delayed eruption of permanent teeth.

Eye abnormalities include strabismus, ophthalmoplegia, microphthalmia, retinal detachment, retinal pigmentation, coloboma, occlusion of the central retinal artery, optic atrophy, and blindness.

Central nervous system manifestations seem to arise from compromised vascularization or from vaso-obliteration in the developing brain. This results in ischemia causing cerebral and cerebellar atrophy, formation of small cavities in the brain white matter, and defects in neuronal migration. The clinical correlate of these neuropathological findings are microcephaly, developmental delay/ mental retardation, cerebral palsy, visual loss, and seizures.

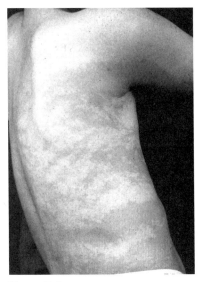

Figure 7-6.
Hyperpigmented skin areas following the dermatome lines (Blaschko lines) in incontinentia pigmenti.

Other clinical findings that can be seen in IP are skull and ear deformities, cleft lip or palate, spina bifida, incomplete development of one side of the spinal bones, extra ribs, atrophy on one side of the body, congenital dislocation of the hip, club foot, webbed fingers, nail dystrophy, alopecia, abnormal development of cartilage, and short stature.

The male phenotype has clinical features similar to those of the female phenotype. Unilateral presentation is a distinct occurrence in boys, especially in early stages.

Physical Examination

The examination of patients with IP should focus on describing the skin, teeth, and eye lesions typical of the condition. A detailed evaluation of their psychomotor development and neurologic status is important to suspect associated neurologic abnormalities.

Diagnosis

The diagnosis of IP is based on clinical examination (Table 7-1). A careful family history in a suspect patient is crucial for confirmation of the diagnosis and future genetic counseling.

Some of the clinical findings may generate a differential diagnosis. Thus the vesicular rash in the newborn period needs to be differentiated from herpes simplex infection at this age. Blaschko hyperpigmentation lines, although very typical of IP, can also be seen in other skin disorders like hypomelanosis of Ito (HI).

Brain MRI is indicated if the neurologic examination is abnormal or if vascular retinopathy is detected. It will demonstrate the cerebral abnormalities associated with IP, as described previously. Electroencephalography will be necessary for the diagnosis and management of seizures.

Testing of *NEMO* gene mutations may be helpful to confirm the diagnosis.

Treatment

With the exception of hyperplastic retinopathy, there are no treatable features. Therapies should be provided by a multidisciplinary group of doctors to alleviate the associated problems (teeth abnormalities, orthopedic deformities) and clinical symptoms (early intervention for developmental delay, antiepileptic drugs for seizures).

Natural History and Prognosis

The usual natural history of the skin lesions has been described previously. However, bullous and verrucous lesions do not always resolve during the first or second year of life, and may recur throughout childhood.

The neurologic prognosis depends on the associated neuropathology lesions and seizures. Although most patients with IP are of normal intelligence, those with neonatal seizures and brain abnormalities have a poor prognosis for normal development.

Hypomelanosis of Ito

Hypomelanosis of Ito, also termed *IP achromians* or *IP type 1,* is a sporadic multisystemic neurocutaneous disorder characterized by the presence during the first few months of life of skin hypopigmentation along the lines of

Table 7-1. Diagnostic Criteria for Incontinentia Pigmenti (IP)[a]	
No Incidence of IP in at Least 1 First-Degree Female Relative	**Evidence of IP in at Least 1 First-Degree Female Relative**
Major Criteria	
Typical neonatal rash	History or evidence of typical rash
Erythema, vesicles, eosinophilia	Skin manifestations of IP
Typical hyperpigmentation	Hyperpigmentation
Mainly on trunk	Scarring
Following Blaschko lines	Hairless streaks
Fading in adolescence	Alopecia at vertex
Linear, atrophic, hairless lesions	Anomalous dentition
	Wooly hair
	Retinal disease
	Miscarriages of male fetuses
Minor Criteria (Supportive Evidence)	
Dental involvement	
Alopecia	
Wooly hair, abnormal nails	
Diagnosis of sporadic IP: At least one major criterion.	Diagnosis of IP in a first-degree relative of an affected female patient: likely if any of the mentioned minor criteria are present, alone or combined
Minor criteria, if present, will support the diagnosis; complete absence would make the diagnosis uncertain	

[a]Reprinted from Landy SJ, Donnai D. Incontinentia pigmenti (Bloch-Sulzberger syndrome). *J Med Genet.* 1993;30:53–59, with permission from BMJ Publishing Group, Ltd.

Blaschko, frequent involvement of the CNS in the first decade of life, and associated extra-neurologic complications.

Epidemiology and Genetics

The incidence of HI has been reported to be 1 in 7,500 to 40,000 births, 1 in every 8,000 to 10,000 new patients in a hospital, and 1 in every 1,000 new patients in a pediatric neurology service. It is the third most frequent neurocutaneous disorder, after NF and TSC. The female to male ratio varies according to the different series, ranging from 0.7 to 1.7.

Chromosome abnormalities have been reported in about half of the patients. The most common ones are trisomy 18, diploidy, mosaicism for sex chromosomes, aneuploidy and tetrasomy 12p, and balance X autosome translocations with break points in the juxtacentromeric region of the X chromosome at Xp11. The recognition of chromosomal mosaicism in many cases of HI explains the variable clinical findings and the often asymmetrical expression.

There have been a number of single case reports suggesting familial occurrence and single gene inheritance, but none has been proved.

Clinical Characteristics

Hypomelanosis of Ito presents with hypomelanotic whirls in the newborn period or shortly thereafter. These lesions are clearly seen by visual inspection, but the Wood light may be used to better identify them. In some cases, zones of diffuse alopecia in the scalp may precede the presence of hypopigmented skin. Overall, pigmentation in HI can be decreased or increased, and there is no preceding vesicular or verrucous phase. Histopathological analysis of the depigmented lesions shows decreased number of melanocytes and decreased number and size of melanosomes in the basal layer of the epidermis with selective decrease in eumelanin. Other minor skin abnormalities that can be seen in HI include café-au-lait spots, cutis marmorata, angiomatous nevi, nevus of Ota, Mongolian blue spots, abnormal sweating, icthyosis, and morphea.

About 50% of patients with HI have white matter changes seen on MRI as high signal on T2-weighted images in the periventricular and subcortical regions, corresponding to delayed myelination or to dilated Virchow-Robin spaces. Other brain abnormalities include megalencephaly or micrencephaly; cerebral, cerebellar or brain stem atrophy; hemimegalencephaly; agenesis or dysplasia of the corpus callosum; gray matter heterotopias; lissencephaly; pachygyria; polymicrogyria; porencephaly; Dandy-Walker malformation; periventricular cystic lesions; moyamoya disease; arteriovenus malformations; and stroke. The most common neurologic manifestations are mental retardation and seizures. IQ is borderline in 20% of patients and below 70 in 60% (40% <50). Among the children who are cognitive deficient, approximately 10% have autistic-like behavior, most of whom had previously suffered infantile spasms or refractory epilepsy. Seizures are present in up to 50% of patients, more frequently generalized tonic-clonic, followed by partial, infantile spasms and myoclonic. Other neurologic manifestations are hypotonia or hypertonia, hyperactivity, nystagmus, ataxia, neuropathy, sensorineural deafness, and speech delay. The severity of the neurologic manifestations does not correlate with the extent of the hypopigmented skin lesion.

Other clinical findings seen in HI are craniofacial abnormalities (macrocephaly or microcephaly, hypertelorism or hypotelorism, low-set ears, frontonasal dysplasia), skeletal anomalies (congenital hip dyslocation, small hands and feet, pes valgus or varus, genu varus, pectus carinatum or excavatum, kyphoscoliosis), eye problems (strabismus, nystagmus, iris heterochromia or coloboma, hypopigmented retina, retinal detachment, optic atrophy), and cardiac or urogenital malformations. Growth and bone maturation may be compromised in some patients.

Some patients with HI have been reported who developed tumors (benign tumors like cystic teratoma, sacrococcygeal dysembryonal tumor, choroid plexus papilloma, dental hamartomatous tumor and, rarely, malignant tumors like acute lymphoblastic leukemia, medulloblastoma, neuroblastoma, or meningeal rhabdomyosrcoma). The risk of tumors is increased in the patients with chromosome abnormalities.

Physical Examination

The examination of patients with HI should focus on the description of the skin hypopigmented lesions and on the demonstration of other associated clinical findings described previously. A detailed neurologic examination and assessment of the psychomotor and cognitive development should also be performed.

Diagnosis

The diagnosis of HI is a clinical (Box 7-5). Brain CT or MRI scans will demonstrate the associated cerebral neuropathological abnormalities in patients with clinical neurologic findings. Electroencephalography will be necessary in the diagnostic evaluation of patients with seizures. Chromosome analysis in peripheral lymphocytes and, if normal, in skin fibroblasts, keratinocytes, or melanocytes should be performed. The differential diagnosis should be established with other conditions that present with patchy depigmentation of the skin (IP in the fourth stage of the disease, isolated hypomelanotic nevus, or nevus depigmentosus).

Box 7-5. Diagnostic Criteria for Hypomelanosis of Ito[a]

1. *Sine qua non*
   Congenital, or early acquired nonhereditary cutaneous hypopigmentation in linear streaks or patches involving more than 2 body segments

2. *Major criteria*
   One or more nervous system anomalies
   One or more musculoskeletal anomalies

3. *Minor criteria*
   Two or more congenital malformations other than nervous system or musculoskeletal
   Chromosome abnormalities

Definite diagnosis
Criterion 1 plus one or more criterion 2 or 2 or more criterion 3

Presumptive diagnosis
Criterion 1 alone, or in association with one minor criteria

---

[a]*From Ruiz-Maldonado R, Toussaint S, Tamayo L, Hypomelanosis of Ito: diagnostic criteria and report of 41 cases. Pediatr Dermatol. 1992;9:2. Reproduced with permission of Blackwell Publishing Ltd.*

Genetic counseling should be provided to the parents, indicating that the risk of recurrence of the disease in another pregnancy is low. However, chromosome studies should be performed not only in the patient, but also in his or her parents.

Treatment

No special treatment is indicted for the skin lesions, and no precautions need to be taken with regard to sun exposure or cream applications. Treatment is symptomatic and should be provided by a multidisciplinary group of doctors to improve the signs and symptoms of the associated conditions (orthopedic problems, seizures, developmental delay). The recommended follow-up protocol requires an annual clinical review, unless the presence of complications requires otherwise.

Natural History and Prognosis

Long-term follow-up of patients has shown that the skin lesion shows a general increase in hypopigmentation or hyperpigmentation in infancy, but later on it remains constant. After adolescence there is a decrease in hypopigmentation or hyperpigmentation, but lesions remain evident in adulthood.

Complications, if present, usually manifest early in infancy. Malignant transformation of a hypomelanocytic zone of the skin has been reported, but it is very rare. The chance of the patient developing a tumor is basically the same as in the general population. Patients with the most marked cutaneous phenotype tend to have the most severe extracutaneous phenotype as well and, therefore, are at risk for a worse prognosis.

Other Neurocutaneous Disorders

Other less frequent neurocutaneous disorders include the following:

Cerebrotendinous xanthomatosis: Autosomal recessive disorder with tendon xanthomas, cataracts, and progressive neurologic deterioration (dementia, ataxia, nystagmus, peripheral neuropathy, parkinsonism, cataracts). There are abnormal deposits of cholesterol in all tissues.

Encephalocutaneous lipomatosis: Sporadic condition characterized by hairless lipomatous scalp mass ipsilateral to brain malformation. Neurologic manifestations include mental retardation and epilepsy.

Epidermal nevus syndrome: A group of disorders with patchy, cutaneous hamartomatous lesions and neurologic manifestations like seizures, brain malformations, and cerebrovascular anomalies, including arteriovenous malformations. Although most cases occur sporadically, autosomal dominant transmission has also been reported.

Kinky hair syndrome: Also known as *Menkes syndrome,* an X-linked disorder of copper metabolism. Patients have brittle, light-colored hair, pilli torti (kinky hair), and trichorrexis nodosa (hair fractures). Other clinical findings are bladder diverticulae and skeletal abnormalities. Neurologic manifestations include temperature instability, hypotonia, seizures, quadriparesis, and mental retardation.

Klippel-Trénaunay-Weber syndrome: Classic features include subcutaneous hemangiomas (distinctive port-wine stain with sharp borders), varicose veins, abnormally developed lymphatic system, and hypertrophy of bony and soft tissues that causes unilateral limb hypertrophy.

Maffucci syndrome: Mesenchymal dysplasia characterized by dyschondrodysplasia (Ollier disease), and vascular abnormalities in the form of cavernous hemangiomata and phlebectasia.

Neurocutaneous melanosis: Disorder of melanotic cell development that involves primarily the meninges and the skin. There is usually a dark nevi present at birth (>6 cm in the body or >9 cm in the scalp) and multiple small nevi. Neurologic manifestations include hydrocephalus, cranial nerve deficits, seizures, and mental retardation. Patients may develop leptomeningeal melanoma,

Osler-Weber-Rendu disease: Also called *hereditary hemorrhagic telangiectasia.* Autosomal dominant disorder with telangiectasias of the skin and internal organs, including vascular malformations of the brain. Patients may develop meningitis and brain abscess.

Pseudoxanthoma elasticum: Characterized by cutaneous signs (yellowish plaques affecting neck, axilla, abdomen, inguinal, cubital, or popliteal areas) and neurologic vaso-occlusive manifestations resembling severe atherosclerosis.

Von Hippel-Lindau disease: This is an autosomal dominant disorder characterized by hemangioblastomas of the retina and CNS (cerebellum most common site). Patients also exhibit other visceral cysts (pancreas) and tumors. Neurologic symptoms are explained by the location and slow growth of the lesions.

Wyburn-Mason syndrome: A rare disorder without clear inheritance characterized by retinal, facial, and intracranial arteriovenous malformations. Neurologic and visual symptoms usually begin in adulthood.

Xeroderma pigmentosum: Group of autosomal recessive diseases characterized by susceptibility to sun-induced skin disorders and progressive neurologic deterioration. Skin manifestations include sunlight sensitivity, freckling, atrophy, xerosis, scaling, telangiectasia, keratosis, angioma, and melanoma. Neurologic symptoms include progressive dementia, sensorineural hearing loss, tremor, choreoathetosis, and ataxia.

Web Sites

National Neurofibromatosis Foundation: www.nf.org

Neurofibromatosis, Inc: www.nfinc.org

Tuberous Sclerosis Alliance: www.tsalliance.org

Sturge-Weber Foundation: www.sturge-weber.com

Ataxia Telangiectasia Children's Project: www.atcp.org

National Incontinentia Pigmenti Foundation: http://imgen.bcm.tmc.edu/
nipf

National Foundation for Ectodermal Dysplasias: www.nfed.org

Bibliography

Neurocutaneous Disorders

Barbagallo JS, Kolodzieh MS, Silverberg NB, Weinberg JM. Neurocutaneous disorders.
Dermatol Clin. 2002;20:547–560

Jentarra G, Snyder SL, Narayanan V. Genetic aspects of neurocutaneous disorders. *Semin
Pediatr Neurol.* 2006;13:43–47

Nowak CB. The phakomatoses: dermatologic clues to neurologic anomalies. *Semin Pediatr
Neurol.* 2007;14:140–149

Roach ES. Neurocutaneous syndromes. *Continuum.* 2000;6:35–58

Thiele EA, Korf BR. Phakomatoses and allied conditions. In: Swaiman KF, Ashwal S, Ferriero
DM, eds. *Pediatric Neurology. Principles & Practice.* Philadelphia, PA: Mosby Elsevier;
2006:771–796

Neurofibromatosis

Babovic-Vuksanovic D, Ballman K, Michels V, et al. Phase II trial of pirfenidone in adults with
neurofibromatosis type 1. *Neurology.* 2006;67:1860–1862

Evans DG, Baser ME, McGaughran J, Sharif S, Howard E, Moran A. Malignant peripheral nerve
sheath tumors in neurofibromatosis 1. *J Med Genet.* 2002;39:311–314

Evans DG, Huson SM, Donnai D, et al. A genetic study of type 2 neurofibromatosis in the
United Kingdom. I. Prevalence, mutation rate, fitness, and confirmation of maternal transmission effect on severity. *J Med Genet.* 1992;29:841–846

Falsini B, Ziccardi L, Lazzareschi I, et al. Longitudinal assessment of childhood optic gliomas:
relationship between flicker visual evoked potentials and magnetic resonance imaging.
J Neurooncol. 2008;88:87–96

Ferner RE, Huson SE, Thomas N, et al. Guidelines for the diagnosis and management of
individuals with neurofibromatosis 1. *J Med Genet.* 2007;44:81–88

Gupta A, Cohen BH, Ruggieri P, Packer RJ, Phillips PC. Phase I study of thalidomide for the
treatment of plexiform neurofibroma in neurofibromatosis 1. *Neurology.* 2003;60:130–132

Gutmann DH, Aylsworth A, Carey JC, et al. The diagnostic evaluation and multidisciplinary
management of neurofibromatosis 1 and neurofibromatosis 2. *JAMA.* 1997;278:51–57

Korf BR. Diagnostic outcome in children with multiple cafe au lait spots. *Pediatrics.*
1992;90:924–927

Lama G, Esposito-Salsano M, Grassia C, et al. Neurofibromatosis type 1 and optic pathway glioma. A long-term follow-up. *Minerva Pediatr.* 2007;59:13–21

Mautner VF, Tatagiba T, Guthoff R, Samii M, Pulst SM. Neurofibromatosis 2 in the pediatric age group. *Neurosurgery.* 1993;33:92–96

Messiaen LM, Callens T, Mortier G, et al. Exhaustive mutation analysis of the NF1 gene allows identification of 95% of mutations and reveals a high frequency of unusual splicing defects. *Hum Mutat.* 2000;15:541–555

Nunes F, MacCollin M. Neurofibromatosis 2 in the pediatric population. *J Child Neurol.* 2003;18:718–724

Parry DM, Eldridge R, Kaiser-Kupfer MI, Bouzas EA, Pikus A, Patronas N. Neurofibromatosis 2 (NF2): clinical characteristics of 63 affected individuals and clinical evidence for heterogeneity. *Am J Med Genet.* 1994;52:450–461

Zeid JL, Charrow J, Sandu M, Goldman S, Listernick R. Orbital optic nerve gliomas in children with neurofibromatosis type 1. *J AAPOS.* 2006;10:534–539

Tuberous Sclerosis Complex

Au KS, Williams AT, Gambello MJ, Northrup H. Molecular genetic basis of tuberous sclerosis complex: from bench to bedside. *J Child Neurol.* 2004;19:699–709

Boer K, Jansen F, Nellist M, et al. Inflammatory processes in cortical tubers and subependymal giant cell tumors of tuberous sclerosis. *Epilepsy Res.* 2008;78:7–21

Crino, PB, Nathanson KL, Henske EP. The tuberous sclerosis complex. *N Engl J Med.* 2006;355:1345–1356

Datta AN, Hahn CD, Sahin M. Clinical presentation and diagnosis of tuberous sclerosis complex in infancy. *J Child Neurol.* 2008;23:268–273

Devlin LA, Shepherd CH, Crawford H, Morrison PJ. Tuberous sclerosis complex: clinical features, diagnosis, and prevalence within Northern Ireland. *Dev Med Child Neurol.* 2006;48:495–499

Gómez MR, Sampson JR, Wittemore VH. *Tuberous Sclerosis Complex.* New York, NY: Oxford University Press; 1999

Husain AM, Foley CM, Legido A, Chandler DA, Miles DK, Grover WD. Tuberous sclerosis complex and epilepsy: prognostic significance of electroencephalography and magnetic resonance imaging. *J Child Neurol.* 2000;15:81–83

Jueste SS, Sahin M, Bolton P, Ploubidis GB, Humphrey A. Characterization of autism in young children with tuberous sclerosis complex. *J Child Neurol.* 2008;23:520–525

Jóźwiak S, Schwartz RA, Janniger CK, Bielicka-Cymerman J. Usefulness of diagnostic criteria of tuberous sclerosis complex y pediatric patients. *J Child Neurol.* 2000;15:652–659

Jóźwiak S, Kotulska K, Kasprzyk-Obara J, et al. Clinical and genotype studies of cardiac tumors in 154 patients with tuberous sclerosis complex. *Pediatrics.* 2006;118:e1146–e1151

Jóźwiak S, Kwiatkowski D, Kotulska K, et al. Tuberin and hamartin expression is reduced in the majority of subependymal giant cell astrocytomas in tuberous sclerosis complex consistent with a two-hit model of pathogenesis. *J Child Neurol.* 2004;19:102–106

Maria BL, Deidrick KM, Roach ES, Gutmann DH. Tuberous sclerosis complex: pathogenesis, diagnosis, strategies, therapies, and future research directions. *J Child Neurol.* 2004;19:632–642

Prather P, de Vries PJ. Behavioral and cognitive aspects of tuberous sclerosis complex. *J Child Neurol.* 2004;19:666–674

Roach ES, MR Gómez MR, Northrup N. Tuberous sclerosis complex consensus conference: revised clinical diagnostic criteria. *J Child Neurol.* 1998;13:624–628

Roach ES, Sparagana SP. Diagnosis of tuberous sclerosis complex. *J Child Neurol.* 2004;19: 643–649

Valencia I, Legido A, Yelin K, Khurana D, Kothare SV, Katsetos CD. Anomalous inhibitory circuits in cortical tubers of human tuberous sclerosis complex associated with refractory epilepsy: aberrant expression of parvalbumin and calbindin-D28k in dysplastic cortex. *J Child Neurol.* 2006;21:1058-1063

Wong V. Study of the relationship between tuberous sclerosis complex and autistic disorder. *J Child Neurol.* 2006;21:199–204

Sturge-Weber Syndrome

Bodensteiner JB. Sturge-Weber syndrome. *Facial Plast Surg Clin North Am.* 2001;9:569–576

Bourgeois M, Crimmins DW, de Oliveira RS, et al. Surgical treatment of epilepsy in Sturge-Weber syndrome in children. *J Neurosurg.* 2007;106:20–28

Chapieski L, Friedman A, Lachar D. Psychological functioning in children and adolescents with Sturge-Weber syndrome. *J Child Neurol.* 2000;15:660–665

Comati A, Beck H, Halliday W, Snipes GJ, Plate KH, Acker T. Upregulation of hypoxia-inducible growth factor (HIF)-1alpha and HIF-2alpha in leptomeningeal vascular malformations of Sturge Weber syndrome. *J Neuropathol Exp Neurol.* 2007;66:86–97

Comi AM. Pathophysiology of Sturge-Weber syndrome. *J Child Neurol.* 2003;18:509–516

Comi AM. Update on Sturge-Weber syndrome: diagnosis, treatment, quantitative measures and controversies. *Lymphat Res Biol.* 2007;5:257–264

Comi AM, Weisz CJ, Highest BH, Skolasky RL, Hess EJ. Sturge-Weber syndrome: altered blood vessel fibronectin expression and morphology. *J Child Neurol.* 2005;20:572–577

Pascual-Castroviejo I, Pascual-Pascual SI, Velázquez-Fragua R, Viaño J. Sturge-Weber syndrome. Study of 55 patients. *Can J Neurol Sci.* 2008;302–307

Sperner J, Schmauser I, Bittner R, Henkes, et al. MR-imaging findings in children with Sturge-Weber syndrome. *Neuropediatrics.* 1990;21:146–152

Sujansky E, Conradi S. Outcome of Sturge-Weber syndrome in 52 adults. *Am J Med Genet.* 1995;57:35–45

Sujansky E, Conradi S. Sturge-Weber syndrome: age of onset of seizures and glaucoma and the prognosis for affected children. *J Child Neurol.* 1995;10:49–58

Thomas-Sohl KA, Vaslow DF, Maria BL. Sturge-Weber syndrome: a review. *Pediatr Neurol.* 2003;30:303–310

van Emelen C, Goethals M, Dralands L, Casteels L. Treatment of glaucoma in children with Sturge-Weber syndrome. *J Pediatr Ophthalmol Strabismus.* 2000;37:29–34

Ataxia Telangiectasia

Bott L, Thumerelle C, Cuvellier JC, Deschildre A, Vallée L, Sardet A. Ataxia-telangiectasia: a review[in French]. *Arch Pediatr.* 2006;13:293–298

Chun HH, Gatti RA. Ataxia-telangiectasia, an evolving phenotype. *DNA Repair.* 2004;3: 1187–1196

Frappart PO, McKinnon PJ. Ataxia-telangiectasia and related diseases *Neuromolecular Med.* 2004;8:495–511

Mavrou A, Tsangaris GTH, Roma E, Kolialexi A. The ATM gene and ataxia telangiectasia. *Anticancer Res.* 2008;28:401–406

McKinnon PJ. ATM and ataxia telangiectasia. *EMBO Reports.* 2004;5:772–776

Stray-Pedersen A, Borresen-Dale AL, Paus E, Lindman CR, Burgers T, Abrahamsen TG. Alpha fetoprotein is increasing with age in ataxia-telangiectasia. *Eur J Paediatr Neurol.* 2007;11:375–380

Taylor AM, Byrd PJ. Molecular pathology of ataxia telangiectasia. *J Clin Pathol.* 2005;58: 1009–1010

Incontinentia Pigmenti

Ardelean D, Pope E. Incontinentia pigmenti in boys: a series and review of the literature. *Pediatr Dermatol.* 2006;23:523–527

Berlin AL, Paller AS, Chan LS. Incontinentia pigmenti: a review and update on the molecular basis of pathology. *J Am Acad Dermatol.* 2002;47:169–187

Carney RG Jr. Incontinentia pigmenti: a world statistical analysis. *Arch Dermatol.* 1076;112: 535–542

Fusco F, Fimiani G, Tadini G, Michele D, Ursini MV. Clinical diagnosis of incontinentia pigmenti in a cohort of male patients. *J Am Acad Dermatol.* 2007;56:264–267

Hadj-Rabia S, Froidevaux D, Bodak N, et al. Clinical study of 40 cases of incontinentia pigmenti. *Arch Dermatol.* 2003;139:1163–1170

Kim BJ, Shin HS, Won CH, et al. Incontinentia pigmenti: clinical observation of 40 Korean cases. *J Korean Med Sci.* 2006;21:474–477

Landy SJ, Donnai D. Incontinentia pigmenti (Bloch-Sulzberger syndrome). *J Med Genet.* 1993;30:53–59

Mangano S, Barbagallo A. Incontinentia pigmenti: clinical and neuroradiologic features. *Brain Dev.* 1993;15:362–366

Nelson DL. NEMO, NFkB signaling and Incontinentia pigmenti. *Curr Opin Genet Dev.* 2006;6:282–288

O'Brian JE, Feingold M. Incontinentia pigmenti: a longitudinal study. *Am J Dis Child.* 1985;139:711–712

Phan TA, Wargon O, Turner AM. Incontinentia pigmenti case series: clinical spectrum of incontinentia pigmenti in 53 female patients and their relatives. *Clin Exp Dermatol.* 2005;30:474–480

Tanboga I, Kargul B, Ergeneli S, Aydin MY, Atasu M. Clinical features of incontinentia pigmenti with emphasis on dermatoglyphic findings. *J Clin Pediatr Dent.* 2001;25:161–165

Hypomelanosis of Ito

Lenzini E, Bertoli P, Artifoni L,. Battistella PA, Baccichetti C, Peserito A. Hypomelanosis of Ito: involvement of chromosome aberrations in this syndrome. *Ann Genet.* 1991;34:30–32

Pascual-Castroviejo I, López-Rodríguez L, de la Cruz Medina M, Salamanca-Maesso C, Roche Herrero C. Hypomelanosis of Ito. Neurological complications in 34 cases. *Can J Neurol Sci.* 1988;15:124–129

Quigg M, Rust RS, Miller JQ. Clinical findings of the phakomatoses: hypomelanosis of Ito. *Neurology.* 2006;66:e45

Ruggieri M, Pavone L. Hypomelanosis of Ito: clinical syndrome or just phenotype? *J Child Neurol.* 2000;15:635–644

Ruiz-Maldonado R, Toussaint S, Tamayo L, Hypomelanosis of Ito: diagnostic criteria and report of 41 cases. *Pediatr Dermatol.* 1992;9:1–10

Chapter 8

Febrile Seizures

Ignacio Valencia, MD

Introduction

Febrile seizures are the most common seizure disorder in childhood, occurring in 2% to 9% of all children in Europe, North America, or Japan. The National Institutes of Health consensus statement defines a febrile seizure as "an event in infancy or childhood usually occurring between 3 months and 5 years of age, associated with fever but without evidence of intracranial infection or defined cause for seizure." The International League Against Epilepsy defines a febrile seizure as "a seizure occurring in childhood after age 1 month, associated with a febrile illness not caused by an infection of the central nervous system (CNS), without previous neonatal seizures or a previous unprovoked seizure, and not meeting criteria for other acute symptomatic seizures."

Most febrile seizures occur between the ages of 6 months and 3 years, but some children may have them up to age 6 years, with a peak incidence around 18 months. A febrile seizure in the first few months of life or after age 6 years should warrant a differential diagnosis. However, there has been described a subgroup of children in whom febrile seizures persist beyond the age of 5 years or who have their first febrile seizure after the age of 5 years. All of them have a normal neurologic examination and normal psychomotor development, but they have a high risk of developing unprovoked seizures. These patients are very similar to, and probably overlap with, those with generalized epilepsy with febrile seizures plus (GEFS+), which is a genetically determined epilepsy with autosomal dominant inheritance related to mutations on sodium channels. Children with GEFS+ may start having febrile seizures, but may continue suffering febrile and afebrile seizures after 6 years of age, including myoclonic, focal, or absence seizures.

Etiopathogenesis

Febrile seizures have a strong genetic basis. They are more likely to occur with a high frequency in families where there is a documented history of febrile seizures; thus, a positive history is present in 25% to 40% of patients. There is an increased risk of first febrile seizure when there is a history of a first- or second-degree relative with febrile seizures. The incidence of febrile seizures in siblings is also increased from 10% to 25% if parents had febrile seizures. Although there is clear evidence for a genetic basis of febrile seizures, the mode of inheritance is unclear; polygenic, autosomal dominant, and autosomal recessive models have been formulated. Six susceptibility febrile seizure loci have been identified on chromosomes 8q13-q21 *(FEB1)*, 19p *(FEB2)*, 2q23-q24 *(FEB3)*, 5q14-q15 *(FEB4)*, 6q22-q24 *(FEB5)*, and 18p11 *(FEB6)*. Furthermore, mutations in the voltage-gated sodium channel α-1, α-2, and β-1 subunit genes *(SCN1A, SCN2A,* and *SCN1B)* and the $GABA_A$ receptor γ-2 subunit gene *(GABRG2)* have been identified in families with GEFS+. Despite the identification of multiple febrile seizure loci and mutated genes, little evidence points to their direct contribution toward most febrile seizures reported in most affected individuals. This probably reflects the genetic heterogeneity, because most causes of febrile seizures are considered multifactorial; they may depend on 2, 3, or more genetic factors, with additional contribution from environmental factors.

Febrile seizures typically are associated with common childhood illnesses, most frequently viral upper respiratory tract, middle ear, and gastrointestinal infections. Specific microorganisms associated with febrile seizures include influenza A, human herpesvirus 6, and human metapneumovirus. Shigellosis may present with diarrhea, fever, and seizures but, in this case, the mechanism of the seizure included not only the fever, but metabolic complications like hyponatremia and hypoglycemia, and the toxic effect of Shiga toxin and other toxic products of *Shigella* organisms. Child care attendance and iron deficiency anemia are considered risk factors. Previous reports have indicated also an elevated risk in children with underlying brain disorders associated with premature birth, delayed discharge from the neonatal intensive care unit, and developmental delay. However, a causal link between these factors and febrile seizures has not yet been established, and the evidence may be hampered by selection bias.

The risk of initial febrile seizures is increased after pediatric immunization: there is an increase in the risk of febrile seizures of 4-fold within 1 to 3 days of receipt of DTP (diphtheria, tetanus, pertussis) vaccination, and 1.5- to 3.0-fold within 1 to 2 weeks following administration of MMR (measles, mumps, rubella). Preliminary results of MMR plus varicella (MMRV) vaccine follow-up, presented in February 2008 by the Advisory Committee on Immunization Practice (ACIP) of the Centers for Disease Control and Prevention reported a rate of febrile seizure of 9 per 10,000 vacccinations, among MMRV recipients compared with 4 per 10,000 vaccinations among MMR and varicella vaccine recipients. However, ACIP did not express a preference for use of MMRV vaccine over separate injections of equivalent component vaccines.

Despite the common belief that the rise on temperature per se is more important for the development of febrile seizures than the actual temperature achieved, there is no evidence to support that view. Although the average level of fever in children with febrile seizures is high (39.8°C), the seizure itself is the first sign of febrile illness in 25% to 50% of all cases.

Infection-associated metabolic changes occur in patients with febrile seizures in response to the release of pyrogenic, proinflammatory cytokines (ie, IFN-γ, IL-1, Il-6, and TNF-α). They have been implicated in the pathogenesis of the seizures, because their levels have been found to be elevated in the cerebrospinal fluid (CSF) of patients. And there is an increased frequency of allele promoting IL-1β production in children with febrile seizures. Also, increased secretion of IL-6 and IL-10 by liposaccharide-stimulated mononuclear cells is higher in patients with a history of previous febrile seizures.

Clinical Manifestations

A seizure can be classified as febrile if the following characteristics are present: (1) the patient is in the peak age range (a few months of age to about 6 years), (2) fever is present and is at least 38.0°C, (3) there is no evidence of CNS infection, (4) there is no history of epilepsy or prior non-febrile seizure, and (5) there is no other known cause of seizure.

Febrile seizures can be further classified into simple or complex. Simple febrile seizures last less than 15 minutes and spontaneously resolve, are non-focal, do not recur during a 24-hour period, and/or occur in a neurologically normal child. Complex febrile seizures last longer than 15 minutes, have focal features, repeat within a 24-hour period or within the same febrile illness, or occur in a patient with a previous neurologic impairment such as cerebral palsy or developmental delay. Between 80% and 90% of all febrile seizures are simple.

In general, febrile seizures are predominantly brief, generalized tonic-clonic seizures, and 4% to 16% have focal features. More recently, febrile myoclonic seizures have been recognized. In 87% of children, the duration of the febrile seizures is less than 10 minutes; seizures last more than 15 minutes in 9% of children. Febrile status epilepticus (>30 minutes' duration) occurs in 5% of children and is more likely to have focal features.

Diagnosis

Physical Examination
A detailed history and a targeted physical examination are essential and can eliminate several serious conditions. The examination should be focused to detect the fever source and other neurologic abnormalities. In a patient with febrile seizures, the physical examination should be normal. Specifically, the physician should look for physical findings suggestive of infectious illnesses such as upper respiratory infection, otitis media, pharyngitis, pneumonia, gastroenteritis, urinary tract infection, or pyelonephritis. Other neurologic signs indicating focality may be present, such as weakness in one side of the body. (If the weakness resolves within 24 hours, it is termed the *Todd phenomenon*.) Serial examinations should be performed to ensure that the patient returns to his or her baseline after the postictal state.

Differential Diagnosis
The diagnosis of febrile seizures is based on the definition and clinical manifestations previously described. In addition, it is important to establish a differential diagnosis, which should include convulsive syncope (no postictal period, vasovagal episode, orthostasis), breath-holding spells (elicited by fear, pain, temper tantrum, apnea episode; can alter level of consciousness), tic disorders, and Sandifer syndrome (due to gastroesophageal reflux, with posturing, associated with feeding).

Fever is so prevalent in young children that seizures that would be otherwise afebrile may coincide with febrile illnesses, making the diagnosis of febrile seizure and epilepsy more difficult.

Other causes of seizures associated with fever in infancy include shaking chills (common in highly febrile children with fine rhythmic movements without loss of consciousness); toxic ingestions (such as anticholinergic agents, which can cause fever and seizures); metabolic abnormalities (such as hypernatremia, hyponatremia, and hypoglycemia); and children with vomiting, diarrhea, abnormal fluid intake, or electrolyte disturbances. Meningitis and encephalitis are 2 life-threatening conditions that should always be excluded, clinically or with the appropriate testing.

Laboratory Studies

Unnecessary routine laboratory studies should be avoided in most patients with febrile seizures. Laboratory studies should be ordered to identify the source of fever if necessary, not as part of the seizure evaluation. Specific blood work should be ordered when clinical indications exist, such as electrolytes in the setting of dehydration, blood glucose in young children with prolonged postictal states, cell blood count, and blood culture when it is indicated independent of the presence of seizures. This is supported by the 1996 American Academy of Pediatrics (AAP) practice parameter recommendations on the evaluation of children with a first simple febrile seizure.

Lumbar Puncture

The National Institutes of Health consensus statement published in 1980 states that an LP is indicated when CNS infection is suspected, though signs of infection may be absent in young infants. The AAP strongly recommends an LP in infants younger than 12 months and consideration for children between 12 and 18 months presenting with seizures and fever.

Bacterial meningitis occurs in up to 18% of children with febrile status epilepticus. Meningitis is very unlikely in children older than 2 years in the absence of a complex febrile seizure, meningeal irritation, or petechiae. Children younger than 2 years with meningitis without meningismus usually show other signs such as not being well for a few days, vomiting, drowsiness, poor feeding, or complex febrile seizures. Nonetheless, close surveillance for meningitis is needed in young children who may not show meningismus or in any child who presents repeatedly for medical attention.

Therefore, an LP should be performed in patients at risk for menigitis: focal, prolonged, multiple febrile seizures or prolonged postictal period, history of irritability, poor feeding, or lethargy in young children, meningismus, and pretreatment with oral antibiotics. When in doubt, it is better to err on the side of an aggressive workup to rule out a life-threatening condition.

In interpreting the results of the LP, one should take into consideration that seizures per se may increase the number of white blood cells in the CSF. If herpes encephalitis is considered in the differential diagnosis, the first and last tube of CSF should be sent for cell count to differentiate traumatic from hemorrhagic spinal tap, and herpes polymerase chain reaction (PCR) should be ordered.

Neuroimaging

Computed tomography (CT) or magnetic resonance imaging (MRI) should be deferred in uncomplicated first or recurrent febrile seizures. Most children with febrile seizures do not have clinically important intracranial pathology. A CT or MRI may be indicated in children with abnormally large heads, complicated seizures (status epilepticus, persistent focality), suspicion of trauma, signs of increased intracranial pressure, cerebrospinal shunts, and those immunocompromised due to increased risk for abscesses. Other radiologic studies such as chest or sinus radiographs should be done as needed for evaluation of the origin of the fever. The AAP supports the recommendation that neuroimaging not be performed in the routine evaluation of children with a first simple febrile seizure. The yield of positive findings in emergency neuroimaging studies for complex febrile seizures is also very low.

Electroencephalogram

Routine electroencephalography (EEG) should also be deferred in children with febrile seizures. Routine EEGs are not predictive of future febrile seizures or epilepsy. The AAP recommends that EEGs not be performed in the evaluation of a normal child with a first simple febrile seizure.

Treatment

Antipyretics such as acetaminophen or ibuprofen at the time of febrile illnesses should be administered around the clock to make children more comfortable, but they may not prevent recurrence of febrile seizures. Cooling measures that may cause a quick drop in the body's temperature should be avoided because they can trigger seizures. Appropriate management of hydration is necessary to avoid further metabolic complications, such as hyponatremia.

Chronic treatment with antiepileptic (AED) medications is currently not recommended for children with febrile seizures. Although some AEDs are effective in controlling febrile seizures (ie, phenobarbital, valproate), they do not prevent epilepsy and their risks outweigh their benefits. Thus chronic treatment with phenobarbital for febrile seizure prophylaxis has been shown to cause a significant drop in IQ that persists 6 months after discontinuation of the medication. Valproate may have significant side effects in young children.

Most febrile seizures are brief and resolve on their own. Otherwise, AEDs should be administered acutely, such as rectal diazepam gel (Diastat), 0.3 mg/kg if at home, or intravenous (IV) lorazepam, 0.1 mg/kg if in the hospital. Intranasal midazolam (0.2 mg/kg) is also effective, although it can also be used through intramuscular, IV, or oral routes. Oral or rectal diazepam, administered intermittently at the time of fever detection, has demonstrated to be effective in decreasing the rate of seizure recurrence.

In prolonged febrile seizures and febrile status epilepticus, airway management and ABC resuscitation should be performed as in patients with afebrile status epilepticus. The treatment of febrile status epilepticus should follow a sequence of AED treatment similar to the one recommended in afebrile status. Benzodiazepines should be repeated 5 to 10 minutes after the first dose if this was ineffective. Other therapies for status include fosphenytoin, phenobarbital, valproate, levetiracetam, midazolam, and general anesthesia if seizures are refractory.

A multidisciplinary effort is essential for the treatment of children with prolonged seizures including physicians and nurses from the emergency department and the intensive care unit, and anesthesia and neurology specialists. A pediatric neurology consultation should be obtained for the acute management of patients with prolonged febrile seizures or status epilepticus, or with seizures accompanied by persistent focality, abnormal neurologic examination, suspected intracranial structural abnormalities, or unclear diagnosis.

Treatment with antibiotics or antivirals should be started for underlying infectious causes of febrile seizures. Antibiotics should be prescribed when treating bacterial infections that routinely would be treated in febrile patients without seizures. Broad-spectrum antibiotics should be used in patients with febrile status epilepticus, in whom a reliable examination cannot be obtained or in patients too ill for a lumbar puncture. Bacterial meningitis may be more common in cases of febrile status compared with simple febrile seizures; therefore, early LP and antibiotics are indicated. In children younger than 2 years, particularly if presenting with focal seizures, a frequent differential diagnosis includes herpes encephalitis. In these cases, an LP should be performed and initiation of treatment with acyclovir until herpes PCR results are available should be considered.

Children with simple febrile seizures with no suspicion of serious under-lying illness who are older than 18 months do not need to be routinely admitted to a hospital ward. The decision to admit should be individualized. Criteria for admission are age younger than 18 months, lethargy beyond the postictal state, unstable clinical status, complex febrile seizures, parental anxiety, and/or uncertain home situation. Diagnostic uncertainty is often more common in the first event of febrile seizures than in forthcoming events, but it is important to remember that a history of previous febrile seizures does not rule out the possibility of, for example, meningitis with later febrile seizures. Any child in whom there is the slightest suspicion of menin-gitis should be admitted.

Parental education and counseling is an important aspect of the treat-ment. Many parents or other caretakers faced for the first time with a febrile seizure may believe that the child is dying, and they develop serious anxiety, fear, and fever phobia. High levels of anxiety are more often found in parents with little or no knowledge of febrile seizures and with a low level of educa-tion. Adequate information on the nature and prognosis of febrile seizures should be provided and repeated. In those cases for which prophylactic treatment with diazepam is recommended, careful instructions regarding its use must also be provided and most probably repeated.

Prognosis

The recurrence rate of febrile seizures is 30% overall, and increases to 50% if the initial febrile seizure occurs in a child younger than 1 year. Of those who experience a second febrile seizure, the risk of recurrence increases 2-fold. Predictors of recurrent febrile seizures include family history of febrile sei-zures, previous complex seizures (focal, prolonged or multiple), influenza A viral infection, onset of febrile seizures younger than 12 months, and tem-perature less than 40°C at time of seizure.

Some patients with febrile seizures will develop afebrile seizures or epilepsy. Risk factors of developing epilepsy after febrile seizure include complex febrile seizures, neurologic abnormality, family history of epilepsy, and short duration of fever (<1 hour) before the seizure. Children with no risk factors have a 2.4% chance of developing afebrile seizures by age 25 years compared with 1.4% for the general population. Children with a history of at least one complex feature, a neurologic abnormality, and a family history have a 10% risk of developing epilepsy by age 7 years. Prolonged febrile seizures increase the incidence of epilepsy to 21%. For children with all 3 features of a complex febrile seizure, the risk increases to 49%.

Epilepsy following febrile seizures can be focal or generalized. In some cases, retrospectively, one can establish the diagnosis of the initial febrile seizure as the first epileptic seizure triggered by fever, because it is followed by afebrile seizures. Another type of epilepsy, the first manifestation of which may be a febrile seizure, is GEFS+, previously mentioned. Dravet syndrome or "severe myoclonic epilepsy of infancy" may also begin with febrile seizures during the first year of life in infants with normal psychomotor development. They further develop either generalized or unilateral clonic seizures, myoclonic jerks, and partial seizures, which are accompanied by psychomotor retardation and other neurologic deficits.

Some patients with a history of febrile seizures develop focal temporal lobe epilepsy, which is frequently refractory to treatment and is associated with the underlying pathological finding of hippocampal sclerosis (atrophic hippocampus).

The association between prolonged febrile seizures and hippocampal sclerosis continues to be controversial. Studies of patients with epilepsy and history of prolonged first febrile seizure have shown no decrease in hippocampal volume compared with patients with a simple febrile seizure who did not develop epilepsy. These results contradict several well-documented, individual prospective case studies linking prolonged febrile seizures to subsequent hippocampal swelling, atrophy, and sclerosis. Prolonged febrile seizures that predispose individuals to hippocampal sclerosis occur in clusters of unilateral or generalized febrile status epilepticus with unilateral ictal EEG discharges and prolonged postictal unresponsiveness.

Neuroimaging studies further support the concept of selective hippocampal vulnerability to prolonged or recurrent febrile seizures in susceptible individuals. Hippocampal volumetry reveals smaller total volumes and a larger right-to-left ratio in children with complex febrile seizures than in controls.

Some authors believe that the hippocampus is abnormal before the seizure with fever, predisposing the child to prolonged seizures and subsequent development of hippocampal sclerosis. Alternatively, it is possible that prolonged febrile seizures act in combination with later afebrile seizures to influence the development of hippocampal sclerosis.

Overall, febrile seizures have an excellent outcome. Population studies show normal intellect and behavior, even for children with complex febrile seizures. There is an increased risk of having impaired psychomotor development or cognitive outcome only in patients with a preexisting neurologic abnormality or those who subsequently developed epilepsy.

Web Sites

National Institute of Neurological Disorders and Stroke. Febrile seizures fact sheet: www.ninds.nih.gov/disorders/febrile_seizures/detail_febrile_seizures.htm/

Mayo Clinic: www.mayoclinic.com/health/febrile-seizure/DS00346

Bibliography

American Academy of Pediatrics Committee on Quality Improvement, Subcommittee on Febrile Seizures. Practice parameter: long-term treatment of the child with simple febrile seizures. *Pediatrics.* 1999;103:1307–1309

American Academy of Pediatrics Provisional Committee on Quality Improvement, Subcommittee on Febrile Seizures. Practice parameter: the neurodiagnostic evaluation of the child with a first simple febrile seizure. *Pediatrics.* 1996;97:769–772; discussion 773–775

Annegers JF, Hauser WA, Shirts SB, Kurland LT. Factors prognostic of unprovoked seizures after febrile convulsions. *N Engl J Med.* 1987;316:493–498

Audenaert D, Van Broeckhoven C, De Jonghe P. Genes and loci involved in febrile seizures and related epileptic syndromes. *Hum Mutat.* 2006;27:391–401

Baram TZ, Shinnar S. Febrile seizures. San Diego, CA: Academic Press; 2002:327

Berg AT, Shinnar S. Complex febrile seizures. *Epilepsia.* 1996;37:126–133

Berg AT, Shinnar S, Darefsky AS, et al. Predictors of recurrent febrile seizures. A prospective cohort study. *Arch Pediatr Adolesc Med.* 1997;151:371–378

Bethune P, Gordon K, Dooley J, Camfield C, Camfield P. Which child will have a febrile seizure? *Am J Dis Child.* 1993;147:35–39

Camfield PR, Camfield CS, Shapiro SH, Cummings C. The first febrile seizure—antipyretic instruction plus either phenobarbital or placebo to prevent recurrence. *J Pediatr.* 1980;97:16–21

Carroll W, Brookfield D. Lumbar puncture following febrile convulsion. *Arch Dis Child.* 2002;87:238–240

Chin RF, Neville BG, Scott RC. Meningitis is a common cause of convulsive status epilepticus with fever. *Arch Dis Child.* 2005;90:66–69

Commission on Epidemiology and Prognosis, International League Against Epilepsy. Guidelines for epidemiologic studies on epilepsy. *Epilepsia.* 1993;34:592–596

Consensus statement. Febrile seizures: long-term management of children with fever-associated seizures. *Pediatrics.* 1980;66:1009–1012

Dubé CM, Brewster AL, Richichi C, Zha Q, Baram TZ. Fever, febrile seizures and epilepsy. *Trends Neurosci.* 2007;30:490–496

Duchowny M. Febrile seizures. In: Wyllie E, Gupta A, Lachhwani DK, eds. *The Treatment of Epilepsy: Principles & Practice.* 4th ed. Philadelphia, PA: Lippincott Williams & Wilkins 2006:511–520

Fetveit A. Assessment of febrile seizures in children. *Eur J Pediatr.* 2008;167:17–27

Freeman JM, Vining EP. Febrile seizures: a decision-making analysis. *Am Fam Physician.* 1995;52:1409–1410

Green SM, Rothrock SG, Clem KJ, Zurcher RF, Mellick L. Can seizures be the sole manifestation of meningitis in febrile children? *Pediatrics.* 1993;92:527–534

Hoption Cann SA. Febrile seizures in young children: role of fluid intake and conservation. *Med Sci Monit.* 2007;13:RA159–RA167

Jones T, Jacobsen SJ. Childhood febrile seizures: overview and implications. *Int J Med Sci.* 2007;4:110–114

Kenney RD, Taylor JA. Absence of serum chemistry abnormalities in pediatric patients presenting with seizures. *Pediatr Emerg Care.* 1992;8:65–66

Maytal J, Steele R, Eviatar L, Novak G. The value of early postictal EEG in children with complex febrile seizures. *Epilepsia.* 2000;41:219–221

Meremikwu M, Oyo-Ita A. Paracetamol for treating fever in children. *Cochrane Database Syst Rev.* 2002; CD003676

Mewasingh LD. Febrile seizures. *Clin Evid.* 2006;15:415–422

Nakayama J, Arinami T. Molecular genetics of febrile seizures. *Epilepsy Res* 2006;70(S1): S190–S198.

Nelson KB, Ellenberg JH. Prenatal and perinatal antecedents of febrile seizures. *Ann Neurol.* 1990;27:127–131

Nelson KB, Ellenberg JH. Prognosis in children with febrile seizures. *Pediatrics.* 1978;61: 720–727

Nypaver MM, Reynolds SL, Tanz RR, Davis AT. Emergency department laboratory evaluation of children with seizures: dogma or dilemma? *Pediatr Emerg Care.* 1992;8:13–16

Offringa M, Bossuyt PM, Lubsen J, et al. Risk factors for seizure recurrence in children with febrile seizures: a pooled analysis of individual patient data from five studies. *J Pediatr.* 1994;124:574–584

Rosman NP, Colton T, Labazzo J, et al. A controlled trial of diazepam administered during febrile illnesses to prevent recurrence of febrile seizures. *N Engl J Med.* 1993;329:79–84

Sadleir LG, Scheffer IE. Febrile seizures. *BMJ.* 2007;334:307–311

Teach SJ, Geil PA. Incidence of bacteremia, urinary tract infections, and unsuspected bacterial meningitis in children with febrile seizures. *Pediatr Emerg Care.* 1999;15:9–12

Teng, D, Dayan, P, Tyler, S, et al. Risk of intracranial pathologic conditions requiring emergency intervention after a first complex febrile seizure episode among children. *Pediatrics.* 2006;117:304–308

Trainor JL, Hampers LC, Krug SE, Listernick R. Children with first-time simple febrile seizures are at low risk of serious bacterial illness. *Acad Emerg Med.* 2001;8:781–787

van Esch A, Steyerberg EW, van Duijn CM, Offringa M, Derksen-Lubsen G, van Steensel-Moll HA. Prediction of febrile seizures in siblings: a practical approach. *Eur J Pediatr.* 1998;157: 340–344

van Stuijvenberg M, Derksen-Lubsen G, Steyerberg EW, Habbema JD, Moll HA. Randomized, controlled trial of ibuprofen syrup administered during febrile illnesses to prevent febrile seizure recurrences. *Pediatrics.* 1998;102:e51

Verity CM, Greenwood R, Golding J. Long-term intellectual and behavioral outcomes of children with febrile convulsions. *N Engl J Med.* 1998;338:1723–1728

Verrotti A, Giuva T, Cutarella R, Morgese G, Chiarelli F. Febrile convulsions after 5 years of age: long-term follow-up. *J Child Neurol.* 2000;15:811–813

Wallace SJ, Smith JA. Successful prophylaxis against febrile convulsions with valproic acid or phenobarbitone. *Br Med J.* 1980;280:353–354

Waruiru C, Appleton R. Febrile seizures: an update. *Arch Dis Child.* 2004;89:751–756

Chapter 9

Epilepsy

Sanjeev V. Kothare, MD
Divya S. Khurana, MD
Joseph Madsen, MD
Alexander Papanastassiou, MD

Introduction

Epilepsy is the term given to recurrent convulsive or non-convulsive seizures caused by partial or generalized epileptogenic discharges in the cerebrum. It has been defined by the International League Against Epilepsy (ILAE) as "a transient occurrence of signs and/or symptoms due to abnormal excessive or synchronous neuronal activity in the brain."

To establish the diagnosis of epilepsy the patient must have at least 2 seizures (non-febrile). Until recently, 2 or mores seizures occurring within 24 hours were considered "one seizure episode," but epidemiological studies have shown that the risk of further developing epilepsy is the same as for 2 or more seizures occurring days apart.

Recent estimates of the prevalence of single and recurrent non-febrile seizures in children younger than 10 years range from 5.2 to 8.1 per 1,000. By age 40 the cumulative incidence is 1.7% to 1.9%.

Classification

The epilepsies can be classified as primary (idiopathic), secondary (symptomatic), or reactive. The term *primary* implies that, with current knowledge, no structural or biochemical cause for recurrent seizures can be identified. In general, the primary epilepsies are genetically transmitted and tend to have a better prognosis for seizure control. The term *secondary* or *symptomatic* epilepsy indicates that the cause of the seizure is known. Such seizures occur as a manifestation of many congenital or acquired conditions of the nervous system or can complicate systemic disease. Epilepsy can also be designated as cryptogenic, implying that the underlying etiology is symptomatic but not readily demonstrable by available diagnostic techniques. In reactive epilepsies, seizures are due to the abnormal reaction of an otherwise normal brain to physiological stress or transient insult.

The ILAE divides the clinical manifestations into partial seizures, which begin in a part of one hemisphere, and generalized seizures, which begin in both hemispheres simultaneously (Box 9-1). Localization-related (partial or focal) seizures are classified into simple, complex and secondarily generalized. During simple partial seizures, consciousness is preserved, whereas during complex partial seizures, there is alteration or impairment of consciousness. Abnormal discharges that begin in a discrete area of the brain give rise to partial epileptic seizures and can propagate over time. Thus simple partial seizures can evolve into complex partial seizures, and both can evolve into secondarily generalized convulsive seizures.

The descriptive classification of epilepsy syndromes is extremely useful clinically, especially in pediatric epilepsy. Epilepsy syndromes are classified by a combination of distinctive features: age of onset, seizure types, electroencephalographic (EEG) features, and prognosis. Childhood epilepsy syndromes can be considered as benign or catastrophic based on their responsiveness to treatment, possibility of seizure remission, and long-term prognosis for cognitive development (Table 9-1).

Common Epilepsy Syndromes in Children

Catastrophic Epilepsy Syndromes of Childhood Associated With an Epileptic Encephalopathy

Infantile Spasms (West Syndrome)

Infantile spasms are classified as symptomatic or cryptogenic. A variety of prenatal and perinatal insults such as intrauterine infections, complications of prematurity, neuronal migrational disorders, perinatal asphyxia, and traumatic brain injury account for the symptomatic group. Tuberous sclerosis is also a major etiologic factor; therefore, a careful examination of the skin for hypomelanotic skin lesions is mandated. Recent reports have described patients with deletion in chromosome 7q11.23-q21.11, involving the MAGI2 gene, which encodes the synaptic scaffolding protein membrane-associated guanylate kinase inverted-2 that interacts with stargazin, a protein also associated with epilepsy in the stargazer mouse.

Box 9-1. Classification of Epileptic Seizures[a]

1. Partial (focal or local) seizures
   Simple partial seizures
       Seizures with motor signs
       Seizures with somatosensory or special sensory symptoms
       Seizures with autonomic symptoms or signs
       Seizures with psychic symptoms
   Complex partial (psychomotor) seizures
       Simple partial onset followed by impairment of consciousness
       Seizures with impairment of consciousness at onset
   Partial seizures evolving to secondarily generalized (tonic-clonic) seizures
       Simple partial evolving to generalized seizures
       Complex partial evolving to generalized seizures
   Simple partial seizures evolving to complex partial seizures evolving to generalized seizures

2. Generalized seizures (convulsive and non-convulsive)
   Absence seizures
       Typical absence seizures (petit mal attacks)
       Atypical absence seizures (atypical petit mal attacks)
   Myoclonic seizures
   Clonic seizures
   Tonic seizures
   Tonic-clonic seizures (grand mal seizures)
   Atonic seizures (akinetic or astatic seizures)

3. Unclassified epileptic seizures

[a]*From Commission on Classification and Terminology of the International League Against Epilepsy. Proposal for revised clinical and electroencephalographic classification of epileptic seizures.* Epilepsia. *1981;22:489.*

Infantile spasms most commonly develop between 3 and 8 months of age. Attacks can be either flexor with repeated episodes of head and trunk flexion (also known as *salaam spells*), extensor with extension of the arms and head, or mixed flexor and extensor. A cry or giggling can precede or follow the seizure; therefore, they are at times misdiagnosed as attacks of infantile colic. Clusters of seizures occur typically on awakening or with onset of drowsiness, and some children can have 50 to 100 per day. With onset of spasms, there is usually regression or plateau in acquisition of developmental milestones. In most patients, the electroencephalogram (EEG) will show the characteristic pattern of hypsarrhythmia (Figure 9-1), namely slowing and disorganization of background rhythms with high voltage

Table 9-1. Classification of Epilepsies and Epilepsy Syndromes[a]		
	With Generalized Seizures	**With Partial (focal seizures)**
Primary (idiopathic) epilepsies Without structural lesions, benign, genetic	Childhood absence epilepsy Juvenile absence epilepsy Juvenile myoclonic epilepsy	Benign epilepsy with centro-temporal spikes (rolandic epilepsy) Childhood epilepsy with occipital spikes
Secondary (symptomatic) epilepsies with anatomical or known biochemical lesions	Infantile spasms Lennox-Gastaut syndrome	Temporal lobe epilepsy caused by mesial temporal sclerosis Epilepsies caused by gray matter heterotopias, polymicrogyria Epilepsies caused by focal post-asphyxial gliosis
Conditions with reactive seizures Abnormal reaction of an otherwise normal brain to physiological stress or transient epileptogenic insult	Febrile seizures Most toxic and metabolic induced seizures Many isolated tonic-clonic seizures Early posttraumatic seizures	Head trauma, hypernatremia, hypoglycemia

[a]Adapted from Engel J. *Seizures and Epilepsy*. Philadelphia, PA; FA Davis; 1989.

slow waves and multiple spike-wave discharges. In some infants, the typical changes are most evident in non–rapid eye movement (REM) sleep, with the EEG appearing normal in wakefulness and REM sleep.

Cryptogenic spasms tend to be associated with a better prognosis. However, in most children, the outlook for normal cognitive development is poor, even though in approximately 50%, spasms cease by 3 years of age or are replaced by other seizure types.

Management of infantile spasms requires referral to a specialist.

Lennox Gastaut Syndrome

This epilepsy syndrome is characterized by an early age of onset (two-thirds with onset between 2 and 14 years of age), an EEG characterized by slow spike wave forms at 1 to 2 Hz (Figure 9-2), and a poor prognosis both for seizure control and ultimate cognitive development.

There are multiple causes for Lennox-Gastaut syndrome (LGS). Prenatal causes appear to be the most frequent, followed by perinatal asphyxia,

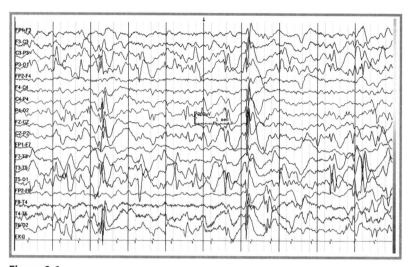

Figure 9-1.
Electroencephalogram showing hypsarrhythmia with a disorganized background and multifocal spike wave epileptiform activity.

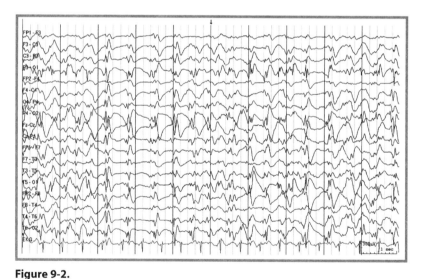

Figure 9-2.
Electroencephalogram of Lennox-Gastaut syndrome with repetitive slow spike wave epileptiform activity.

infections, and genetic factors. Children with infantile spasms often go on to develop LGS.

Seizure types are multiple and include atonic, tonic, myoclonic, and atypical absence seizures. Atonic or akinetic seizures are characterized by a sudden, momentary loss of posture or muscle tone and in older children can cause sudden falls to the ground with injuries to the face and head. Tonic seizures are characterized by a brief, generalized increase in muscle tone and are generally the most common seizure type in LGS, as well as the type most resistant to anticonvulsant treatment. Atypical absence seizures are episodes of absence-like seizures that, unlike true absence seizures, tend to last longer than a few seconds to a few minutes and occur in cycles. Myoclonic seizures are episodes of single or repetitive muscle contractions associated with EEG changes of frontally predominant discharges.

Episodes of non-convulsive status epilepticus are frequent. Commonly they are characterized by alternation of tonic attacks and episodes of confused behavior and can last from hours to days. Mental retardation is present before onset of seizures in 20% to 60% of cases and in 90% 5 years after onset.

Management of LGS requires referral to a specialist.

Benign Epilepsy Syndromes

Childhood Absence Epilepsy

This is a generalized epilepsy that is inherited as an autosomal dominant trait. The locus for childhood absence epilepsy persisting with tonic-clonic seizures has been mapped to chromosome 8q24. Several studies have suggested specific genes as candidates for susceptibility to develop this type of epilepsy: TASK3 potassium channel gene *KCNK9* on chromosome 8q24, chloride channel gene *CLCN2* located on chromosome 3q26, voltage-gated calcium channel gene *CACNG3* on chromosome 16p12-p13.1, and T-type calcium channel gene *CACNA1H* on chromosome 16p.

Typical absence seizures usually are seen in children between the ages of 5 to 9 years. They are characterized by brief episodes of arrest of consciousness lasting 5 to 10 seconds, appearing without warning or aura. The seizure terminates abruptly and the child is often unaware of the event. Onset of seizures is usually abrupt, and children can develop 20 or more episodes daily. Some absence attacks can involve behavioral automatisms such as lip smacking and eye rolling and can be mistaken for complex partial seizures. The EEG of absence epilepsy is characteristic and during a typical event, which is usually easily elicited by hyperventilation, shows high amplitude 3 Hz spike and wave discharges (Figure 9-3).

The most common differential is episodes of daydreaming or attention-deficit disorder, which can also occur multiple times daily and can last several seconds to minutes. Attacks are not induced by hyperventilation, and the EEG is normal. Sometimes, complex partial seizures need to be considered in the differential diagnosis; in this case, there is usually an aura, the ictal event lasts minutes instead of seconds, there is postictal lethargy, and the EEG shows focal epileptiform discharges.

While most children with absence epilepsy respond to treatment, absences may persist into adulthood in a small proportion of cases, and generalized tonic-clonic (GTC) seizures develop in about 10% to 30% of patients followed into adulthood.

Juvenile Absence and Juvenile Myoclonic Epilepsy

Childhood absence epilepsy can be a prelude to juvenile absence epilepsy (JAE). Typical features of JAE are episodes of absence seen with age of onset later than typical childhood absence epilepsy. Brief myoclonic jerks that

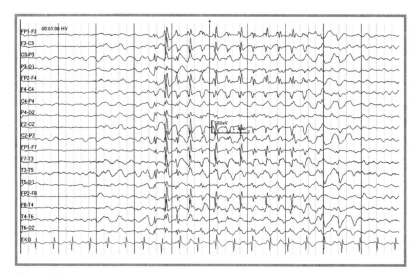

Figure 9-3.
Electroencephalogram of absence epilepsy showing 3 Hz spike and wave activity. (Heavier vertical bars represent 1 second intervals.)

generally occur on awakening develop around 15 years of age, and tonic-clonic seizures develop some months thereafter. Attacks occur much less frequently than in absence seizures. The interictal EEG in JAE can show epileptiform discharges at 3Hz as well as at 4 to 6 Hz. Features of JAE often overlap with juvenile myoclonic epilepsy (JME).

Juvenile myoclonic epilepsy has a prevalence of 0.5 to 1.0 per 1,000 and represents 4% of the primary generalized epilepsies. A genetic contribution to JME has long been established, although the mode of inheritance is unclear. Autosomal dominant, autosomal recessive, 2 loci, and multifactorial models have been proposed.

Symptoms in JME usually appear in adolescence and are characterized by episodes of myoclonic jerks on awakening. More than 90% also experience GTC seizures, and 30% have absence seizures. The interictal EEG is characteristic and displays 4- to 6-Hz polyspike and wave complexes (Figure 9-4) with photosensitivity at 30%. Valproic acid is effective in up to 90% of patients but typically has to be continued for the remainder of the patient's life, because withdrawal of anticonvulsants results in seizure recurrence in 90% of patients.

Benign Rolandic Epilepsy With Centro-Temporal Spikes

This is the most common idiopathic focal epilepsy. Age of onset is typically between 5 and 10 years. It has been postulated that classic benign rolandic epilepsy (BRE) is partially determined by genetic factors, mediated to some extent via the centro-temporal spikes (CTS) trait. However, recent studies in monozygous and dizygous twin pairs have shown that the genetic influence in BRE is far less than that of the other major idiopathic generalized epilepsies. The obligatory CTS trait is likely to have a polygenic or multifactorial basis. A full understanding of the cause of BRE must look beyond traditional genetics and consider mechanisms such as environmental factors, somatic mutations, and epigenetic influences.

Seizures are infrequent, occurring less than 3 to 4 times a year in most. Attacks begin with a somatosensory aura, usually referred to as the *tongue and cheek,* followed by speech arrest, excessive salivation, and tonic-clonic movements involving the face. The interictal EEG shows midtemporal and CTS and, in 30%, spikes are seen only during sleep (Figure 9-5). The prognosis in this condition is excellent, with most children responding to antiepileptic medications. Most patients stop having seizures in their teens.

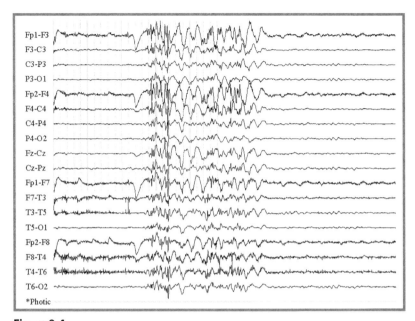

Figure 9-4.

Electroencephalogram of juvenile myoclonic epilepsy with generalized polyspike wave discharges.

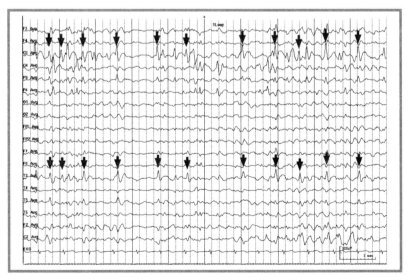

Figure 9-5.

Electroencephalogram with centro-temporal spikes (black arrowheads) seen during sleep in a child with benign rolandic epilepsy. In this epoch the spikes were most prominent in the left central (C3) and mid temporal (T3) regions.

Some studies have shown that the treatment of seizures does not affect the outcome and, therefore, in patients with infrequent seizures, the use of rectal diazepam to treat the acute events and avoiding chronic antiepileptic drug (AED) treatment may be an acceptable management choice.

Benign Epilepsy of Childhood With Occipital Spikes (Panayiotopoulos Syndrome)

This is less frequently seen than rolandic epilepsy, accounting for 6% of all children with seizures. Age of onset is in younger children, with the peak age being 5 years. Seizures are infrequent. Attacks can begin with hemianopia, visual hallucinations, or phosphenes (white or colored luminous spots) and can be followed by unilateral convulsions, automatisms, or GTC seizures. Ictal eye deviation and vomiting can be seen, and postictal migraine can be seen in up to one half of patients. The interictal EEG shows frequent unilateral or bilateral high-voltage spike wave discharges from the occipital of posterior temporal regions. The prognosis is excellent, and 89% to 100% of children gain remission by age 9 to 13 years.

Localization-Related Epilepsies in Children

Temporal Lobe Epilepsy

Temporal lobe epilepsy is the most common cause of complex partial seizures. In older children and adolescents, the most common syndrome is that of mesial temporal lobe epilepsy. The syndrome is associated with atrophy and gliosis of the hippocampus and of the amygdala. A history of febrile seizures is found in approximately 40% to 60% of patients. Partial seizures start in the first 10 years of life and tend to become more severe with by automatisms such as lip smacking, licking, and swallowing. Dystonic posturing of the arm is often seen. The EEG usually shows an interictal anterior temporal spike focus. Magnetic resonance imaging (MRI) shows atrophy of the hippocampus, loss of its internal structure, and increased T2 signal. The outcome of this syndrome following surgery is usually good.

Frontal Lobe Epilepsy

Frontal lobe epilepsy can be secondary to structural lesions or it can be transmitted as an autosomal dominant trait with a reduced penetrance of 70% to 80% (autosomal dominant nocturnal frontal lobe epilepsy). It has been associated with mutations of the genes coding for the β-4 (CHRNA4), β-2 (CHRNB2), and β-2 (CHRNA2) subunits of the neuronal nicotinic ace-tylcholine receptors, and for the corticotrophin-releasing hormone.

Seizures of frontal lobe origin may look like complex partial seizures. These children are often misdiagnosed as having psychogenic events, because associated automatisms can be complex and often violent, with rocking, kicking, and dystonic activity. Seizures tend to be primarily noc-turnal, frequently repeated, of brief duration, and with only a brief or no postictal period. Electroencephalogram abnormalities are frequently absent interictally and sometimes ictally.

Neonatal Seizures

The main types of neonatal seizures are shown in Table 9-2. Only some of the behaviors described as neonatal seizures are associated with rhythmic epileptogenic EEG discharges. Other behaviors, which include most tonic, and subtle seizures, are not accompanied by EEG correlates. It has been proposed that these represent brain stem "release" phenomena from corti-cal inhibition. Most neonatal seizures are either symptomatic of underlying cerebral injury or provoked by a metabolic derangement. Box 9-2 lists the main causes of neonatal seizures.

Table 9-2. Features of Neonatal Seizures		
Type of Seizure	**Clinical Features**	**Ictal EEG Discharges**
Tonic, generalized	Sustained posturing of neck and trunk sometimes provoked by stimulation	Rarely present
Tonic, focal	Sustained posturing of single limb, sustained eye deviation not suppressed by restraint	Present in some cases
Clonic, focal, or multifocal	Rhythmic jerks, focal or multifocal. Not suppressed by restraint.	Almost always present
Myoclonic	Arrhythmical, non-repetitive jerks, gener-alized, focal or fragmentary	Frequently present in generalized forms
Subtle or minimal seizures or motor automatisms	Roving eye movements, blinking, grimac-ing, sucking, chewing, tongue thrusting, swimming, boxing, or cycling movements, suppressed by restraint and precipitated by stimulation	Seldom present

Abbreviation: EEG, electroencephalogram.

Box 9-2. Causes of Neonatal Seizures

Hypoxic-ischemic encephalopathy (may produce epileptic and non-epileptic seizures)

Intracranial hemorrhage

   Subarachnoid hemorrhage (clonic seizures in term infants 1–5 days of age)

Intraventricular hemorrhage (mainly tonic seizures and episodes of apnea without electroencephalogram (EEG) correlates, occasionally typical EEG discharges)

Intracerebral hematoma (fixed, localized clonic seizures)

Intracranial infections

   Bacterial meningitis

   Viral meningoencephalitis

Cerebral malformations

   Myoclonic and focal tonic seizures

Metabolic causes

   Hypocalcemia (clonic, multifocal seizures)

   Hypoglycemia

   Hyponatremia

   Inborn errors of amino acids or organic acids and urea cycle disorders

   Pyridoxine dependency

   Biotinidase deficiency

   Folinic acid–responsive seizures

   Molybdenum cofactor deficiency

   Bilirubin encephalopathy

   Carbohydrate-deficient glycoprotein syndrome

   Glucose transporter defect

Toxic or withdrawal seizures

Familial neonatal convulsions

   Clonic localized, shifting seizures with EEG correlates

Benign neonatal seizures of unknown origin (fifth-day fits)

   Clonic and apneic seizures with typical EEG correlates

Status Epilepticus

Status epilepticus is defined as a seizure lasting more than 30 minutes or recurrent seizures lasting more than 30 minutes from which the patient does not regain consciousness (ILAE 1981). The classification of status epilepticus is based on the observation of clinical events combined with EEG information whenever possible (Box 9-3).

Differential Diagnosis

A thorough history is essential for arriving at the diagnosis of an epileptic seizure. Generalized tonic-clonic seizures are usually easy to identify, although psychogenic seizures should be kept in mind. Grand mal seizures should also be distinguished from syncope (typically more common in female adolescents) and from breath-holding spells in younger children. Box 9-4 lists a variety of conditions that can mimic seizures.

Box 9-3. Classification of Status Epilepticus

Partial

Convulsive

Tonic: hemiclonic status epilepticus, hemiconvulsion-hemiplegia epilepsy

Clonic: hemi-grand mal status epilepticus

Non-convulsive

Simple: focal motor status, focal sensory, epilepsia partialis continua, adversive status epilepticus

Complex partial: epileptic fugue state, prolonged epileptic stupor, temporal lobe status epilepticus

Generalized

Convulsive

Tonic-clonic: grand mal, status epilepticus convulsivus

Tonic

Clonic

Myoclonic: myoclonic status epilepticus

Non-convulsive

Absence

Spike and wave stupor, petit mal epileptic fugue

Undetermined

Subtle: epileptic coma

Neonatal

Box 9-4. Episodic Disorders That Mimic Seizures

Benign neonatal sleep myoclonus

Jitteriness of newborns (including drug withdrawal in maternal addiction)

Breath-holding spells

Gastroesophageal reflux (Sandifer syndrome)

Sleep disorders including pavor nocturnus, sleep myoclonus, and narcolepsy

Abnormal startle reaction (hyperekplexia)

Infantile shuddering attacks

Nocturnal paroxysmal dystonia

Migraine and syncope

Habit spasms, tics, Tourette syndrome

Pseudoseizures

Benign paroxysmal vertigo of childhood

Diagnostic Workup

Blood Chemistries

In our experience, the routine request of blood chemistries, including glucose and electrolytes, in the workup of an acute seizure in young infants and children is not cost-effective, because they are abnormal only in 15% of cases. We recommend performance of these tests in children younger than 2 years presenting with a first seizure or when accompanied by gastrointestinal or diffuse neurologic symptoms. Renal function should be obtained in neonates. Serum hyponatremia (sodium <125 mEq/L) is frequently associated with seizures, particularly if there is a suspicious history of excessive water intake. Serum and urine toxicology screen are frequently indicated for all first-time seizures, particularly when no other cause is apparent.

Electroencephalogram

The EEG is useful in confirming the diagnosis of seizures, because "not everything that shakes is epilepsy," and there is a broad differential diagnosis of non-epileptic events. It also helps to determine the seizure type of a particular patient; for example, it differentiates between complex partial and absence seizures, or between typical and atypical absence attacks. It is the best predictor of the likelihood of seizure recurrence. The EEG needs to be interpreted in conjunction with the child's history. A normal EEG can be seen in one-half of patients with epilepsy, so it does not exclude the diagnosis of epilepsy. Conversely, an abnormal EEG does not necessarily establish the diagnosis of epilepsy either. An EEG obtained within 24 hours of a seizure is more likely to show epileptiform abnormalities. A sleep-deprived EEG can increase the yield of abnormal findings. If typical events occur frequently enough and a routine EEG is unremarkable, prolonged EEG monitoring done either inpatient or outpatient for up to 3 days at a time can be useful in capturing typical events and distinguishing epileptic from non-epileptic events, as well as in characterizing epileptic seizures.

Lumbar Puncture

While lumbar puncture is not performed routinely in patients with epilepsy, it is usually indicated in children with their first febrile seizure and in all infants with their first seizure. Obviously, it is the diagnostic test in cases of suspected meningitis or encephalitis.

Neuroimaging Studies

Neuroimaging studies should be obtained for children who present with a first seizure and are at risk for an intracranial abnormality. Risk factors include an abnormal neurologic examination, dysmorphic features, skin lesions suggestive of phakomatoses, history of malignancy, sickle cell disease, bleeding disorder, closed head injury or travel to an area endemic for cysticercosis, history of neonatal seizures or seizures compatible with partial onset, and focal EEG abnormalities, including children with benign rolandic epilepsy. Patients with a normal neurologic examination and a normal EEG have a low yield of positive scan results as do children with primary generalized seizures, particularly those with absence epilepsy.

In children younger than 33 months with focal seizures, computed tomography (CT) scans may be abnormal in up to 29%. In children with non-focal seizures and no predisposing conditions, only approximately 2% of CTs are abnormal. However, MRI is the preferred initial screening procedure in the evaluation of a child with seizures. Magnetic resonance imaging detects congenital malformations of the cortex, gray matter heterotopias, arteriovenous malformations, and neoplasms, while CT scans are more sensitive to foci of calcification or hemorrhage.

The Management of Epilepsy in Children and Teenagers

Epilepsy is defined as more than one unprovoked seizure. The goal of epilepsy management is to achieve seizure freedom with minimum side effects. Treatment of a first unprovoked seizure does decrease the risk of a second seizure. However, AED treatment does not seem to prevent the development of epilepsy and may carry the unnecessary risks of side effects, drug interactions, social stigmatization, and psychological burdens of chronic drug therapy. Also, once initiated, the AED is usually given for several years.

Although numerous guidelines and consensus statements are available, choosing an appropriate AED can pose a challenge to the treating physician. In addition, these guidelines may be inadequate for specific epilepsy syndromes or in age-specific patient populations like children and teenagers. In general, initial treatment of epilepsy should begin with AED monotherapy. Selection of an appropriate AED should be based on careful consideration of age, sex, epilepsy type and syndrome, coexisting comorbidities, concomitant medications, and lifestyle of the patient, in addition to the efficacy, tolerability, and side effect profile of the AED. If the patient fails the initial trial, the next step is to try monotherapy with a second AED. Combination therapy (rational polytherapy) should be considered only if the patient fails at least 2 monotherapy trials. The ultimate goal of any epilepsy therapy is to maintain optimal quality of life by achieving complete seizure freedom with no drug-induced side effects.

Choice of Antiepileptic Drugs

Antiepileptic drugs remain the mainstay of the treatment of epilepsy. Since 1857, when potassium bromide was first recognized as the first effective chemical for controlling seizures, multiple agents have been discovered. Antiepileptic drugs introduced in the US market before 1980 are referred to as *older (first generation)* AEDs, while 10 new agents approved since 1993 are called *newer (second generation)* AEDs. The older AEDs have multiple advantages, including familiarity, well-documented efficacy, long-term experience, lower cost, and effectiveness against a broad range of seizure types. However, their use is limited by adverse effects, complex pharmacokinetics, and significant effects on liver cytochrome P450 enzymes. Even though clinical studies have demonstrated that older and newer AEDs have similar efficacy when given as monotherapy, newer AEDs have less impact on hepatic metabolism, simpler pharmacokinetics, less frequent drug inter-actions, better tolerability, and fewer side effects. However, they are significantly more expensive and therefore face difficulty in approval from many third-party payers.

Older Antiepileptic Drugs

Phenobarbital

Introduced in 1912, it is indicated for the treatment of GTC and partial seizures. It remains the first choice of drugs in the treatment of neonatal seizures and is an important AED in the treatment of status epilepticus. It binds to the barbiturate site at the γ-aminobutyric acid (GABA) receptor complex, enhancing inhibitory activity. Side effects include impact on behavior and cognition, paradoxical excitement, hyperkinetic activity, decreased attention span, sedation, rash, folate deficiency, bone loss.

Phenytoin

Discovered by Merritt and Putnam in 1938, it is indicated for the treatment of GTC and partial seizures, and it is the second line of treatment for status epilepticus after benzodiazepines (diazepam or lorazepam). Phosphenytoin, an ester of phenytoin, was introduced in 1996 to reduce the risk of intrave-nous thrombophlebitis while maintaining equal efficacy to phenytoin. It acts on the sodium channel. It is not effective for and may worsen myoclonic, absence, and tonic/atonic drop attacks. Due to nonlinear elimination phar-macokinetics, frequent monitoring of serum levels is necessary after changes in dosage or if there is potential for drug interaction with use of other medi-cations to avoid toxicity. Side effects include early non–dose-related hyper-sensitivity reactions including Stevens-Johnson syndrome, and dose-related ataxia, lethargy, sedation, and encephalopathy. Chronic effects include gin-gival hyperplasia, hirsutism, hematologic abnormalities, neurologic effects, such as cerebellar atrophy, and systemic manifestations, such as lupus, thy-roiditis, and bone loss.

Ethosuximide

Marketed in 1960, it is still considered first-line treatment of absence sei-zures; it does not, however, work against associated GTC seizures. It alters thalamocortical signals through the inhibition of thalamic T-type calcium currents, which have a role in the generation of the 3-second spike-wave activity. Side effects include mild gastrointestinal complaints, sedation or insomnia, headaches, dizziness, and suppression of bone marrow.

Benzodiazepines

Since diazepam was introduced in 1968, several other benzodiazepines like clonazepam, lorazepam, and midazolam are also available. They act via inhibition of neuronal excitation at the level of chloride channels, through specific binding to GABA-A receptors. Rectal diazepam is approved to abort prolonged seizures; intravenous lorazepam as first-line treatment of status epilepticus; intravenous midazolam for treatment of refractory status epilepticus; and clonazepam as adjunctive therapy of myoclonic seizures, drop attacks of LGS, and infantile spasms. Side effects include sedation, tolerance, and cardiovascular and respiratory depression.

Carbamazepine

It was approved as an AED in 1974 and is indicated for the treatment of partial and secondary GTC seizures. It may worsen myoclonic and absence seizures. Similar to phenytoin, it acts on the sodium channel. Common adverse events include drowsiness, nausea, diplopia, headache, dizziness, ataxia, leukopenia, skin rash, and hyponatremia.

Valproate

Approved for the treatment of epilepsy in 1978, it has broad-spectrum activity against many seizure types. It is a highly efficacious AED, and it is considered first-line treatment for primary generalized epilepsy such as absences, GTC seizures, and myoclonic seizures. It also has proven efficacy in the treatment of partial seizures and infantile spasms, and in the various seizure types seen in patients with LGS. Valproate potentiates GABA activity, reduces glutamate excitation, and inhibits voltage-sensitive sodium channels. Adverse events include dose-dependent tremors, nausea, vomiting, weight gain, drowsiness, thrombocytopenia, bleeding dyscrasias, hyperammonemia, encephalopathy, and alopecia. The most feared side effects include hepatotoxicity and hemorrhagic pancreatitis. Hepatotoxicity is linked to age younger than 2 years, polytherapy, mental retardation, organic brain disease, or congenital metabolic disorders. The role of valproate in the development of polycystic ovarian disease and its teratogenic effects on the developing fetus has received attention in recent years.

Newer Antiepileptic Drugs

Felbamate

Introduced in 1993, it is approved to be used as adjunctive therapy in patients with LGS with drop attacks. It has dual mechanisms related to both excitatory N-methyl-D-aspartate and inhibitory GABA receptors. Its common side effects include anorexia, insomnia, and weight loss. Its rare but potential life-threatening side effects include aplastic anemia and hepatic failure. It is also a drug with significant drug interactions, and periodic drug level monitoring along with complete blood count and liver function testing are essential with its use in clinical practice.

Gabapentin

It has been in use since 1994 as an AED, and it is approved for treatment of partial seizures as adjunctive therapy in patients older than 3 years. It has also been used to treat patients with benign rolandic epilepsy. It has no drug interactions and no fatal (black box warning) side effects. Although it is structurally related to GABA, the exact mechanism of action is unclear. In recent years, it has been more widely used off-label to treat various pain syndromes. Adverse events include somnolence, dizziness, ataxia, behavioral effects, weight gain, and movement disorders.

Lamotrigine

Marketed since 1994, it is a broad-spectrum AED. It is approved to be used as adjunctive therapy in patients older than 2 years with partial epilepsy and for the drop attacks seen in LGS, and it is also effective in various generalized epilepsy syndromes including absences and JME. However, it may worsen the myoclonic seizures in patients with JME and severe myoclonic epilepsy of infancy. It acts by blockade of the sodium channel, resulting in inhibition of glutamate release. The slow titration of the drug is one of its limitations; even more so in patients with concomitant valproate therapy. Faster escalation may lead to a serious drug rash including Stevens-Johnsons syndrome. Other adverse effects include dizziness, sedation, headache, diplopia, ataxia, and insomnia.

Topiramate

It has been available since 1997, and it is indicated for children older than 2 years as adjunctive therapy of partial seizures and drop attacks of LGS.

It is also useful in various generalized epilepsy syndromes including JME, absences, and infantile spasms. Topiramate has also been widely used for prophylaxis against migraine and other pain syndromes. It is a weak carbonic anhydrase inhibitor, although other mechanisms of action include blockade of sodium channels, potentiation of GABA inhibition, and blockade of glutamate-mediated neuron excitation. Common adverse effects include weight loss, paresthesias, cognitive deficits, sedation, oligohydrosis, metabolic acidosis, glaucoma, and nephrolithiasis.

Tiagabine
Also approved in 1997, it is indicated as adjunctive therapy in children older than 12 years with partial seizures. It inhibits synaptic reuptake of GABA. Its use in patients with epilepsy has declined in recent years, maybe related to lack of efficacy and the possibility of developing non-convulsive status epilepticus. Side effects include dizziness, asthenia, and tremors. Buckling of the knees has been associated with use of tiagabine and may represent a negative myoclonus. It has found some use in the reduction of spasticity seen in patients with cerebral palsy and improving slow-wave sleep in patients with insomnia.

Levetiracetam
It was approved at the end of 1999, and it is indicated to be used as adjunctive therapy in partial epilepsy in children older than 4 years. It has recently also received approval for use in JME and primary generalized epilepsy. It is a broad-spectrum AED with no drug interactions or black box warnings. It has been used first line in patients with brain tumors and patients with HIV with seizures because it does not interfere with the metabolism of the chemotherapeutic agents and anti-AIDS medications. It acts on specific binding sites within the brain on a specific receptor (SV22 protein), leading to reduction in high-voltage–activated calcium currents. Side effects include mood and behavioral changes, somnolence, asthenia, and dizziness.

Oxcarbazepine
Approved as an AED in 2000, it is indicated as first-line monotherapy in patients older than 2 years with partial seizures. The active metabolite of oxcarbazepine is a 10-mono-hydroxy derivative that blocks the sodium channel like carbamazepine. Unlike carbamazepine; however, it does not

involve the epoxide metabolite, which is responsible for some of the neurologic side effects of carbamazepine. It also does not induce the cytochrome P450 enzyme system. Side effects include hyponatremia and drug rash, the 2 most important ones; asthenia; sedation; ataxia; and drowsiness.

Zonisamide

Also approved for the treatment of epilepsy in 2000, it is indicated to be used as adjunctive therapy in patients older than 16 years with partial epilepsy. However, it has been widely used in Japan prior to its release in the United States and has been found to be efficacious in patients with infantile spasms and various primary generalized epilepsies, including JME, and absences, and also in the drop attacks associated with LGS. It is a sulfonamide derivative that acts by blocking the T-type calcium channels. Because it is a carbonic anhydrase inhibitor, side effects are similar to those of topiramate.

Other Antiepileptic Drugs

Some AEDs are not yet available in the United States, but can be purchased from neighboring Mexico and Canada for compassionate use, like vigabatrin in patients with tuberous sclerosis with infantile spasms and clobazam, a benzodiazepine effective as an add-on for various refractory epilepsy syndromes.

Pregabalin is a new AED approved in the United States since 2005 as adjunctive therapy in patients older than16 years with partial epilepsy and has also received approval for use in pain syndromes.

Adrenocorticotropic hormone is very useful in patients with infantile spasms.

Intravenous IgG can be used successfully in some patients with refractory epilepsy.

Dosage and formulations of the AEDs are summarized in Table 9-3. The choice of AEDs in the treatment of various epilepsy syndromes in the pediatric population is summarized in Table 9-4. The treatment of status epilepticus is summarized in Table 9-5.

Reasonable Expectations of Initial Therapy

In a pivotal study in which more than 500 patients with epilepsy were followed after initiation with an AED, 47% achieved seizure freedom with use of the first-choice AED, and 14% of additional patients achieved seizure

Table 9-3. Dosage and Formulations for Various AEDs Available for Children			
AED	**Dosage**	**Serum Level**	**Formulation**
Phenobarbital	3–8 mg/kg/d	15–45 µg/mL	20 mg/5 mL PO; 15, 30, 60 mg tabs, 200 mg/mL IV
Phenytoin	5 mg/kg/d	10–20 µg/mL	125 mg/5mL PO; 30, 50, 100 mg tab; 100 mg/mL IV
Ethosuximide	15–20 mg/kg/d	40–100 µg/mL	250 mg/5mL; 250 mg tab
Diazepam	0.3–1 mg/kg/d	Not known	2, 5, 10 mg tabs 2.5–20 mg rectal syringe 5 mg/mL, 1, 2, 10 mL, IV, IM
Lorazepam	0.1 mg/kg/d	Not known	2 mg/mL
Clonazepam	0.1 mg/kg/d	Not known	0.5, 1, 2, mg tab; 0.1 mg/mL suspension
Carbamazepine	20 mg/kg/d	4–12 µg/mL	100 mg/5 mL suspension; 100, 200, 300 mg capsules
Valproate	20-30 mg/kg/d	50–100 µg/mL	250/5 mL suspension 125 mg sprinkles 100 mg/100 mg IV
Felbamate	30–45 mg/kg/d	40–100 µg/mL	600 mg/5 mL suspension 400, 600 mg tabs
Gabapentin	30–100 mg/kg/d	4–16 µg/mL	300 mg/5 mL suspension 100, 300, 400, 600 mg tabs
Lamotrigine	5–15 mg/kg/d	5–15 µg/mL	5, 25, 50, 100, 150, 200 mg tabs
Topiramate	5–10 mg/kg/d	2–25 µg/mL	15, 25, 50, 100, 200 mg tabs/ sprinkles
Tiagabine	1 mg/kg/d	5–70 µg/mL	2, 4, 12, 16, 20 mg tabs
Levetiracetam	40–60 mg/kg/d	20–60 µg/mL	500 mg/5 mL suspension; 250, 500, 750 mg tabs, 500 mg/5 mL IV
Oxcarbazepine	30 mg/kg/d	10–30 µg/mL	300 mg/5 mL; 150, 300, 600 mg tabs
Zonisamide	5–10 mg/kg/d	20–30 µg/mL	25, 50, 100 mg tabs

Abbreviations: AEDs, antiepileptic drugs; PO, orally; tabs, tablets; IV, intravenously; IM, intramuscularly.

Table 9-4. Choice of AED in Children Based on Seizure Type and Syndrome

Seizure Type/Syndrome	First Choice	Second Choice	Others
Partial epilepsy	OXC, CBZ	LTG, VPA, LEV, TPM, BZD	ZNS, PB, PHT,
Primary GTC	VPA, TPM, LTG	CBZ, OXC, PHT	PB, GBP, ZNS, LEV
Childhood absence	ESM, VPA	LTG, LEV	ZNS, TPM
Juvenile absence	VPA	LTG, TPM	LEV, ZNS
JME	VPA	LTG, TPM, LEV	ZNS
BREC	CBZ, OXC	GBP	Sulthiame
IS	ACTH, VGB	VPA	BZD, TPM, ZNS
LGS	TPM, LTG	VPA, LEV,	FBM, KD, ZNS
Neonatal seizures	PB	PHT	BZD, TPM, LEV

Abbreviations: AED, antiepileptic drug; OXC, oxcarbazepine; CBZ, carbamazepine; LTG, lamotrgine; VPA, valproate; LEV, levetiracetam; TPM, topiramate; BZD, benzodiazepines; ZNS, zonisamide; PB, phenobarbital; PHT, phenytoin; GTC, generalized tonic-clonic; GBP, gabapentin; ESM, ethosuximde; JME, juvenile myoclonic epilepsy; BREC, benign rolandic epilepsy; IS, infantile spasms; ACTH, adrenocorticotropic hormone; LGS, Lennox-Gastaut syndrome; FBM, felbamate; KD, ketogenic diet.

Table 9-5. Management of Status Epilepticus

Time	Procedure
0–5 min	Perform airway, breathing, circulation assessment. Get vitals, start oxygen, and procure IV access, draw blood for CBC, chemistry, glucose, AED levels, toxicology screen if necessary.
6–9 min	Administer 2 mL/kg of intravenous 50% glucose.
10–30 min	IV lorazepam 0.1 mg/kg at 1-2 mg/min to a maximum of 8 mg. This is followed by IV phosphenytoin at 20 mg/kg of phenytoin equivalent (PE) at 3 mg/kg/min. May repeat an additional 10 mg/kg PE of phosphenytoin before proceeding to the next step.
31–59 min	If seizures continue, administer 20 mg/kg of Phenobarbital IV.
61–80 min[a]	Intubate, and transfer to the ICU for either pentobarbital or midazolam infusion to induce burst suppression on EEG, under very close monitoring of blood pressure.
>80 min	If seizures are still uncontrolled, consider using general anesthesia.

Abbreviations: IV, intravenous; CBC, complete blood count; AED, antiepileptic drug; PE, phenytoin equivalent; ICU, intensive care unit; EEG, electrocardiogram.

[a]Consider imaging of the head with computed tomographic scan or if possible magnetic resonance imaging of the brain, and spinal tap if considering an infectious or para-infectious etiology.

freedom with the use of second- or third-choice AED. Only 3% additional achieved seizure freedom with polytherapy. Higher seizure counts prior to initiating therapy, symptomatic etiology, and abnormal neurologic examination and development were predictors for failure of seizure freedom on AED therapy. Hence a third of the population with epilepsy will be inadequately controlled on AEDs. Failure to respond to more than 2 AEDs used in combination is defined as medically refractory epilepsy.

When to Discontinue Therapy

Two years of seizure freedom may be considered a safe time interval to attempt weaning of the AED. Normal EEG, neurologic examination, and development prior to withdrawal of the AED are important favorable prognostic factors, which predict prolonged periods of remission or cure. After 2 years have passed without a seizure, and if an EEG is normal, AEDs should be tapered over a period of 2 to 4 months. If the EEG is abnormal, it is recommended to continue AED treatment for a third year before reconsidering tapering of treatment. However, almost 24% of patients going off AEDs eventually have recurrence of seizures.

Adverse Effects of Antiepileptic Drugs

Efficacy of AEDs is often equivalent, hence selection of an AED is often determined by the adverse effects. They are observed in over a third of patients on AEDs and affect the ultimate quality of life and drop-out rates in patients with epilepsy, independent of their seizure control. The development of neurocognitive adverse effects is almost inevitable with the use of AEDs, especially in high-risk groups. Teratogenesis with major or minor malformations is of great concern during the first trimester of pregnancy, but an increasing body of information suggests that potential neurocognitive developmental delay may also occur with use of AEDs in the latter part of pregnancy. Valproate has been found to have the highest risk of both neurocognitive effects on the brain of the developing fetus and fetal malformations, including neural tube defects. Decreased bone mineral density has been found in adults and children receiving both enzyme-inducing AEDs and valproate, an enzyme-inhibiting drug. Adrenocorticotropic hormones may influence the lipid profile, body weight, reproductive, hormones and other endocrine functions, and sleep architecture. There also are age-specific adverse effects related to pharmacokinetic differences, such as higher risk of developing valproate induced hepatotoxicity and lamotrigine-induced skin rash in children younger than 2 years. Table 9-6 summarizes the adverse effects of all the AEDs.

Non-Pharmacologic Approaches to the Management of Epilepsy

Ketogenic Diet

The ketogenic diet may be helpful in refractory cases of LGS, infantile spasms, and progressive myoclonic epilepsy in the pediatric population. It is also the treatment of choice for patients with glucose transporter deficiency. The exact mechanism of action of this high-fat, low-carbohydrate, and protein diet is unknown, but it can reduce seizure frequency and intensity in patients with refractory epilepsy. Compliance is an issue, and it is not without risks, which include metabolic acidosis, renal stones, and weight loss.

Vagus Nerve Stimulation

Vagus nerve stimulation (VNS) consists of intermittent stimulation of the left vagus nerve in the neck to reduce the frequency and intensity of seizures. A small, programmable stimulus generator is implanted under the skin below the clavicle, and electrode leads pass subcutaneously to a second incision in the neck. Vagus nerve stimulation is recommended for the treatment of medically refractory partial and generalized epilepsy in patients older than 12 years who are not candidates for resective epilepsy surgery; however, it has been widely used in children as young as 1 year. Vagus nerve stimulation achieves 50% seizure reduction in a third of patients with refractory epilepsy; its efficacy is comparable to addition of a new AED in these patients. The surgery is relatively simple, and complications and side effects are infrequent and minor: hoarseness of voice, cough, pain, and infection. Although only the exceptional patient enjoys complete remission of seizures, VNS is an extremely flexible therapy applicable to a wide range of epileptic syndromes.

Epilepsy Surgery

There are 3 principal steps in the surgical evaluation of patients with epilepsy: (1) determining that the patient has medically refractory epilepsy,

Table 9-6. Antiepileptic Drug Side Effects

AED	CNS	Blood	Rash	Liver	BW	Miscellaneous	Serious and Life-Threatening
Phenobarbital	Sedation, irritability, hyperactivity, ↓ cognition and concentration	+	+	+		Exacerbation of porphyria, ↓ vit A, D, and folic acid	SJS, AHS
Phenytoin	Nystagmus, ataxia, drowsiness, lethargy, sedation	+	+	+		Gingival hypertrophy, hirsutism, osteoporosis, SLE	SJS, AHS, renal and hepatic failure
Benzodiazepine	Sedation, ataxia, drowsiness, hyperactivity ↓ cognition, depression	+	+	+	←	Exacerbation of seizures, tolerance and withdrawal syndrome	No
Ethosuximide	Sedation, dizziness, headaches, photophobia movement disorders	+	+		→	Gastric upset, anorexia, vomiting, SLE	SJS, AHS, renal and hepatic failure
Carbamazepine	Sedation, ataxia, headache, nystagmus, diplopia, tremor, movement disorders	+	+	+	←	Hyponatremia, osteomalacia, lupus, atrio-ventricular blockade, arrhythmias,	SJS, AHS, hepatic failure
Valproate	Tremor, sedation, fatigue, ataxia, behavioral changes	+	+	++	←	GI irritation PCOS, alopecia	Hepatic and pancreatic failure
Vigabatrin	Fatigue, sedation, change mood, psychosis				←		Irreversible visual field defects
Felbamate	Headache, dizziness, tremor, diplopia	++	+		→	Urolithiasis Hyponatremia	Aplastic anemia, hepatic failure
Lamotrigine	Headache, asthenia, dizziness, insomnia Mild hand tremor, tics		++	+		Gastrointestinal disturbances Pseudolymphoma	SJS DIC, Multiorgan or hepatic failure

Table 9-6. Antiepileptic Drug Side Effects, continued

AED	CNS	Blood	Rash	Liver	BW	Miscellaneous	Serious and Life-Threatening
Gabapentin	Somnolence, dizziness, nystagmus diplopia, tremor, memory difficulties, fatigue, behavioral changes, exacerbation of psychosis				↑	Aggravation of absences and precipitation myoclonus Movement disorders GI effects	No
Topiramate	Somnolence, dizziness, ataxia, diplopia, difficulty in memory and concentration, speech problems				→	Parasthesias Kidney stones Oligohydrosis	Hepatic failure
Oxcarbazepine	Dizziness, nausea, headache, drowsiness, ataxia, diplopia, fatigue		+			Hyponatremia	AHS, hematologic
Zonisamide	Somnolence, ataxia dizziness, fatigue, difficulty in concentration and language, psychosis	+			→	Kidney stones Oligohydrosis and hyperthermia	SJS, AHS, aplastic anemia
Levetiracetam	Irritability, behavioral changes, dizziness, insomnia					Increase seizure frequency	No

Abbreviations: AED, antiepileptic drugs; CNS, central nervous system; BW, body weight; SJS, Stevens-Johnson syndrome; AHS, anticonvulsant hypersensitivity syndrome; SLE, systemic lupus erythematosus; PCOS, polycystic ovary syndrome, DIC, disseminated intravascular coagulation; GI, gastrointestinal.

(2) determining whether the epilepsy arises from a single focus and whether that focus is resectable without risk of an unacceptable neurologic deficit, and (3) considering non-resective palliative treatments if resection is not an option. The ultimate treatment goal for surgery is freedom from seizures. Anything less than freedom from seizures generally does not lead to a significant improvement in the patient's overall daily life.

Is the epilepsy refractory? The recognition of failure of medical management must trigger consideration for surgical treatment. As described previously, 61% of patients will achieve adequate control of their seizures during the trial of 3 AEDs, but only an additional 3% will respond to further medical treatment. Thus, as previously mentioned, medically refractory epilepsy is defined as failure to achieve seizure control with at least 2 AEDs in combination, usually over 1 year.

Patients whose epilepsy is likely due to focal brain abnormalities should also undergo further evaluation even if seizures are well controlled medically. In such cases resection of the responsible focal brain lesion will likely render the patient seizure-free, thereby allowing discontinuation of AEDs and relief from their associated side effects.

Early referral for surgical evaluation is critical for 2 reasons. First, medically refractory epilepsy carries a small but not negligible mortality rate from status epilepticus. Second, intractable epilepsy is a self-aggravating process: uncontrolled seizures over time cause progressive brain injury that, in turn, exacerbates the severity of the epilepsy.

Do the seizures arise from a single focus, and is that focus resectable without neurologic morbidity? The tools available for noninvasive localization of the focus of seizure onset are history, physical examination, including neuropsychological testing, EEG, and brain imaging. The phenomenology of the seizure may point reliably to a specific brain location. For instance, a partial complex seizure preceded by an aura of an unpleasant taste or smell or the sensation of déjà vu very likely originates in the mesial temporal lobe. A focal neurologic abnormality may be indicative of a localized brain injury responsible for the epilepsy. The interictal EEG may similarly draw attention to a localized region of brain injury, but actual capture of the onset of a typical seizure on EEG is a much more valuable datum and often necessitates prolonged inpatient monitoring with concurrent video recordings. Likewise, a focal brain imaging abnormality may provide important confirmation.

Contemporary brain imaging is not only anatomical, such as CT scanning and MRI, but also functional, such as single photon emission computed tomography, positron emission tomography, and functional MRI. When all the data from history, physical examination, EEG, and imaging are concordant, that is, when all the data implicate a single, discrete focus of seizure onset, they can form the basis for a confident recommendation for surgery.

If after the initial evaluation uncertainty remains about the location of seizure onset or about the proximity of the locus of seizure onset to so-called eloquent cortex, brain structures that cannot be resected without disabling neurologic morbidity, then invasive monitoring is necessary for further consideration of surgical treatment. Available equipment for invasive monitoring includes depth electrodes and surface grid and strip electrodes. Depth electrodes are commonly inserted into the medial temporal lobe structures, but may also be used to survey other regions. Grid and strip electrodes are inserted over the cortical surface. Electrodes are implanted for about 7 days, which is usually enough time to record intracranial EEG during several seizures and to perform functional mapping.

Grid and strip electrodes may also be used for stimulation mapping of eloquent cortex with higher spatial resolution than noninvasive techniques. The principle is that stimulation inactivates the cortex around the stimulating electrodes, and this momentary interruption of normal function serves to localize small regions of cortex responsible for language, movement, or sensation. Cortical mapping can be performed intraoperatively under local anesthesia in the awake and cooperative patient; however, for children and for many adolescents, extraoperative mapping is safer and more productive. Extraoperative mapping is usually undertaken in conjunction with prolonged invasive monitoring to detect the precise locus of onset of typical seizures.

There are several localization-related epileptic syndromes for which surgery is the presumptive treatment of choice. The best example is temporal lobe epilepsy, the most common cause of complex partial seizures. In 2001 Wiebe et al reported the results of a randomized controlled trial providing Class I evidence that surgery is superior to continued medical treatment in patients with refractory temporal lobe epilepsy. In this trial, patients were selected who had seizures consistent clinically with temporal lobe origin for at least 1 year and were experiencing at least one seizure per month on average despite medical treatment with at least 2 AEDs, one of which was phenytoin, valproate, or carbamazepine. Patients were randomized to anterior temporal lobectomy or continued medical therapy. On follow-up, 58% of those who randomized to surgery (64% of those who underwent surgery) were free of seizures impairing awareness compared with 8% of the medical group. In this trial, 4 surgical patients (10%) experienced serious complications. These results are consistent with numerous other nonrandomized studies. Although this trial was performed in patients at least 16 years old, similar results have been reported in younger patients. A practice parameter issued by the American Academy of Neurology, the American Epilepsy Society, and the American Association of Neurological Surgeons recommends anteromedial temporal lobe resection for disabling complex partial seizures.

Localization-related epilepsy associated with a structural brain lesion, such as cortical dysplasia, brain tumor, or vascular malformation, is likely to benefit from resection of the lesion and the neighboring epileptogenic cortex. About 60% of such patients become free of disabling seizures with surgery. Resection of extratemporal epileptic foci not associated with structural lesions but identified by electrophysiological investigations yields less predictable outcomes.

The most dramatic surgical intervention for intractable localization-related epilepsy is hemispherectomy. This term encompasses a spectrum of surgical procedures that combine cortical resections with interruptions of white matter fiber tracts in varying proportions to isolate one hemisphere from the rest of the brain. Hemispherectomy is indicated for a small number of pathological entities commonly presenting in childhood that affect one cerebral hemisphere diffusely, such as hemimegalencephaly, chronic focal encephalitis (Rasmussen syndrome), Sturge-Weber syndrome, and hemiplegia-hemiconvulsion-epilepsy syndrome. Typically these conditions are catastrophically disabling, and hemispherectomy renders 60% to 90% of patients free or nearly free of seizures. The neurologic morbidity is surprisingly low. Patients experience a homonymous hemianopsia and a contralateral hemiparesis. Almost all patients recover independent ambulation, and the paretic upper limb is useful for most. Speech and language function have often developed in the uninvolved hemisphere and, if not, among the young patients who comprise most of the candidates for hemispherectomy, it often relocates.

If a single site of seizure onset cannot be identified, or if resection of epileptogenic cortex is not possible without unacceptable neurologic morbidity, are there alternative, non-resective surgical strategies? There are options that offer some hope of palliation to patients with a wide range of intractable epileptic syndromes.

Invasive investigation of patients with intractable localization-related epilepsy may define an epileptogenic zone that encroaches on eloquent cortex responsible for speech and language function or for voluntary movement. Resection of such a zone can be curative for the epilepsy but disabling for the patient. Multiple subpial transections (MTS) may be a useful surgical tactic in selected instances. The concept for MTS is based on the architecture of the cerebral cortical gyrus: The projection fibers that connect cortex with subcortical nuclear structures, with the brain stem, and with the spinal cord are oriented perpendicular to the cortical surface. Preservation of these fibers is necessary for preservation of function. On the other hand, the fibers responsible for the initial spread of epileptic activity from the epileptogenic zone to adjacent cortical regions are oriented parallel to the cortical surface, and interruption of these fibers can block the propagation and generalization of a seizure. Multiple subpial transections creates a series of parallel slices of the involved cortex perpendicular to the gyral surface that in principle cut intracortical fibers while leaving the projection fibers and the cortical vasculature undisturbed. In practice, MTS often impairs function to some degree and seldom completely abolishes seizures, but it can serve as a useful adjunct for extension of the reach of resective therapy.

Many patients with epileptic encephalopathies such as the LGS have multiple foci of seizure onset and therefore cannot be managed by cortical resection. Such patients often experience very rapid seizure propagation with sudden loss of consciousness and atonia, so-called drop attacks. Their frequent falls cause lacerations, fractures, and even traumatic brain injuries that can exacerbate the underlying encephalopathy. For such patients and their caretakers, the drop attacks become a major aggravating factor impairing quality of life above and beyond the burden of the epilepsy itself. About 70% of patients with atonic seizures or drop attacks benefit from corpus callosotomy. A common practice is to section of the anterior two-thirds of the corpus callosum, although complete corpus callosotomy may be undertaken either as a second stage or primarily. Roughly half of patients are completely relieved of drop attacks, and another 20% will experience a 50% or greater reduction in attack frequency. Long-term sequelae of corpus callosotomy include an interhemispheric sensory dissociation that is usually not troublesome for patients. Subtle changes in attention and memory may be detectable as well. The effect of callosotomy is to convert generalized seizures into partial seizures, which occasionally increase in frequency after surgery, so corpus callosotomy is indicated only for patients in who control of drop attacks is the dominant clinical objective.

Web Sites

American Epilepsy Society: www.aesnet.org

The Epilepsy Foundation: www.epilepsyfoundation.org

MedlinePlus: National Library of Medicine and the National Institutes of Health: www.nlm.nih.gov/medlineplus/epilepsy.html

National Institute of Neurological Disorders and Stroke: www.ninds.nih. gov/disorders/epilepsy/epilepsy.htm

THRESHOLD—Intractable Seizure Disorder Support Group & Newsletter: www.fscnj.org

Bibliography

Classification and Syndromes

Beaussart M, Faou R. Evolution of epilepsy with rolandic paroxysmal foci: a study of 324 cases. *Epilepsia.* 1978;19:337–342

Commission on Classification and Terminology of the International League Against Epilepsy. Proposal for revised classification of epilepsies and epileptic syndromes. *Epilepsia.* 1989;30: 389–399

Engel J Jr. ILAE classification of epilepsy syndromes. *Epilepsy Res.* 2006;70(suppl 1):5–10

Fisher RS, van Emde Boas W, Blume W, et al. Epileptic seizures and epilepsy: definitions proposed by the International League Against Epilepsy (ILAE) and the International Bureau for Epilepsy (IBE). *Epilepsia.* 2005;46:470–472

Gardiner M. Genetics of idiopathic generalized epilepsies. *Epilepsia.* 2005;46(suppl 9):15–20

Hirose S, Mitsudome A, Okada M, Kaneko S, on behalf of The Epilepsy Genetic Study Group, Japan. Genetics of idiopathic epilepsies. *Epilepsia.* 2005;46(suppl 1):38–43

Nabbout R, Dulac O. Epileptic syndromes in infancy and childhood. *Curr Opin Neurol.* 2008;21:161–166

Panayiotopoulos CP. Benign childhood epilepsy with occipital paroxysms: a 15-year prospective study. *Ann Neurol.* 1989;26:51–56

Riikonen R. A long-term follow-up study of 214 children with the syndrome of infantile spasms. *Neuropediatrics.* 1982;13:14–23

Scher MS. Neonatal seizure classification: a fetal perspective concerning childhood epilepsy. *Epilepsy Res.* 2006;70(suppl 1):41–57

Seino M. Classification criteria of epileptic seizures and syndromes. *Epilepsy Res.* 2006; 70(suppl 1):27–33

Sisodiya S, Cross JH, Blümcke I, et al. Genetics of epilepsy: epilepsy research foundation workshop report. *Epileptic Disord.* 2007;9:194–236

Steinlein OK. Genetics and epilepsy. *Dialogues Clin Neurosci.* 2008;10:29–38

Natural History and Antiepileptic Drug Management

Abend NS, Dlugos DJ. Treatment of refractory status epilepticus: literature review and a proposed protocol. *Pediatr Neurol.* 2008;38:377–390

Berg AT. Risk of seizure recurrence after a first unprovoked seizure. *Epilepsia.* 2008;49(suppl 1):13–18

Berg AT, Shinnar S. Relapse following discontinuation of antiepileptic drugs: a meta-analysis. *Neurology.* 1994;44:601–608

Berg AT, Shinnar S, Levy SR, et al. Two-year remission and subsequent relapse in children with newly diagnosed epilepsy. *Epilepsia.* 2001;42:1553–1562

Berg AT, Shinnar S, Testa FM, et al. Status epilepticus after the initial diagnosis of epilepsy in children. *Neurology.* 2004;63:1027–1034

Elger CE, Schmidt D. Modern management of epilepsy: a practical approach. *Epilepsy Behav.* 2008;12:501–539

French JA, Kanner AM, Bautista J, et al. Efficacy and tolerability of the new antiepileptic drugs I: treatment of new onset epilepsy: report of the Therapeutics and Technology Assessment Subcommittee and Quality Standards Subcommittee of the American Academy of Neurology and the American Epilepsy Society. *Neurology.* 2004;62:1252–1260

French JA, Kanner AM, Bautista J, et al. Efficacy and tolerability of the new antiepileptic drugs II: treatment of refractory epilepsy: report of the Therapeutics and Technology Assessment Subcommittee and Quality Standards Subcommittee of the American Academy of Neurology and the American Epilepsy Society. *Neurology.* 2004;62:1261–1273

Goodridge DM, Shorvon SD. Epileptic seizures in a population of 6000. I: demography, diagnosis and classification, and role of the hospital services. *Br Med J (Clin Res Ed).* 1983;287:641–644

Goodridge DM, Shorvon SD. Epileptic seizures in a population of 6000. II: treatment and prognosis. *Br Med J (Clin Res Ed)*. 1983;287:645–647

Hirtz D, Ashwal S, Berg A, et al. Practice parameter: evaluating a first nonfebrile seizure in children: report of the Quality Standards Subcommittee of the American Academy of Neurology, the Child Neurology Society, and the American Epilepsy Society. *Neurology*. 2000;55:616–623

Hirtz D, Berg A, Bettis D, et al. Practice parameter: treatment of the child with a first unprovoked seizure: report of the Quality Standards Subcommittee of the American Academy of Neurology and the Practice Committee of the Child Neurology Society. *Neurology*. 2003;60:166–175

Kwan P, Brodie MJ. Early identification of refractory epilepsy. *N Engl J Med*. 2000;342:314–319

LaRoche SM, Helmers SL. The new antiepileptic drugs: clinical applications. *JAMA*. 2004;291:615–620

LaRoche SM, Helmers SL. The new antiepileptic drugs: scientific review. *JAMA*. 2004;291: 605–614

Loiseau P, Pestre M, Dartigues JF, Commenges D, Barberger-Gateau C, Cohadon S. Long-term prognosis in two forms of childhood epilepsy: typical absence seizures and epilepsy with rolandic (centrotemporal) EEG foci. *Ann Neurol*. 1983;13:642–648

Mohanraj R, Brodie MJ. Pharmacological outcomes in newly diagnosed epilepsy. *Epilepsy Behav*. 2005;6:382–387

Patsalos PN, Berry DJ, Bourgeois BF, et al. Antiepileptic drugs best-practice guidelines for therapeutic drug monitoring: a position paper by the Subcommission on Therapeutic Drug Monitoring, ILAE Commission on Therapeutic Strategies. *Epilepsia*. 2008;49:1239–1276

Raspall-Chaure M, Neville BG, Scott RC. The medical management of the epilepsies in children: conceptual and practical considerations. *Lancet Neurol*. 2008;7:57–69

Sharma S, Riviello JJ, Harper MB, Baskin MN. The role of emergent neuroimaging in children with new-onset afebrile seizures. *Pediatrics*. 2003;111:1–5

Shinnar S, O'Dell C, Berg AT. Mortality following a first unprovoked seizure in children: a prospective study. *Neurology*. 2005;64:880–882

Sillanpää M, Jalava M, Kaleva O, Shinnar S. Long-term prognosis of seizures with onset in childhood. *N Engl J Med*. 1998;338:1715–1722

Wheless JW, Clarke DF, Arimanoglou A, Carpenter D. Treatment of pediatric epilepsy: European expert opinion. *Epileptic Disord*. 2007;9:353–412

Wheless JW, Clarke DF, Carpenter D. Treatment of pediatric epilepsy: expert opinion, 2005. *J Child Neurol*. 2005;20(suppl 1):1–56

Wiebe S, Téllez-Zenteno JF, Shapiro M. An evidence-based approach to first seizure. *Epilepsia*. 2008;49(suppl 1):50–57

Surgical Management

Engel J Jr, Wiebe S, French J, et al. Practice parameter: temporal lobe and localized neocortical resections for epilepsy: report of the Quality Standards Subcommittee of the American Academy of Neurology, in association with the American Epilepsy Society and the American Association of Neurological Surgeons. *Neurology.* 2003;60:538–547

Fisher RS, Handforth A. Reassessment: vagus nerve stimulation for epilepsy: a report of the Therapeutics and Technology Assessment Subcommittee of the American Academy of Neurology. *Neurology.* 1999;53:666–669

Langfitt JT, Holloway RG, McDermott MP, et al. Health care costs decline after successful epilepsy surgery. *Neurology.* 2007;68:1290–1298

Morris GL III, Mueller WM. Long-term treatment with vagus nerve stimulation in patients with refractory epilepsy. The vagus nerve stimulation study group E01-E05. *Neurology.* 1999;53:1731–1735

Spencer SS, Berg AT, Vickrey BG, et al. Initial outcomes in the Multicenter Study of Epilepsy Surgery. *Neurology.* 2003;61:1680–1685

Spencer SS, Berg AT, Vickrey BG, et al. Predicting long-term seizure outcome after resective epilepsy surgery: the Multicenter Study. *Neurology.* 2005;65:912–918

Tharin S, Golby A. Functional brain mapping and its applications to neurosurgery. *Neurosurgery.* 2007;60:185–201; discussion 201–202

Wiebe S, Blume WT, Girvin JP, Eliasziw M. A randomized, controlled trial of surgery for temporal-lobe epilepsy. *N Engl J Med.* 2001;345:311–318

Chapter 10

Headaches

Marcos Cruz, MD
Agustín Legido, MD, PhD, MBA

Introduction

Headaches are very common during childhood and become increasingly more frequent during the teenage years. By age 3 years, headaches occur in 3% to 8% of children; at age 5 years, 19.5% have headaches; and by 7 years, 37% to 51.5% have headaches. In 7- to 15-year-olds, headache prevalence ranges from 57% to 82%. Before puberty, reports indicate that boys are affected more frequently than girls, but following the onset of puberty, headaches are reported to occur more frequently in girls.

Classification

From a practical viewpoint, it is useful to classify headaches into primary headaches, or primary entities whose only clinical relevance is the discomfort itself (ie, migraine, tension headaches), and secondary headaches, those that are symptomatic of other intracranial disease (ie, brain tumors, increased intracranial pressure, drug intoxication, sinusitis, or febrile illnesses). Box 10-1 enumerates the most frequent types of headaches in children.

Primary Headaches

Migraine

Migraine is the most frequent type of headache in children. Its prevalence at age 7 ranges from 1.2% to 3.2% and, from age 7 to 15 years, it ranges from 4% to 11%. In prepubertal children, boys and girls are affected equally, but, following puberty, migraine is more frequent in girls. There is a positive family history of migraine in 80% to 90% of children who present with this type of headache.

Box 10-1. Headaches in Children

Primary headaches

Migraine
  Migraine without aura
  Migraine with aura
    Typical aura with migraine headache
    Typical aura with non-migraine headache
    Familial hemiplegic migraine
    Sporadic hemiplegic migraine
    Basilar-artery migraine

Precursors of migraine
    Benign paroxysmal vertigo
    Cyclic vomiting
    Abdominal migraine
    Benign paroxysmal torticollis

Migraine variants
    Alice in Wonderland
    Confusional migraine
    Ophthalmoplegic migraine
    Alternating hemiplegia of childhood

Cluster headache

Tension headache

Analgesic rebound headache

Chronic daily headache

Secondary headaches

Intracranial problems
    Brain tumors
    Cerebral vascular lesions
    Central nervous system infection
    Brain injury
    Pseudotumor cerebri

Extracranial problems
    Visual defects
    Sinus disease
    Dental problems
    Temporomandibular joint syndrome

Pathogenesis

The mechanisms underlying migraine attacks can be explained on the basis of 2 theories: that migraine is primarily of vascular or neuronal origin.

The vascular theory suggests that migraine is a disorder of cerebrovascular regulation. During a significant number of migraine attacks, pulsations in the superficial temporal artery can be demonstrated, and pain can be relieved either by physical compression or by the vasoconstrictor agent ergotamine. The proposed sequence of events in migraine begins with the release of a neurotransmitter such as substance P, serotonin, or both. These substances precipitate platelet aggregation, which in turn leads to release of platelet serotonin and thromboxane A2, activation of prostaglandins and kinins, and the production of a localized sterile arteritis that causes symptomatic focal vasoconstriction. Reactive vasodilatation follows, largely in the extracranial cerebral circulation, stretching the pain-sensitive arterioles and producing the familiar throbbing headache of migraine.

The neurogenic theory of migraine is currently the prevalent theory. According to this theory, the fundamental physiological substrate for migraine is hyperexcitability of the cerebral cortex. Multiple genetic influences cause disturbances of neuronal ion channels (eg, calcium channels), which lead to a lowered threshold for a variety of external or internal factors that then trigger episodes of regional neuronal excitation followed by "cortical spreading depression." The latter is a slowly propagating wave (2–6 mm/min) of neuronal depolarization and is likely the key initial phase that is responsible for the aura of migraine and for activation of the trigeminovascular system. This process may be involved not only in the transmission of painful sensory stimuli but, possibly, in the initiation of a sterile neurogenic inflammation. It consists of vascular dilation, enhanced leakage or extravasation of plasma proteins across the endothelium with subsequent edema formation in vessel walls, and a complex chain of chemical and physiological events that excite, sensitize, and lower the threshold of the trigeminal nociceptive terminals in the vessels of the dura and large vessels equipped with vasa vasorum. The consequence of activation of a nociceptive terminal is the release of neuropeptides including substance P, neurokinin A, and calcitonin gene-related peptide (CGRP), which induce vasodilation and extravasation. Substance P also causes the release of histamine and other substances from mast cells and serotonin from platelets.

There is evidence that the brain stem nuclei locus coeruleus, the origin of noradrenergic neurons, and the raphe nuclei, the origin of serotonergic neurons, innervate the intracranial vasculature and can initiate the process of neurogenic inflammation in migraine attacks. These brain stem mechanisms may be triggered from the cerebral cortex in response to emotion or stress; from the thalamus in response to excessive afferent stimulation, glare, noise, or smells; from the hypothalamus, in response to "internal clocks," or from vascular changes in the internal or external carotid territories.

Clinical Symptoms

Classic migraine accounts for less than one-third of migraine cases in childhood. It is a biphasic illness with the vasoconstriction phase associated with an aura, usually visual (blurred vision, scotomata, flashing lights, and hemianopsia), and the subsequent vasodilation phase associated with a throbbing hemicranial headache. The onset of the visual aura is gradual and lasts minutes. Sudden images and complicated visual perceptions should prompt consideration of complex partial seizures, even if followed by headache. Transient visual obscurations, brief episodes of near-complete blindness, are also features of pseudotumor cerebri.

Common migraine is the most frequent form of migraine in childhood. There is no aura but, prior to the onset of the headache, the child often complains of malaise, dizziness or nausea, mood changes, irritability, lethargy, food cravings, or increased thirst. The headache may be unilateral and pounding, but it may also be generalized, bifrontal, or bitemporal in location. It is aggravated by routine physical activity. The onset of the pain is usually gradual, peaks, and then subsides within 2 to 48 hours in children. Box 10-2 shows the diagnostic criteria according to the International Headache Society.

Complicated migraine is the association of migraine with transient neurologic deficits due to prolonged aura of vasoconstriction and ischemia in the affected brain areas. It includes the following syndromes:

- Hemiplegic or hemisensory: hemiparesis or hemisensory loss, sometimes accompanied by aphasia, paresthesias, or seizure
- Ophthalmoplegic: unilateral eye pain and ipsilateral III, IV, or V cranial nerve palsy

---

Box 10-2. Diagnostic Criteria for Pediatric and Adolescent Migraine[a]

A. At least 5 attacks fulfilling criteria B–D (below)

B. Headache attacks lasting 1–72 hours

C. Headache has at least 2 of the following characteristics:
1. Unilateral location, may be bilateral, frontotemporal (not occipital)
2. Pulsatile quality
3. Moderate or severe pain intensity
4. Aggravation by or causing avoidance of routine physical activity (ie, walking or climbing upstairs)

D. During the headache, at least one of the following:
1. Nausea and/or vomiting
2. Photophobia and phonophobia

E. Not attributed to any other disorder

---

[a]*International Headache Society, 2004.*

- Basilar artery migraine: visual symptoms, dizziness, ataxia, loss of consciousness, and drop attacks
- Acute confusional state: acute altered mental status
- Alice in Wonderland syndrome: distortion of body image, spatial relations, and time sense
- Familial hemiplegic migraine: migraine with aura causing some degree of hemiparesis due to a missense mutation in the calcium channel gene (CACNA1A) mapping to chromosome 19p13 or 1q31

Migraine Variants or Precursors of Migraine

- Benign paroxysmal vertigo: occurs in young children and manifests with abrupt episodes of unsteadiness and ataxia
- Cyclic vomiting syndrome: characterized by recurrent episodes of severe vomiting with asymptomatic interval periods
- Benign paroxysmal torticollis: presents during infancy with episodes of head tilt or torticollis accompanied by vomiting and ataxia that may last hours or days
- Abdominal migraine: manifests in school-aged children with recurrent episodes of vague, periumbilical abdominal pain

Cluster Headache

Cluster headache is often included among migraine syndromes. It is uncommon in children, with onset occurring almost exclusively after age 10 years. Attacks are characterized by intense, non-throbbing periorbital pain that may generalize to the hemicranium. They may awaken the patient in the middle of the night. Unilateral conjunctival injection, lacrimation, rhinorrhea, diaphoresis, and transient Horner syndrome may be accompanying signs. Attacks are brief and occur in clusters, followed by periods of remission of 1 year or more.

Tension Headache

Tension headache is usually associated with stress. Patients complain of a dull, bilateral, diffuse pain of variable intensity. Sometimes the pain is described as "a band around the head." It is generally present on awakening and may continue all day, but tends not to be aggravated by routine physical activity in contrast to migraine headaches. Most children describe long periods in which headache occurs almost every day and shorter intervals when they are headache-free. Classically, chronic tension headache is not associated with nausea, vomiting, photophobia, phonophobia, or transient neurologic disturbances, as happens in migraine. The presence of these symptoms suggests the diagnosis of migraine headaches within a background of chronic tension headaches. There is a higher incidence of depressive symptoms in these patients.

Analgesic Rebound Headache

This type of headache occurs in children using over-the-counter analgesics frequently. When the analgesic effects wear off, the underlying headache requires further analgesic administration, and a cycle of headache-analgesic-headache becomes established. Sometimes patients with migraine overuse analgesics, and the rebound headache becomes more frequent, even daily, evolving into the so-called transformed migraine. Analgesic rebound headache tends to be described as frequent or daily, generalized, mild, and dull, and is not aggravated by exercise.

Chronic Daily Headache

This syndrome is frequent among adolescents, and it is defined as greater than 4 months during which the patient has more than 15 headaches per month, with the headaches lasting more than 4 hours. Patients can evolve into a chronic daily headache pattern from chronic migraine or chronic tension headache. Sometimes the headache may start de novo and persist for weeks or months on a daily basis. Hemicranium continuum is another form of chronic daily headache, which basically is a persistent form of cluster headache.

Secondary Headaches

The processes that cause symptomatic headaches most frequently in children are tumor, trauma, infection, vascular disease (arteriovenous malformation, aneurysm, vasculitis), and toxin exposure. In general, these headaches do not follow a typical pattern of any of the primary headaches and are accompanied by other suspicious signs: nausea, vomiting, papilledema, fever, change in mental status, focal neurologic signs, or meningismus. Many of these headaches have a subacute or chronic progressive course.

Idiopathic Intracranial Hypertension or Pseudotumor Cerebri

This is a condition characterized by increased intracranial pressure with a normal cerebrospinal (CSF) evaluation and normal neuroimaging studies. It may be idiopathic or secondary to multiple causes (Box 10-3). The common physiological disturbance seems to be elevated dural venous sinus pressures. Clinically, patients complain of a headache that is usually daily, constant, diffuse, worse at night, and often wakes them up from their sleep in the early hours of the morning. Often, many nonspecific symptoms of meningeal irritation may be present, including photophobia, nausea, and vomiting. Sudden movements, such as coughing, or the Valsalva maneuver can aggravate the headache. Transient visual obscuration, especially with sudden changes in position, is a common complaint. Visual loss is a serious complication and should be investigated promptly as it may be rapid, severe, and permanent.

Patient Evaluation

The evaluation of a child with headache begins with a thorough medical history. Box 10-4 enumerates important questions to ask in the evaluation of children with headaches.

Box 10-3. Causes of Idiopathic Intracranial Hypertension

Drugs
- Treatment with corticosteroids
- Corticosteroid withdrawal
- Oral contraceptives
- Tetracycline
- Thyroid replacement
- Vitamin A
- Anabolic steroids
- Lithium

Systemic disorders
- Chronic obstructive pulmonary disease
- Right heart failure with pulmonary hypertension
- Sleep apnea
- Guillain-Barré syndrome
- Iron deficiency anemia
- Leukemia
- Polycythemia vera
- Protein malnutrition
- Systemic lupus erythematosus
- Vitamin A and D deficiency

Head trauma

Infections
- Otitis media
- Sinusitis

Metabolic disorders
- Adrenal insufficiency
- Diabetic ketoacidosis (treatment)
- Galactosemia
- Hyperadrenalism
- Hyperthyroidism
- Hypoparathyroidism
- Pregnancy

Obstruction to venous drainage
- Cerebral venous thrombosis
- Jugular vein thrombosis

Box 10-4. Information to Seek in the History of a Child With Headache

Age of onset

Severity

Frequency

Duration

Warning sings

Time of onset

Mode of onset

Localization

Characterization of the pain

Symptoms accompanying the headache

Effect on daily activities

What makes the headache better

What makes the headache worse

Possible triggers (foods, odors, heat, etc)

Family history of headaches

Family history of brain tumors or aneurysms

Fever

General health

Sleep hygiene

Change in school, home, or work environment

The analysis of the headache pattern is very useful as, according to Fenichel, it often leads to recognition of either the source or the mechanism of pain.

- A continuous, low-intensity, chronic headache, in the absence of associated symptoms or signs, is unlikely to indicate a serious intracranial disease.
- Intermittent headaches, especially those that make the child look and feel sick, from which the child recovers completely and between which the child is normal, are likely to be migraine.
- A severe headache of recent onset, different from anything previously experienced, from which the child never returns to a normal baseline, is probably due to significant intracranial disease.

- Diagnostic investigation of brief, intense pain lasting for seconds in an otherwise normal child is seldom fruitful.
- Periosteal pain, especially inflammation of the sinuses, localizes in an area that is tender to palpation. Sinusitis as a cause of headache is overstated. Evidence of sinusitis is a common feature of computed tomography (CT) in children evaluated for other reasons.
- Cervical root and cranial nerve pain has a radiating or shooting quality.

The diagnosis of primary headache disorders of children rests principally on clinical criteria as set forth by the International Headache Society (2004). Clues to the presence and identification of secondary causes of headache are uncovered through the process of history and physical examination.

Physical examination should be methodical, with measurement of vital signs, particularly blood pressure. The physical examination should also focus on the facial extracranial structures (eyes, sinuses, teeth, temporomandibular junction), which frequently are causes of headache. A complete neurologic examination should focus on identifying subtle changes (ie, facial asymmetry, asymmetrical limb weakness or deep tendon reflexes, mild gait abnormalities, visual field deficits), and it should include a good visualization of the optic fundus.

Box 10-5 shows red flags to be identified in the history or the physical examination of a patient with headache.

The differential diagnostic list of headaches as a symptom is extensive and should be addressed depending on its temporal course, absence or presence of neurologic deficits, and the presence or absence of fever (Box 10-6).

The principal indication for performance of ancillary diagnostic testing rests on information or concerns revealed during the patient's evaluation. A practice parameter of the American Academy of Neurology concluded that there is inadequate documentation in the literature to support any recommendation for routine laboratory studies (ie, hematology or chemistry panels) or performance of lumbar puncture.

Routine electroencephalography was not recommended as part of the headache evaluation. Electroencephalography does not differentiate primary from secondary headaches and is unlikely to determine an etiology of the headache or distinguish migraine from other types of headaches.

The role of neuroimaging is better defined. Obtaining a neuroimaging study on a routine basis is not indicated in children with recurrent

---

Box 10-5. Red Flags in the History or Physical Examination of Children With Headaches[a]

History
- Age <3 years
- Morning or nocturnal headache
- Morning or nocturnal vomiting
- Headache awakens child during sleep
- Headache increased by Valsalva or straining
- Explosive onset
- Chronic progressive pattern
- Cluster headache in any child <6 years
- Declining school performance or personality changes
- Altered mental status
- Migraine and seizure occur in the same episode
- Visual graying out occurring at the peak of a headache
- Brief cough headache

Physical or neurologic examination
- Hypertension
- Head circumference >95%
- Neurocutaneous findings

Meningeal signs

Papilledema

Abnormal eye movements

Motor asymmetry

Ataxia

Gait disturbance

Abnormal deep tendon reflexes

---

[a]*Modified from Lewis DW. Headaches in children and adolescents. Curr Probl Pediatr Adolesc Health Care. 2007;37:210, with permission from Elsevier.*

---

headaches and a normal neurologic examination. Neuroimaging should be considered in children with an abnormal neurologic examination or other physical findings that suggest central nervous system disease. Variables that predict the presence of a space-occupying lesion are (1) headache of less than 1-month duration, (2) absence of family history of migraine, (3) abnormal neurologic findings on examination, (4) gait abnormalities, and (5) occurrence of seizures. The probability of abnormal magnetic resonance imaging (MRI) in the absence of a neurologic deficit is about 16%,

Box 10-6. Differential Diagnosis of Headaches According to Clinical Course and Symptoms

Acute headaches with a normal neurologic examination
- Migraine
- Tension headaches
- Benign exertional headaches
- Chronic paroxysmal hemicrania
- Cluster headaches
- Hypertension
- Caffeine withdrawal

Acute headaches with an abnormal neurologic examination
- Complicated migraine
- Migraine equivalent
- Pseudotumor cerebri
- Stroke
- Intracranial hemorrhage
- Sagittal sinus thrombosis
- Arteriovenous malformation

Acute headaches with fever
- Meningitis
- Encephalitis
- Sinusitis
- Dental abscess
- Viral syndrome
- Pharyngeal abscess

Chronic nonprogressive headaches
- Muscle tension headaches
- Caffeine withdrawal
- Temporomandibular joint syndrome
- Post-concussive syndrome
- Analgesic rebound
- Carbon monoxide poisoning
- Conversion disorder

Chronic progressive headaches
- Tumor
- Hydrocephalus
- Pseudotumor cerebri
- Intracranial hemorrhage
- Arteriovenous malformation
- Abscess
- Cyst (arachnoid, dermoid, third ventricle)
- Chiari malformation type 1

including conditions such as sinus disease, Chiari malformation, or occult vascular malformations, none of which influence management.

In our experience, a positive family history of brain tumors or aneurysms creates enough anxiety in the families that performing neuroimaging is warranted in many cases.

Head CT scan and MRI are very useful in corroborating the diagnosis of pseudotumor cerebri ("full parenchyma" with small ventricles). Frequently in these patients, MRI or magnetic resonance venography is necessary to demonstrate associated venous sinus thrombosis.

Obviously, neuroimaging studies, facial imaging, or spinal tap may be necessary to diagnose the etiology of secondary headaches.

Treatment

Migraine

The approach to the patient with migraine is based on the patient's age, frequency and severity of attacks, presence of an aura, patient reliability, and family's attitude toward the use of medication. Once assured that there is no underlying serious disorder, many patients appear to have fewer and less distressing attacks. Non-pharmacologic methods of dealing with migraine headache include confidence, reassurance, elimination of trigger factors, and modification of stress. Relaxation therapy, counseling, and biofeedback; regular diet; sufficient sleep; removal of triggers; and stabilization of stressful situations may decrease the number of episodes.

The traditional management of migraine in children is based on the "step-care" model, in which all children are started on first-line analgesics, such as acetaminophen or nonsteroidal anti-inflammatory drugs (NSAIDs) at the bottom of the therapeutic pyramid and, as the treatment fails, the therapy is escalated. The fundamental assumption in the step-care model is that children with migraine have the same treatment needs. Although this is a useful and cost-effective model, it may delay referral of patients to specialists, prolong suffering, increase school absences, limit physical activities, and result in increased use of resources with frequent office and emergency department visits and multiple ineffective medication trials. In addition, these delays in appropriate treatment may lead to indiscriminate use of over-the-counter medications with the risk of chronic headaches secondary to analgesic abuse.

There are 6 primary principles for the treatment of acute migraine headache as recommended by the American Academy of Neurology: (1) treat attacks rapidly and consistently without recurrence, (2) restore the patient's ability to function, (3) minimize the use of backup and rescue medications, (4) optimize self-care and reduce subsequent use of resources, (5) be cost-effective for overall management, and (6) have minimal or no adverse events.

There are 3 complementary approaches once the diagnosis of migraine headaches has been established: (1) acute or episodic medication, (2) prophylactic or preventive agents, and (3) non-pharmacologic or biobehavioral interventions.

Acute Treatment (Table 10-1)

There are basically 3 types of medications for acute migraine treatment: acetaminophen or NSAIDs, including Ibuprofen and Naproxen; ergotamine-derived medications; and 5-hydroxytryptamine receptor agonists (5HT1) or triptans.

The conclusions of the American Academy of Neurology regarding acute treatment of migraine headaches in children are that both ibuprofen and acetaminophen have been shown to be safe and effective (class I evidence). Sumatriptan is the only 5HT1 agonist that has proved to be effective for the treatment of children and adolescents with migraine, with the 5-mg and 20-mg nasal spray having the most favorable profile (class I evidence). There is only class IV evidence for the effectiveness of subcutaneous sumatriptan. Oral triptan agents have not demonstrated efficacy in class I studies. There are currently no agents approved by the US Food and Drug Administration for the acute treatment of migraine in children or adolescents.

The current American Academy of Neurology recommendations for acute treatment of migraine in children and adolescents are as follows:

- Ibuprofen is effective and should be considered for the acute treatment of migraine in children (Level A = 2 consistent class I studies).
- Acetaminophen is probably effective and should be considered for the acute treatment of migraine in children (Level B = at least 1 class I study or 2 class II studies).

Table 10-1. Treatment of Acute Migraine in Children[a]		
Drug	**Dose**	**Available**
Acetaminophen	10–15 mg/kg	Tabs 80, 160, 325 mg Syrup 160 mg/tsp
Ibuprofen	10 mg/kg	Tabs 100 mg chewable Tabs 200, 400, 600, 800 mg Syrup 100 mg/tsp
Naproxen sodium	2.5–5 mg/kg	Tabs 220, 250, 375, 500 mg
Metoclopramide	1–2 mg/kg	Tabs 5, 10 mg Syrup 5 mg/tsp
Acetaminophen/aspirin/caffeine (Excedrin)	1–2 tabs qid	
Butalbital, aspirin/acetaminophen/caffeine (Fiorinal, Fioricet, Esgic)	1–2 tabs qid	
Isometheptene, acetaminophen	1–2 cps, <5/day	
Dichloralphenazone (Midrin)		
Dihydroergotamine mesylate (Migranal)	2 mg/dose	Vials 4 mg DHE/cc +10 mg caffeine/cc
Sumatriptan (Imitrex)		Tabs 25, 50, 100 mg 6 mg subcutaneous injection 5, 20 mg nasal spray
Zolmitriptan (Zomig)		Tabs 2.5, 5 mg 2.5, 5 mg oral disintegrating tabs 5 mg nasal spray
Rizatriptan (Maxalt)		Tabs 5, 10 mg 5, 10 mg oral disintegrating tabs

Abbreviations: tabs, tablets; tsp, teaspoon; qid, 4 times a day; cps, capsules; DHE, dihydroergotamine.

[a]Modified from Lewis DW. Headaches in children and adolescents. *Curr Probl Pediatr Adolesc Health Care.* 2007;37:224, with permission from Elsevier.

- Sumatriptan nasal spray is effective and should be considered for the acute treatment of migraine in adolescents (Level A).
- There are no data to support or refute the use of any oral triptan preparations in children or adolescents (Level U).
- There are inadequate data to make a judgment on the efficacy of subcutaneous sumatriptan (Level U).

Other medications for acute treatment of migraine are

- *Ergotamine-derived medications:* They are serotoninergic agonists. Controlled trials of oral ergotamine have failed to show efficacy in the relief of migraine. Dihydroergotamine mesylate (Migranal) is a nasal spray to treat acute migraine, which has proved to be effective in adults. Dihydroergotamine (DHE) is given intravenously and is effective in the treatment of severe migraine with minimal side effects. It also contains caffeine. It is usually saved for treatment of migraine in the emergency department or the inpatient setting. Intravenous DHE 0.25 to 1.0 mg every 8 hours, preceded by 5- to 10-mg of intravenous metoclopramide (Reglan) is an effective treatment protocol for status migranosus. Ergotamine-derived medications should be avoided in patients with complicated migraine (ie, hemiplegic or basilar artery migraine) as it may exaggerate symptoms by increasing vasospasm. They should also be avoided within 24 hours of the administration of triptans.
- *Metoclopramide (Reglan):* In addition to the use in the emergency department setting, as an isolated treatment of migraine or in conjunction with DHE, it can be used as 5- or 10-mg oral tablets to help control migraines in the outpatient setting, particularly in patients who cannot take NSAIDs.
- *Combination medications:* Excedrin (aspirin/acetaminophen, and caffeine); Fiorinal, Fioricet, or Esgic (butalbital, aspirin/acetaminophen, caffeine); and Midrin (isometheptene, acetaminophen, dichloralphenazone).
- *Triptans:* These are serotoninergic agonists like sumatriptan (Imitrex), zolmitriptan (Zomig), and rizatriptan (Maxalt) that block the pathogenetic mechanisms of migraine, and have shown great efficacy in adults, although they are not approved for pediatric use.

In practice, we use acetaminophen; NSAIDs; or Excedrin, for infrequent, mild to moderate headache, with relatively good success. For more severe migraine episodes, we use dihydroergotamine nasal spray (Migranal) and triptans, nasally or orally, and we have the clinical impression that they are effective also in pediatric patients.

Prophylactic Treatment (Table 10-2)

In the judgment of many practitioners, greater than 3 to 4 severe headaches per month is considered to be an indication for prophylactic treatment. Propranolol, cyproheptadine, amitriptyline, nortriptyline, topiramate, valproic acid, and verapamil, among others, have been widely used for the prophylaxis of migraines.

The conclusions by the American Academy of Neurology in its practice parameters regarding treatment of migraine headaches in children and adolescents are that

1) Flunarizine, a calcium channel antagonist, is probably effective for preventive therapy, and can be considered for this purpose but is not available in the United States (Class I evidence, level B).
2) There is insufficient evidence to make any recommendations concerning the use of cyproheptadine, amitriptyline, divalproex sodium, topiramate, or levetiracetam (Level U).
3) Recommendations cannot be made concerning propranolol or trazodone for preventive therapy as the evidence is conflicting (Level U).

Table 10-2. Prophylactic Treatment of Migraine in Children[a]		
Drug	**Dose**	**Available**
Cyproheptadine	0.25–1.5 mg/kg	Tabs 4 mg Syrup, 2 mg/tsp
Propranolol	2–4 mg/kg/d	Tabs10, 20, 40, 80, 120 mg Cps-LA 60, 80, 120, 160 mg
Verapamil	3–5 mg/kg	Tabs 40, 80, 120 mg SR tab 120, 180, 240 mg
Amitriptyline	5–25 mg qhs	Tabs 10, 25, 50 mg
Nortriptyline	10–75 mg qhs	Tabs 10, 25, 50, 75 mg
Topiramate	1–10 mg/kg/d	Sprinkles 15, 25 mg Tabs 25, 100 mg
Valproic acid	20–40 mg/kg/d	Syrup 250 mg/tsp Sprinkles 125 mg Tabs 250, 500 mg ER 250, 500 mg
Naproxen sodium	250–500 mg bid	Tabs 220, 250, 375, 500 mg

Abbreviations: tabs, tablets; tsp, teaspoon; cps, capsules; SR, suspended release; qhs, at bed time; ER, extended release; bid, twice a day.

[a]Modified from Lewis DW. Headaches in children and adolescents. *Curr Probl Pediatr Adolesc Health Care*. 2007;37:224, with permission from Elsevier.

4) Pizotifen and nimodipine (Level B) and clonidine (Level B) did not show efficacy and are not recommended.

In practice, we use cyproheptadine, propranolol, verapamil, amitriptyline, topiramate, and valproic acid for migraine prophylaxis in children and adolescents with reasonable success.

Box 10-7 shows a biobehavioral program that should be discussed with every child and adolescent, and their families, who consult for headaches.

Tension Headache

There are studies that have shown that relaxation training and amitriptyline are effective in the treatment of tension headache. The addition of a muscle relaxant does not seem to add efficacy to the relaxation technique. Overall, biobehavioral therapies, including relaxation treatment, thermal biofeedback, electromyographic biofeedback, and progressive muscle relaxation, should be the basis of a successful treatment of tension headache.

Analgesic Rebound Headache

This headache is difficult to treat because it is based on an acquired behavior, and pharmacologic dependency may contribute. The use of metoclopramide (Reglan) or ondansetron (Zofran) may be helpful to support the withdrawal of analgesics. Behavior modification therapy may also play an important role. The biobehavioral program displayed in Box 10-7 should also be part of the treatment.

Chronic Daily Headache

The approach to the treatment depends on the cause of the headache. If it has evolved from a tension headache, an aggressive relaxation and biobehavioral program should be initiated. If the chronic headache is the progression of a poorly treated migraine, sometimes complicated with analgesic abuse, admission to the hospital and initiation of a Reglan+DHE protocol may break the cycle. Plans for lifestyle changes should be made on hospital discharge. Other chronic daily headaches may respond to the same protocol.

Idiopathic Intracranial Hypertension or Pseudotumor Cerebri

In many cases, lumbar puncture can be therapeutic as well as diagnostic if drainage of CSF is sufficient to normalize the closing CSF pressure. The

---

Box 10-7. Recommended Biobehavioral Program for Children and Adolescents With Migraine[a]

1. Good sleep hygiene
   Regular sleep schedule
   Avoid excess, inadequate, or chaotic sleep
2. Regular aerobic exercise (30 minutes daily)
3. Regular meals, avoid missing meals
4. Caffeine avoidance/moderation
5. Identification of migraine triggers
7. Biobehavioral
   a. Biofeedback
   b. Relaxation therapy
   c. Cognitive therapy/stress management
8. Complementary and alternative
   a. Herbs: feverfew, gingko, valerian root
   b. Minerals: magnesium
   c. Vitamins: riboflavin (B2)
   d. Acupuncture

---

[a]*Modified from Lewis DW. Headaches in children and adolescents. Curr Probl Pediatr Adolesc Health Care. 2007;37:223, with permission from Elsevier.*

---

patient should be carefully monitored the following days after the spinal tap. The development of a severe headache that is exacerbated by upright posture and is ameliorated by recumbency indicates a syndrome of intracranial hypotension due to leakage of CSF at the dural puncture site, and treatment with an epidural blood patch may be required. Pharmacologic treatment to suppress production of CSF requires acetazolamide (Diamox) at a variable daily dose of 250 to 1,000 mg. Treatment of the underlying cause is also necessary (eg, discontinuation of tetracycline or adoption of a weight loss program). The patient must be followed periodically by the pediatric neurologist and the ophthalmologist. Follow-up of the electrolytes is warranted. Pseudotumor cerebri among children often runs a self-limiting, monophasic course, but a continuing requirement for lumbar puncture for symptom control and progressive visual impairment despite appropriate medical therapy are indications for neurosurgical referral. Lumboperitoneal CSF shunt insertion is effective.

Web Sites

The American Headache Society: www.americanheadachesociety.org/

International Headache Society International Headache Classification (ICHD-2): http://ihs-classification.org/en

Bibliography

Brenner M, Oakley C, Lewis DW. Unusual headache syndromes in children. *Curr Pain Headache Rep.* 2007;11:383–389

Dahlöf C. Placebo-controlled clinical trials with ergotamine in the acute treatment of migraine. *Cephalalgia.* 1993;13:166–171

Evans R, Lewis D. Is an MRI scan indicated in a child with new-onset daily headache? *Headache.* 2001;41:905–906

Fenichel G. Headache. In: Fenichel G, ed. *Clinical Pediatric Neurology: A Signs and Symptoms Approach.* 5th ed. Philadelphia, PA: Elsevier Saunders; 2005:77–89

Fleischer DR. The cyclic vomiting syndrome described. *J Pediatr Gastroenterol Nutr.* 1995;21(suppl 1):S1–S5

Forbes D. Differential diagnosis of cyclic vomiting syndrome. *J Pediatr Gastroenterol Nutr.* 1995;21(suppl 1):S11–S14

Friedman D, Jacobson D. Diagnostic criteria for idiopathic intracranial hypertension. *Neurology.* 2002;59:1492–1495

Headache Classification Subcommittee of the International Headache Society. The international classification of headache disorders. *Cephalalgia.* 2004;24(suppl 1):1–151

Hershey AD, Winner P, Kabbouche MA, Powers SW. Headaches. *Curr Opin Pediatr.* 2007;19:663–669

Lewis DW. Headaches in children and adolescents. *Curr Probl Pediatr Adolesc Health Care.* 2007;37:207–246

Lewis D, Ashwal S, Dahl G, et al. Practice parameter: evaluation of children and adolescents with recurrent headaches. *Neurology.* 2002;59:490–498

Lewis DW, Diamond S, Scott D, Jones V. Prophylactic treatment of pediatric migraine. *Headache.* 2004;44:230–237

Lewis D, Ashwal S, Hershey A, Hirtz D, Yonker M, Silberstein S. Practice parameters: pharmacological treatment of migraine headache in children and adolescents. Report of the American Academy of Neurology Quality Standards Subcommittee and the Practice Committee of the Child Neurology Society. *Neurology.* 2004;63:2215–2224

Lewis DW, Gozzo YF, Avner MT. The "other" primary headaches in children and adolescents. *Pediatr Neurol.* 2005;33:303–313

Lewis DW, Qureshi F. Acute headache in children and adolescents presenting to the emergency department. *Headache.* 2000;40:200–203

Lewis DW, Yonker M, Winner P, Sowell M. The treatment of pediatric migraine. *Pediatr Ann.* 2005;34:448–460

Linder SL. Treatment of childhood headache with dihydroergotamine mesylate. *Headache.* 1994;34:578–580

Lipton RB, Bigal ME, Steiner TJ, Silbertein SD, Olesen J. Classification of primary headaches. *Neurology.* 2004;63:427–435

Mack KJ. Episodic and chronic migraine in children. *Semin Neurol.* 2006;26:223–231

Miller A, ed. Headaches. *Continuum.* 2006;12: number 6

Rothner AD, ed. *Pediatric headaches. Semin Pediatr Neurol.* 2001;8:1–51

Silberstein SD. Practice parameter: evidence-based guidelines for migraine headache (an evidence-based review). *Neurology.* 2000;55:754–762

Silberstein SD, Lipton RB, Goadsby PJ, eds. Headache in clinical practice. London, UK: Martin Dunitz LTD; 2002

Sillanpaa M. Changes in the prevalence of migraine and other headaches during the first seven school years. *Headache.* 1983;23:15–19

Sillanpaa M, Piekkala P. Prevalence of migraine and other headaches in early puberty. *Scand J Prim Health Care.* 1984;2:27–32

Symon DNK, Russell G. The relationship between cyclic vomiting syndrome and abdominal migraine. *J Pediatr Gastroenterol Nutr.* 1995;21(suppl 1):S42–S43

Vendrame M, Kaleyias J, Valencia I, Legido A, Kothare SV. Polysomnographic findings in children with headaches. *Pediatr Neurol.* 2008;39:6–11

Zuckerman B, Stevenson J, Bailey V. Stomachaches and headaches in a community sample of preschool children. *Pediatrics.* 1983;23:15–19

Appendix 10-1

American Academy of Neurology Evidence Classification Scheme for a Diagnostic Article

Class I: Evidence provided by a prospective study in a broad spectrum of persons with the suspected condition, using a "gold standard" for case definition, where the test is applied in a blinded evaluation, and enabling the assessment of appropriate tests of diagnostic accuracy.

Class II: Evidence provided by a prospective study of narrow spectrum of persons with the suspected condition, or a well-designed retrospective study of a broad spectrum of persons with an established condition (by "gold standard") compared to a broad spectrum of controls, in which evaluation is blinded and which employs appropriate tests of diagnostic accuracy.

Class III: Evidence provided by a retrospective study in which either persons with the established condition or controls are of a narrow spectrum, and in which each evaluation is blinded.

Class IV: Any design in which each evaluation is blinded OR evidence provided by expert opinion alone OR descriptive case series (without controls).

Appendix 10-2

American Academy of Neurology System for Translation of Evidence to Recommendations

Translation of Evidence to Recommendations

Level A rating requires at least one convincing class I study or at least 2 consistent, convincing class II studies

Level B rating requires at least one convincing class II study or overwhelming class II evidence

Level C rating requires at least 2 convincing class III studies

Rating of Recommendations

A = Established as useful/ predictive or not useful/least predictive for the given population

B = Probably useful/predictive or not useful/predictive for the given condition in the specified population

C = Possibly useful/predictive or not useful/predictive for the given condition in the specified population

U = Data inadequate or conflicting. Given current knowledge, test, predictor is unproven

Chapter 11

Movement Disorders

Karen S. Carvalho, MD

Introduction

Movement disorders are a complex group of neurologic diseases character-ized by abnormal involuntary movements originated in the basal ganglia and their connections. It is a complex group of disorders with great variability of presentation and therefore difficult to characterize and classify. Movement disorders are usually present at rest but can sometimes be present during sleep (sleep myoclonus, periodic limb movement disorders). They can occur isolated or as a manifestation of an underlying neurologic disease.

The overall incidence and prevalence of movement disorders in children are not known. Tic disorders are estimated to occur in 1% to 29% of chil-dren. The incidence of Tourette syndrome ranges from 0.1 to 1 per 1,000 children. Essential tremor is one of the most common neurologic disorders, with an estimated prevalence of up to 40% in some studies. The incidence of rheumatic fever in industrialized and developing countries is estimated to be 0.5 per 100,000 and 100 to 200 per 100,000 school-aged children per year respectively. Approximately 10% of patients with rheumatic fever develop chorea. More rarely, movement disorders can be a presenting or even sole symptom of a progressively degenerative neurologic disease.

Pathophysiology

Movement disorders result from a disturbance of central neurotransmission involving particularly the basal ganglia but also the corticospinal tract, cer-ebellum, thalamus, and hippocampus. Gamma-aminobutyric acid (GABA), acetylcholine, serotonin, and glycine are the key neurotransmitters involved (Figure 11-1).

Classification

The classification of movement disorders is based on the description of the phenomena; therefore, when encountering a patient with involuntary movements, the clinician must first define the characteristics of the movements. Recognition of type and pattern of the involuntary movement is fundamental to reach a specific diagnosis and essential to develop a treatment strategy (Box 11-1). Involuntary movements can be classified in hyperkinetic (excessive movement) or hypokinetic (slowness/difficulty to initiate or maintain a movement) (Box 11-2).

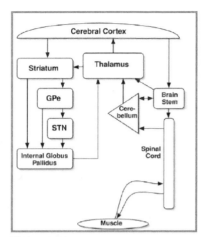

Figure 11-1.
Major systems and pathways involved in the pathophysiology of movement disorders. Abbreviations: GPe, internal globus pallidus; STN, subthalamic nucleus. (Adapted from Sanger TD. Pathophysiology of Pediatric Movement Disorders. *J Child Neurol.* 2003;18[suppl 1]:S9–S24. Reprinted by permission of Sage Publications.)

Tremor

Tremor is a rhythmic, involuntary oscillatory movement with a fixed frequency. Tremor can be classified as

- Resting (occurs at rest)
- Kinetic/action/intentional (occurs during action)
- Postural (occurs with assumption of a posture)

Enhanced Physiological Tremor
Everybody has an unnoticeable physiological tremor. Anxiety, stress, fatigue, and certain drugs can enhance physiological tremor. Hyperthyroidism is also known to enhance physiological tremor.

Essential Tremor
Essential tremor has a bimodal distribution peaking in the second and sixth decades. In children, it has the appearance of restlessness or clumsiness and is enhanced by high, precision movements, anxiety, or fatigue. It can greatly affect schoolwork and cause significant functional impairment. Etiology is poorly understood. This condition can be sporadic or familial. Three gene loci (*ETM1* on 3q13, *ETM2* on 2p24.1, and a locus on 6p23) have been identified in patients and families with the disorder. Essential tremor is a lifelong, benign, usually isolated condition. Treatment is symptomatic. Mild and moderate tremor that does not affect function does not require medical

Box 11-1. Phenomenology of Movement Disorders

Distribution: focal/segmental/generalized

Symmetry: symmetrical/asymmetrical

Nature: stereotyped/non-stereotyped, simple/complex

Amplitude: small/large

Duration: fast/slow

Flowing/continuous/intermittent

Velocity: slow/fast

Rhythm: rhythmic/arrhythmic

Rest/posture/action

Precipitating/aggravating/ameliorating factor

Suppressibility

Box 11-2. Classification and Associated Characteristics of Movement Disorders[a]

Hyperkinetic

Tremor: fast/slow, rhythmic, intermittent/continuous, simple, rest/posture/action

Tics: fast, small, brief, intermittent, simple/complex, rest

Chorea: slow, small, arrhythmic, continuous, "flowing," rest

Dystonia: fast/slow, arrhythmic, brief/sustained, continuous, abnormal posture

Dyskinesias: excessive movement; variable

Myoclonus: fast, small, brief, intermittent, rhythmic/arrhythmic, rest/posture/action

Ballism: large, arrhythmic

Athetosis: slow "wringing movements"

Stereotypies: arrhythmic, repetitive, intermittent, rest

Akathisia: arrhythmic, repetitive, intermittent, complex

Hypokinetic

Spasticity: sustained, velocity-dependent resistance to movement

Rigidity: sustained, uniform, resistance to moment, independent of movement velocity

Bradykinesia: slowness of movement

---

[a]*Modified from Gershanik OS, Koller WC, Tolosa E, eds. Clinical recognition of movement disorders: basal ganglia pathophysiology. In:* Differential Diagnosis and Treatment of Movement Disorders. *Boston, MA: Butterworth-Heinemann; 1997:2, with permission from Elsevier.*

treatment. Pharmacologic treatment is effective in 70% of the patients. Propranolol is thought to be the most efficacious and tolerable drug. Primidone or benzodiazepines (clonazepam, diazepam, lorazepam) can be used; however, sedation is a common limiting side effect. Family reassurance is very important. Occupational therapy may be helpful. Severe cases or patients suspected to have an underlying degenerative neurologic disease should be referred to a neurologist for further investigation.

Intentional Tremor

Intentional tremor is usually seen in diseases affecting the cerebellum and its connections and is an ominous sign of underlying neurologic disorder. Cerebral imaging studies, including brain magnetic resonance imaging (MRI) and computed tomography, are recommended to rule out intracranial tumors and hydrocephalus. Rare neurodegenerative diseases such as juvenile Parkinson disease, Wilson disease, Huntington disease, mitochondrial diseases, and inborn error of metabolism can present with tremor. Tremor can also be present in static encephalopathies like cerebral palsy and posttraumatic brain injury. Any patient with intentional tremor should be immediately referred to a specialist.

Drug-Induced Tremor

Several drugs can precipitate or exacerbate tremor (Box 11-3). It usually improves with reduction or suspension of the affecting agent.

Psychogenic Tremor

Psychogenic etiology should be suspected if the tremor is inconsistent or of sudden onset and if it responds dramatically to placebo. Referral to a child psychologist may be recommended according to the complexity of the psychopathology.

Chorea

Chorea is a sudden, irregular, and arrhythmic purposeless series of movements that flow from one body part to another. Chorea can be inherited or acquired (Box 11-4).

Box 11-3. Drugs and Other Substances Associated With Tremor

Valproate

Lithium

Thyroid hormones

Bronchodilators

Amiodarone

Tricyclic antidepressants

Stimulants (cocaine, amphetamines, methylphenidate)

Caffeine, nicotine

Neuroleptics

Cyclosporine

Mercury, thallium, lead, manganese, arsenic, cyanide

Ethanol

Lindane

Sydenham Chorea

This type of chorea is a late manifestation of rheumatic fever and the most commonly acquired chorea in children. The incidence of rheumatic fever, and therefore Sydenham chorea, has diminished drastically in developed countries because of aggressive antibiotic use; however, a number of outbreaks in the United States have been described in recent years, and the disease is still common in developing countries.

Sydenham chorea typically occurs in children 5 to 15 years old with slight female predominance. Abrupt onset of erratic, jerky, and purposeless movements; muscular weakness; emotional liability; and personality changes between 1 and 6 months after a streptococcal pharyngitis characterize the disease. Psychiatric symptoms can be very debilitating; ranging from emotional liability, anxiety, and inattention to frank obsessive-compulsive disorder (OCD). Sydenham chorea is caused by antibodies against group A beta-hemolytic streptococci cross-reacting with neurons of the basal ganglia, producing an inflammatory response.

PANDAS (pediatric autoimmune neuropsychiatric disorder associated with streptococcal infection), another autoimmune syndrome related to group A beta-hemolytic streptococcal infection, is characterized by abrupt and explosive onset of tics and anxiety/obsessive-compulsive behavior with

Box 11-4. Inherited and Acquired Causes of Chorea

Inherited

Benign hereditary chorea

Ataxias
Ataxia-telangiectasia, spinocerebellar
    ataxias

Inborn errors of metabolism
Glutaric academia, propionic acidemia,
    homocystinuria, phenylketonuria,
    sulfite oxidase deficiency

Mitochondrial encephalomyopathies

Neuroacanthocytosis

Others
    Paroxysmal dyskinesias
    Wilson disease
    Hallervorden-Spatz disease
    Huntington disease
    Familiar paroxysmal dyskinesias

Acquired

Drugs
Anticonvulsants, amphetamines,
    antiemetics, anticholinergics,
    neuroleptics, central nervous system
    stimulants, dopamine agonists/
    antagonists, oral contraceptives

Endocrine
Hyperthyroidism, hypoparathyroidism

Immune/infectious
Sydenham chorea, systemic lupus
    erythematosus, meningoencephalitis

Vascular

Metabolic
Hypocalcemia, hypo/hyperglycemia,
    hypo/hypernatremia

Static encephalopathies
Cerebral palsy, head trauma

Neoplastic

Nutritional
Vitamin B_{12} deficiency

Toxins
Carbon monoxide, manganese,
    organophosphate poisoning
Chorea gravidarum

Hepatic or renal failure

clear temporal correlation with the acute infection. Sydenham chorea can include tics and OCD, whereas children with PANDAS can have choreiform movements, and the 2 entities can clearly overlap.

Cardiac involvement is present in about two-thirds of children with Sydenham chorea; therefore, careful cardiac examination and echocardiogram are recommended. Treatment of rheumatic fever entails preventing recurrence of streptococcal infection with prophylactic penicillin. Oral penicillin has proven to be as effective as intramuscular; however, compliance is an issue. The chorea is usually self-limited and improves after weeks to months. Severe chorea can be treated with neuroleptics and anticonvulsants. Valproate is now recommended as a first-line treatment. Neuroleptics are highly effective, but they are associated with significant extrapyramidal side effects. Psychiatric symptoms often need to be addressed with psychotherapy and selective serotonin reuptake inhibitors (SSRIs). Intravenous methylprednisolone followed by oral prednisone, intravenous immunoglobulin, and plasmapheresis have shown success in refractory patients.

Benign Hereditary Chorea

This is an autosomal dominant nonprogressive chorea of childhood onset without other neurologic manifestations. These patients are usually described as clumsy, with frequent falls beginning around 1 to 2 years of age. Intellectual function is typically normal but low IQ scores have been reported. Children often present to a physician because of delayed motor development. The chorea is initially progressive, but subsequently reaches a plateau with no future progression.

Huntington Disease

This condition is an inherited autosomal dominant disorder caused by expansion of (CAG) repeats in the coding region of the *IT15* gene in locus 4p16.3. Onset is usually in the fourth and fifth decade of life. An early-onset form, juvenile Huntington disease, can occur anytime in childhood. Children present with cognitive decline, psychiatric symptoms, parkinsonism, chorea, myoclonus, and seizures. No treatment is available. Prognosis is poor, with death occurring within years.

Wilson Disease

This is an autosomal recessive disorder caused by the mutation *ATP7B* localized on the chromosome 13q14.3. This genetic mutation results in dysfunction of hepatic copper metabolism with subsequent copper accumulation in hepatocytes and extrahepatic organs (brain, cornea). Patients present in the first and second decade with progressive neuropsychiatric symptoms (chorea, spasticity, psychosis) and or hepatic insufficiency. A characteristic corneal discoloration (copper deposition within the Descemet membrane) seen by slit-lamp examination, known as the *Kayser-Fleischer ring,* is pathognomonic but absent early in the disease. The diagnosis is made by demonstrating decreased serum ceruloplasmin and copper levels and increased 24-hour urine copper excretion. Liver biopsy may be necessary. Life-long treatment of Wilson disease aims to prevent the accumulation of copper or reverse its toxic effects with chelating agents (d-penicillamine, trientine, BAL) and zinc. Neurologic symptoms are often irreversible.

Chorea can be treated with neuroleptics (dopaminergic antagonists), and anticholinergic and anticonvulsant agents (Box 11-5).

Tics

Tics are brief, fast, stereotyped, and repetitive movements typically preceded by an urge to perform them and often followed by a sense of relief after they are completed. Tics can be temporarily suppressed and disappear during sleep. They may be simple, affecting one body part such as the shoulder or face; or complex, involving multiple different noncontiguous muscle groups. Tics are the most frequent involuntary movement in children. Tics have a tendency of improving after puberty but may persist through life. A familial history of tics as well as personal and familial history of neurobehavioral disturbances are common.

Tics are classified as follows:
- Transient tic disorder is the most common form, consisting of single or multiple motor and/or vocal tics that occur for at least 4 weeks, but no longer than 12 months.
- Chronic tic disorder is characterized by tics (motor or vocal, but not both) that persist for more than 1 year.
- Tourette syndrome is a genetically complex disorder that likely arises owing to the effects of multiple genes interacting with environmental components that also influence its onset.

The diagnostic criteria require the presence of multiple motor and at least one vocal tic that (1) occur many times daily nearly every day through a period of more than 1 year (although not necessarily continuously for both types of tics), (2) appear before 18 years of age, and (3) are not directly caused by a general medical condition or substance exposure. The rate of psychiatric comorbidity is higher in Tourette than in other tic disorders. Attention-deficit/hyperactivity disorder (ADHD), anxiety, OCD, and sleep problems are frequently reported. One-third of patients have sleep problems. Dyslexia occurs in 20% of patients and school-related difficulties in 80% of patients.

The approach to a child with tics requires an accurate diagnosis and evaluation of the severity of symptoms and presence of comorbidities. The

---

Box 11-5. Pharmacologic Treatment of Chorea

Dopamine receptor antagonists
　　Haloperidol
　　Pimozide
　　Risperidone
　　Clozapine

Dopamine receptor agonists
　　L-Dopa

Anticholinergics
　　Amantadine
　　Trihexyphenidyl

Anticonvulsants
　　Phenytoin
　　Carbamazepine
　　Valproate
　　Lamotrigine

Alpha adrenergic agonists
　　Clonidine

Tetrabenazine

---

decision to begin pharmacologic treatment is based on whether the target symptoms impair the patient's function at home, at school, or at work. Mild and sometimes moderate tics that do not negatively impact the child's psychosocial functioning do not require treatment.

High-potency neuroleptics (haloperidol, pimozide) have been used for years and are highly effective. Because of high incidence of extrapyramidal side effects, they are now reserved for severe and intractable tics. Pimozide has also been associated with prolonged QT interval and, if used, baseline and follow-up electrocardiography is are recommended. Atypical neuroleptics such as risperidone and olanzapine have fewer extrapyramidal side effects and can be an alternative to classic neuroleptics. Excessive weight gain is common. Guanfacine and clonidine are currently the first-line treatment for tics. They are better tolerated and have the advantage of improving ADHD symptoms. Botulinum toxin can be used for vocal tics; hypophonia is a common side effect.

Cognitive behavioral therapy and SSRIs are effective for anxiety and OCD and may consequently decrease the frequency of tics. Patients should be referred to a neurologist for severe intractable tics and to a behavior specialist (psychologist, psychiatrist) for severe behavior problems. Stimulant medications can potentially trigger and exacerbate tics in predisposed children and should be avoided if possible.

Dystonias

Dystonia is characterized by repetitive, sustained movement that typically produces twisting postures. Most patients have a sensory trick, a maneuver that attenuates the involuntary movement. Dystonia may be classified by the affected body region(s).

- *Focal:* Affects a single body part.
- *Segmental:* Affects one or more contiguous body parts.
- *Multifocal:* Affects 2 or more noncontiguous body parts.
- *Generalized:* Affects one leg and the trunk plus one other body part, or both legs plus one other body part.
- *Hemidystonia:* Affects only one-half of the body.

Dystonia can be the presenting or prominent symptom of a variety of neurodegenerative diseases (Box 11-6). Recently, several chromosomal loci and genes involved in dystonia have been identified, advancing our understanding of the genetic and molecular mechanisms underlying the various dystonias (Table 11-1).

Treatment of dystonia is often challenging, and results are disappointing. Anticholinergic agents seem to be most effective and best tolerated. Other agents can be used alone or in combination with anticholinergic drugs, including antidopaminergics, levodopa, baclofen, carbamazepine, and the benzodiazepines (clonazepam, diazepam, lorazepam). Botulinum toxin can be helpful for focal dystonias. For dystonia in the setting of cerebral palsy, continuous intrathecal baclofen administration by means of an implanted drug pump can be useful for comfort and for facilitation of toileting, dressing, seating, and other caretaking tasks. Deep brain stimulation (DBS) has a role in the management of medically refractory dystonia as well. This therapy involves permanent implantation of precisely positioned electrodes in the globus pallidus internus, the posterior ventral thalamus, or other anatomical targets for long-term electrical stimulation by means of an implanted signal generator. Unilateral DBS deserves consideration for hemidystonia, and it is indicated for the management of dystonia musculorum deformans or primary torsion dystonia, a rare and severely disabling genetic

---

Box 11-6. Etiologic Classification of Childhood Dystonia[a]

Primary (idiopathic)
  Primary torsion dystonia (dystonia musculorum deformans)
  Segmental (cervical/cranial) dystonia
  Sporadic focal dystonia

Secondary dystonia
  Congenital malformations
  Trauma, perinatal cerebral injury (anoxia, kernicterus, trauma)
  Drug-induced (neuroleptics, antiepileptics, levodopa, cocaine)
  Toxic (manganese, cyanide, carbon monoxide)
  Infection (encephalitis, HIV)
  Endocrine (hypoparathyroidism)
  Psychogenic dystonia

Dystonia plus syndromes
  Dopa-responsive dystonia
  Rapid onset dystonia-parkinsonism
  Myoclonus-dystonia syndrome

Inherited degenerative disorders
  Autosomal dominant (juvenile Parkinson disease, Huntington disease)
  Autosomal recessive (Wilson disease, Hallervorden-Spatz syndrome)
  X-linked recessive (dystonia-parkinsonism)
  Mitochondrial (Leigh disease)

---

[a]*Modified from Langlois M, Richer F, Chouinard S. New perspectives on dystonia. Can J Neurol Sci. 2003;30:S34–S44. Reprinted by permission.*

---

condition seen among Ashkenazi Jewish families. Its employment in other forms of dystonia in childhood is a matter of current, active exploration.

Dyskinesias

Paroxysmal Dyskinesias

These are rare neurologic conditions characterized by sudden transient episodes of abnormal involuntary movements followed by a relatively rapid return to normal motor function and behavior. Age of onset is 1 to 20 years; however, infantile cases have been reported. Paroxysmal dyskinesias can be idiopathic (familial or sporadic) or acquired, choreoathetotic, dystonic, or mixed forms. Familial forms can be kinesigenic (movement-induced) and

Table 11-1. Genetic Classification of Dystonias[a]				
Class	Clinical Phenotype	Inheritance	Locus	Gene
DYT1	Primary torsion dystonia	AD	9q34	A
DYT2	Primary torsion dystonia	AD		not mapped
DYT3	Dystonia-parkinsonism	X-linked	Xq13.1	not mapped
DYT4	Whispering dysphonia	AD	not mapped	not mapped
DYT5	Dopa-responsive dystonia	AD AR	14q22.11 11p15.5	GTPCH-1 Tyrosine hydroxylase
DYT6	Torsion dystonia, in adults	AD	8p21	not mapped
DYT7	Familial cervical dystonia	AD	18p	not mapped
DYT8	Paroxysmal dystonic choreoathetosis	AD	2q33	not mapped
DYT9	Paroxysmal dyskinesia with spasticity	AD	1p21	not mapped
DYT10	Paroxysmal kinesigenic dyskinesia	AD	16p11-12	not mapped
12DYT11	Myoclonus-dystonia	AD	7q21	ε-sarcoglycan
DYT12	Dystonia-parkinsonism	AD	19q13	not mapped
DYT13	Cranial-cervical-brachial	AD	1p36	not mapped
DYT14	Dopa-responsive dystonia	AD	14q13	not mapped
DYT15	Myoclonus-dystonia	AD	18p11	not mapped

[a]Modified from Jan MMS. Misdiagnoses in children with dopa-responsive dystonia. *Pediatr Neurol.* 2004;31(4):298–303, with permission from Elsevier.

non-kinesigenic according to precipitating factors that precede or trigger the episodes.

Paroxysmal kinesigenic dyskinesia is the most common type of paroxysmal dyskinesia and is characterized by attacks of brief duration (<5 minutes) triggered by initiation of voluntary movements. Consciousness is usually preserved between attacks, and response to antiepileptic drugs (AEDs) is good. Paroxysmal non-kinesigenic dyskinesia is not precipitated by movement, is longer in duration, and has poor response to AEDs. Other types of paroxysmal dyskinesias include episodes precipitated by prolonged exertion (paroxysmal exertion-induced dyskinesia) or sleep (paroxysmal hypnogenic dyskinesia).

The diagnosis is based on detailed characterization of the event and family history. A thorough neurologic examination is mandatory to rule out other neurologic disorders. A trial with AEDs, usually phenytoin or carba-mazepine, is recommended.

Myoclonus

This involuntary movement is characterized by sudden, brief, jerky, shock-like movements without loss of consciousness. Myoclonus can be idiopathic or secondary to a neurodegenerative, systemic metabolic disorders or central nervous system infections (Box 11-7).

Benign Sleep Myoclonus

This type of myoclonus is a benign, self-limiting condition that presents within a few days of birth as rhythmic, brief jerks during drowsiness and sleep. It usually resolves by 3 to 4 months of age. Neonatal epilepsy must be ruled out, in which case a prolonged video electroencephalogram (EEG) monitoring study is recommended. No treatment is necessary.

Box 11-7. Causes of Myoclonus

Benign sleep myoclonus

Essential myoclonus

Progressive myoclonic epilepsy
   Neuronal ceroid lipofuscinosis
   Lafora body disease
   MERRF (myoclonic epilepsy with ragged red fibers)
   MELAS (mitochondrial encephalomyopathy, lactic acidosis, and stroke)
   Sialidosis
   Unverricht-Lundborg disease

Juvenile myoclonic epilepsy

Post-anoxic myoclonus

Metabolic encephalopathy
   Uremia, liver failure

Associated with other degenerative neurologic disease
   Huntington disease
   Subacute sclerosing panencephalitis

Drugs
   Dopamine agonists and antagonists, anticholinergics, tricyclic antidepressants, selective serotonin reuptake inhibitors, lithium, anticonvulsants, opiates, antine-oplastics, antibiotics

---

Opsoclonus Myoclonus

This condition is a rare neurologic disorder characterized by unsteady, trembling gait; myoclonus; and opsoclonus (rapid, chaotic eye movements). Other symptoms are poorly articulated speech, hypotonia, lethargy, and irritability. The underlying disease mechanism is likely to be immune mediated, either as a postinfectious process or as a neuroimmunologic complication of neuronal/neuroblastic tumors, most commonly neuroblastoma. Treatment includes intravenous or oral corticosteroids, intravenous immunoglobulin, adrenocorticotropic hormone, and plasmapheresis. Trazodone can be useful to treat associated irritability and sleep problems. If a tumor is present, treatment with chemotherapy, surgery, or radiation therapy may be required. The prognosis depends on the underlying disease.

Progressive Myoclonic Epilepsies

Progressive myoclonic epilepsies are a heterogeneous group of inherited disorders characterized by myoclonus, epilepsy, and progressive neurological deterioration (Box 11-7).

Post-anoxic Myoclonus

Myoclonus can be treated with clonazepam, valproate, primidone, and more recently levetiracetam.

Drug-Induced Movement Disorders

Several medications can precipitate or exacerbate movement disorders. Neuroleptics (dopamine antagonists) and antiemetics are the most common cause of drug-induced movement disorder; however, other drugs can also be involved (Table 11-2). The onset of drug-induced movement disorders can be

1) Acute: Acute dystonic reaction, akathisia, and neuroleptic malignant syndrome
2) Chronic: Tardive dyskinesia and drug-induced parkinsonism

Table 11-2. Drug-Induced Movement Disorders[a]	
Medication Class	**Movement Disorder**
Neuroleptics	Tremor, dystonia, parkinsonism, dyskinesias
Antidepressants	Myoclonus, tremor, chorea
Antiemetics	Chorea, akathisia, dystonia
Anticonvulsants	Tremor, chorea, myoclonus
Antibiotics	Chorea, tremor, myoclonus
Antineoplastics	Tremor, chorea, myoclonus
Central nervous system stimulants	Tremor, chorea, myoclonus, dyskinesias
Histamine 2 blockers	Dystonia, chorea

[a]Modified from Pranzatelli MR. Movement disorders in childhood. *Pediatr Rev.* 1996;17(30):388–394.

Acute Dystonic Reaction

This type of dystonia can occur in 2% to 3% of patients treated with neuroleptics, usually within days of therapy initiation. Children and young adults are at a higher risk. Patients may present with trismus, oculogyric crisis, torticollis, or even opisthotonus. It is more common with high-potency neuroleptics, but it can also occur with atypical neuroleptics. Patients respond dramatically to intravenous anticholinergics (benztropine) or antihistamines (diphenhydramine). Treatment should be continued orally for a few days. The use of prophylactic anticholinergics is common but controversial.

Akathisia

This movement disorder is characterized by increased motor activity, consisting of complex, semi-purposeful, stereotypic, and repetitive movements to calm down their urge to move. It usually occurs early in the treatment and subsides shortly after cessation of the medication. If symptoms do not improve, anticholinergic agents (amantadine, benztropine), clonazepam, and clonidine can be used.

Neuroleptic Malignant Syndrome

Neuroleptic malignant syndrome (NMS) is one of the most serious adverse, life-threatening reactions to antipsychotic medications (neuroleptics). Recent studies in Japanese patients have suggested that the cytochrome P450 (CYP) enzyme CYP2D6*5 allele is likely to affect vulnerability to development of NMS. Symptoms can occur at any time during neuroleptic treatment and include hyperthermia, rigidity, rhabdomyolysis, reduced consciousness, and autonomic failure. It can be complicated by pulmonary insufficiency, cardiac arrhythmias, renal failure, and death. Laboratory work shows elevated serum creatine phosphokinase and myoglobinuria. Early recognition and immediate withdrawal of the offending agent are paramount. Treatment includes aggressive supportive care; dantrolene (2–3 mg/kg, 3–4 times/day) and bromocriptine (2.5–30 mg/d) can be used in severe cases.

Neuroleptic-Induced Parkinsonism

This condition is characterized by gradual onset of rigidity, postural abnormalities, and tremor. Bradykinesia is the early and often only sign of the disease. Improvement is noticed a few weeks after the cessation of the treatment, but it may take months to years to resolve.

Tardive Dyskinesia

This movement disorder can occur anytime during neuroleptic treatment or after reduction/cessation of the drug. Patients present with chewing, tongue protrusion, and lip-smacking movements. Limbs and trunk can also be involved. The symptoms respond poorly to pharmacologic therapy. Prevention using low-potency antipsychotics and avoidance of chronic exposure is the best treatment. Clozapine can be used in substitution for patients who developed tardive dyskinesia and need prolonged neuroleptic treatment. Patients on clozapine need to be closely monitored for aplastic anemia.

Other Movement Disorders

Stereotypies

Sterotypies are continuous, repetitive, purposeless or ritualistic movements, postural changes, or utterances. Common stereotypies include body rocking, self-caressing, crossing and uncrossing of legs, and marching in place. They usually occur when the child is playing a game or participating in an activity, but also at times of excitement, stress, fatigue, and boredom. They can last from seconds or minutes to hours, appearing many times per day and can be suppressed by sensory stimuli or distraction. They are usually not bothersome to the child, but they are worrisome to the parents. They can occur in normal children or be associated with pervasive developmental disorder, ADHD, OCD, tics, learning disability, or developmental delay. Treatment is usually not necessary. Severe cases can be treated with benzodiazepines, beta-adrenergic agonists, antipsychotics, and SSRIs.

Excessive Startle Response (Hyperekplexia)

Hyperekplexia is an inherited disorder characterized by an excessive response to auditory, visual, or sensory stimuli and stiffness present during the neonatal period. Nose tapping is particularly effective in eliciting the response. It disappears by late infancy. It has been associated with mutations in the glycine receptor subunit genes *GLRA1* and *GLRB* and within the neuronal glycine transporter 2 gene *GLYT2* or *SLC6A5*. No treatment is necessary.

Jitteriness

Almost half of the normal-term neonates exhibit jitteriness during the first days of life, usually provoked by stimulation. However, it can also occur in anoxic injury, drug withdrawal, and some metabolic derangements (hypocalcemia, hypoglycemia). Jitteriness can be difficult to differentiate from seizures, particularly during the neonatal period. Seizures are usually associated with abnormality of gaze or eye movements and do not stop with touch. Prolonged EEG monitoring is often necessary.

Shuddering

Episodes of shuddering consist of brief bursts of rapid tremor of the head and arms, similar to shiver, occurring several times a day with onset during the first few months of life. The etiology is unknown, although some authors believe shuddering precedes essential tremor. The clinical course is benign. No treatment is necessary.

Spasmus Nutans

This is a self-limiting disorder of infants characterized by a slow head tremor (horizontal, vertical, or rotatory head nodding) associated with nystagmus (unilateral or bilateral, rapid, fine, pendular, and horizontal) and sometimes head tilt. The onset is generally between 4 and 12 months of age and disappears in a few months. Patients should be referred to a pediatric ophthalmologist for evaluation of visual acuity. The main differential diagnosis is congenital nystagmus. Brain MRI is recommended to rule out optic nerve or posterior fossa tumors.

Periodic Limb Movement Disorder

Periodic limb movement disorder (PLMD) is characterized by periodic stereotyped limb movements that occur during the non–rapid eye movement phase of sleep. Periodic limb movement disorder can cause nocturnal awakenings, but patients usually present with poor sleep and daytime somnolence. It can be associated with restless legs syndrome (RLS), a condition with sensory features that manifest during wakefulness. Potential risk factors include sleep apnea, narcolepsy, benzodiazepine/barbiturate withdrawal, neuroleptics/dopaminergic agents, uremia, iron deficiency, spinal cord injury, and diabetes mellitus. A definitive diagnosis requires polysomnography. Treatment includes L-dopa, clonazepam, baclofen, gabapentin, and opioids.

Restless Legs Syndrome

Restless legs syndrome is characterized by unpleasant sensations in the legs and an uncontrollable urge to move them when at rest in an effort to relieve such feelings. Patients describe a burning, creeping, tugging sensation, or like insects crawling inside the legs. The diagnosis is clinical. Children with RLS can present with conduct problems including aggression, inattention, hyperactivity, and daytime somnolence because of inability to sleep or difficulty maintaining sleep. It is often associated with PLMD and ADHD. Treatment includes managing the associated condition, caffeine restriction, and good sleep hygiene. Clonidine, guanfacine, clonazepam, and L-dopa have been tried with some success.

Diagnostic Approach

Isolated occurrence of a nonprogressive movement disorder in an otherwise normal child suggests that the disorder is idiopathic, and referral to a specialist is often unnecessary. When there are other developmental and neurologic abnormalities, the child should be immediately referred to a neurologist for further evaluation. Investigation often starts with complete blood cell count, comprehensive metabolic panel (including renal and hepatic function tests), and thyroid tests. If there is suspicion of an auto-immune disease, antinuclear antibodies, urinalysis, sedimentation rate and C-reactive protein should be obtained. Once metabolic and drug-induced etiologies are excluded, establishing an etiologic diagnosis often relies on ancillary studies such as MRI, MR spectroscopy, and genetic testing. Electro-encephalography sometimes may be necessary to rule out seizures.

Therapeutic Approach

Effective treatment of a patient with a movement disorder is based on understanding the relationship between etiology and clinical symptoms. Certain movement disorders, such as mild tics and essential tremors do not require pharmacologic treatment. They can be managed by the pediatrician or family practitioner. Patients should be referred to a specialist if all revers-ible underlying etiologies have been excluded, the symptoms pose a serious problem to the patient, or a degenerative neurologic disease is suspected.

Treatment of movement disorders is usually symptomatic and includes neuroleptics, anticonvulsants, benzodiazepines, and alpha-adrenergic ago-nists (Table 11-3). Intrathecal baclofen has been used for years for spasticity in patients with cerebral palsy and more recently for generalized dystonia. Botulinum toxin is used for spasticity and focal dystonias, with minimal side effects. Deep brain stimulation has been used in adults with Parkinson dis-ease, tremor, and dystonia with some success; however, there are no data of its use available in children.

While more simple nonprogressive movement disorders can be man-aged by a generalist, more complex and severe cases need to be evaluated by a multidisciplinary team of health care professionals including a physi-cal and occupational therapists, pediatric psychologist, pediatric neurolo-gist, and orthopedic surgeon. Psychological and educational support are also important.

| Table 11-3. Pharmacologic Treatment of Movement Disorders ||
Medications	Suggested Dosing
Dopaminergics	
haloperidol	0.5–5.0 mg/d ÷ bid–tid
pimozide	1–2 mg/kg/d ÷ bid
Benzodiazepines	
clonazepam	0.01–0.03 mg/kg/d ÷ bid–tid
diazepam	0.12–0.8 mg/Kg/d ÷ tid–qid
Anticonvulsants	
phenytoin	3–6 mg/kg/d ÷ bid–tid
carbamazepine	10–40 mg/kg/d ÷ bid–tid
valproate	15–50 mg/kg/d ÷ bid–tid
lamotrigine	2–20 mg/kg/d ÷ bid
primidone	2–10 mg/kg/d ÷ bid
Anticholinergics	
trihexyphenidyl	60–80 mg/d ÷ bid
amantadine	50–200 mg/d ÷ bid
Alpha-adrenergic agonists	
clonidine	0.005 mg/kg/d ÷ tid–qid
guanfacine	0.25–3 mg/d ÷ bid–tid
Alpha-adrenergic antagonists	
propranolol	1–2 mg/kg/d ÷ bid–tid
Baclofen	10–60 mg/d ÷ bid–tid
Dantrolene	0.5 mg–3.0 mg/kg/day ÷ bid–tid
Antiemetics	diphenhydramine 25–100 mg/d
Botulin toxin	100–200 UI every 3–6 months

Abbreviations: bid, twice a day; tid, 3 times a day; qid, 4 times a day.

Web Sites

Tourette Syndrome Association (TSA): www.tsa-usa.org/

Dystonia Medical Research Foundation (DMRF):
www.dystonia-foundation.org

National Institute of Neurological Disorders and Stroke (NINDS):
www.ninds.nih.gov/

**World Wide Education and Awareness for Movement Disorders
(WE MOVE):** www.wemove.org

Bibliography

Agarwal P, Frucht SJ. Myoclonus. *Curr Opin Neurol.* 2003;16:515–521

American Psychiatric Association. *Diagnostic and Statistical Manual-Text Revision (DSM-IV-TRTM, 2000).* 4th ed. Washington, DC: American Psychiatric Association; 2000

Ayoub EM. Resurgence of rheumatic fever in the United States. The changing picture of a preventable illness. *Postgrad Med.* 1992;92:133–136, 139–142

Church AJ, Cardoso F, Dale RC, Lees AJ, Thompson EJ, Giovannoni G. Anti-basal ganglia antibodies in acute and persistent Sydenham's chorea. *Neurology.* 2002;59:227–231

Comings DE. Tourette syndrome: a hereditary neuropsychiatric spectrum disorder. *Ann Clin Psychiatry.* 1994;6:235–247

Dressler D, Bedecked R. Diagnosis and management of acute movement disorders. *J Neurol.* 2005;252:1299–1306

Fenichel GM. Movement disorders. In: Fenichel GM, editor. *Clinical Pediatric Neurology. A Signs and Symptoms Approach.* Philadelphia, PA: Elsevier Saunders; 2005:281–298

Garvey MA, Snider LA, Leitman SF, Werden R, Swedo SE. Treatment of Sydenham's chorea with intravenous immunoglobulin, plasma exchange, or prednisone. *J Child Neurol.* 2005;20:424–429

Gershanik OS, Koller WC, Tolosa E, eds. Clinical recognition of movement disorders: basal ganglia pathophysiology. In: *Differential Diagnosis and Treatment of Movement Disorders.* Boston, MA: Butterworth-Heinemann; 1997:1–6

Gilbert D. Treatment of children and adolescents with tics and Tourette syndrome. *J Child Neurol.* 2006;21:690–700

Goodenough DJ, Fariello RG, Annis BL, Chun RW. Familial and acquired paroxysmal dyskinesias. A proposed classification with delineation of clinical features. *Arch Neurol.* 1978;35:827–831

Goodman WK, Storch EA, Geffken GR, Murphy TK. Obsessive-compulsive disorder in Tourette syndrome. *J Child Neurol.* 2006;21:704–714

Higgins JJ, Pho LT, Nee LE. A gene (ETM) for essential tremor maps to chromosome 2p22-p25. *Mov Disord.* 1997;12:859–864

Huntington's Disease Collaborative Research Group. A novel gene containing a trinucleotide repeats that is expanded and unstable on Huntington's disease chromosome. *Cell.* 1993;72:971–983

Jankovic J, Madisetty J, Vuong KD. Essential tremor among children. *Pediatrics.* 2004;114:1203–1205

Keen-Kim D, Freimer NB. Genetics and epidemiology of Tourette syndrome. *J Child Neurol.* 2006;21:665–671

Khalifa N, von Knorring AL. Psychopathology in a Swedish population of school children with tic disorders. *J Am Acad Child Adolesc Psychiatry.* 2006;45:1346–1353

Langlois M, Richer F, Chouinard S. New perspectives on dystonia. *Can J Neurol Sci.* 2003;30: S34–S44

Loudianos G, Gitlin JD. Wilson's disease. *Semin Liver Dis.* 2000;20:353–364

Louis ED, Ottman R, Hauser WA. How common is the most common adult movement disorder? Estimates of the prevalence of essential tremor throughout the world. *Mov Disord.* 1998;13:5–10

Mohammed MS. Misdiagnoses in children with dopa-responsive dystonia. *Pediatr Neurol.* 2004;31:298–303

Olson LL, Singer HS, Goodman WK, Maria BL. Tourette syndrome: diagnosis, strategies, therapies, pathogenesis, and future research directions. *J Child Neurol.* 2006;21:630–641

Pavone P, Parano E, Rizzo R, Trifiletti RR. Autoimmune neuropsychiatric disorders associated with streptococcal infection: Sydenham's chorea, PANDAS, and PANDAS variants. *J Child Neurol.* 2006;21:727–736

Pena J, Mora E, Cardozo J, Molina O, Montiel C. Comparison of the efficacy of carbamazepine, haloperidol and valproic acid in the treatment of children with Sydenham's chorea: clinical follow-up of 18 patients. *Arq Neuropsiquiatr.* 2002;60:374–377

Pranzatelli MR. Movement Disorders in childhood. *Pediatr Rev.* 1996;17:388–394

Sandor P. Pharmacological management of tics in patients with TS. *J Psychosom Res.* 2003;55: 41–48

Sanger TD. Pathophysiology of pediatric movement disorders. *J Child Neurol.* 2003;18 (suppl 1):S9–S24

Sanger TD, Delgado MR, Gaebler-Spira D, Hallett M, Mink JW. Classification and definition of disorders causing hypertonia in childhood. *Pediatrics.* 2003;111:e89–e97

Swedo SE, Leonard HL, Schapiro MB,et al. Sydenham's chorea: physical and psychological symptoms of St Vitus dance. *Pediatrics.* 1993;91:706–713

Wheeler PG, Weaver DD, Dobyns WB. Benign hereditary chorea. *Pediatr Neurol.* 1993;9: 337–340

Chapter 12

Ataxias

Karen S. Carvalho, MD
Joseph J. Melvin, DO

Definition

Ataxia is defined as impaired balance and incoordination of intentional movements. It is a specific clinical manifestation that usually implies dysfunction of the cerebellum and its connections.

The most prominent feature of ataxia is abnormal gait, characterized by a wide-based, unsteady, staggering gait. Other signs and symptoms of ataxia include slurred speech, difficulty with fine-motor tasks, slow eye movements, and difficulty swallowing.

A thorough history and physical examination followed by appropriate laboratory studies will distinguish among a wide variety of etiologies, some of which can be treated by specific therapies.

Pathophysiology

The presence of ataxia usually implies involvement of the cerebellum and its connections. Afferent and efferent pathways connect the cerebellum to the brain stem and the rest of the central nervous system (CNS). Afferent connections originating from position sense in muscles and tendons ascend through the spinal cord. Other afferent connections also originate from the inner ear and cerebral cortex. Efferents return to the cerebral cortex by way of the thalamus. The anatomy and physiology of the cerebellum and its efferent and afferent connections is complex, and a full description is beyond the scope of this book (for a review see *The Global Cerebellum* by John K. Harting (www.neuroanatomy.wisc.edu/cere/text/cere/contents.htm).

Classification

Ataxias can be classified according to presentation and progression of the disease as acute, intermittent, progressive chronic, or nonprogressive chronic ataxias.

Acute Ataxias

Acute ataxias are characterized by sudden disturbance of gait and balance, and they have quite diverse etiologies. Acute cerebellar ataxia, ingestion, and Guillain-Barré syndrome (GBS) encompass 80% of all acute childhood ataxias. The differential diagnosis of acute and intermittent ataxias is shown in Boxes 12-1 and 12-2, respectively.

Acute Cerebellar Ataxia

Acute cerebellar ataxia, formerly known as *cerebellitis,* is the most common cause of acute ataxia in childhood. It typically occurs in association with a primary infection, postinfectious, or postvaccination. A history of recent viral illness is found in two-thirds of patients.

Acute postinfectious cerebellar ataxia usually occurs in children between 2 and 5 years of age and is rare in adolescents and adults. The ataxia may appear any time up to 6 weeks after the inciting illness. Symptoms worsen during a 24-hour period and then slowly resolve within several days. Varicella is a common cause in the younger patients, whereas Epstein-Barr virus (EBV) infection and immunizations are the most common causes in older patients (Box 12-3). Transient behavioral alterations and school difficulties are seen in at least one-third of children. Laboratory studies may reveal a mild cerebrospinal fluid pleocytosis. Neuroimaging studies are usually normal; occasionally, an abnormal signal can be seen in the cerebellum with magnetic resonance imaging.

Meningoencephalitis, particularly involving the brain stem, can produce ataxia; however, most patients have additional neurologic abnormalities such as stiff neck, fever, lethargy, focal deficit, and seizures. Magnetic resonance imaging may show leptomeningeal enhancement. Cerebrospinal fluid analysis demonstrates elevated cell count and protein.

Brain stem encephalitis in children has been associated with several microorganisms including mycoplasma, EBV, mumps, herpes simplex virus, enterovirus 71, and *Listeria monocytogenes* among others.

Drug Ingestion

Drug ingestion is the second most common cause of acute ataxias in children, accounting for as much as 32.5% of cases. Ataxia is often accompanied by changes in mental status, such as lethargy, confusion, and inappropriate speech or behavior. Ataxia commonly follows ingestion of anticonvulsants,

Box 12-1. Acute Ataxias

Postinfectious cerebellitis
  Varicella
  Enterovirus
  Influenza
  Mycoplasma

Drug ingestion
  Anticonvulsants (phenytoin, barbiturates)
  Carbamazepine
  Sedatives
  Hypnotics

Autoimmune
  Guillain-Barré syndrome/Miller Fisher variant
  Multiple sclerosis
  Acute disseminated encephalomyelitis

Meningitis/encephalitis (bacterial or viral)

Head trauma

Cerebrovascular diseases

Hydrocephalus

Vestibular disturbances
  Otitis
  Labyrinthitis
  Endolymphatic hydrops
  Perilymphatic fistula

Seizures

Toxins
  Alcohol
  Ethylene glycol
  Hydrocarbonates
  Lead
  Mercury
  Thallium

Paraneoplastic
  Opsoclonus-myoclonus syndrome

Metabolic
  Hypoglycemia
  Hyponatremia
  Hyperammonemia

Psychogenic

Box 12-2. Episodic or Intermittent Ataxias[a]

Recurrence of acute cerebellar ataxia

Vestibular dysfunction

Multiple sclerosis

Hydrocephalus

Migraine or migraine equivalents
    Basilar migraine
    Benign paroxysmal vertigo
    Benign paroxysmal torticollis of infancy

Metabolic disorders
    Mitochondrial disorders
        Pyruvate decarboxylase deficiency
        Pyruvate dehydrogenase deficiency
        Leigh disease

    Amino acidopathies
        Maple syrup urine disease, intermittent form
        Hartnup disease
        γ-Glutamylcysteine synthetase deficiency

    Urea cycle disorders
        Carbamoyl phosphate synthetase type 1 deficiency
        Ornithine transcarbamylase deficiency
        Citrullinemia
        Argininosuccinic aciduria

    Organic acidopathies
        Holocarboxylase deficiency
        Biotinidase deficiency
        Isovaleric acidemia

    Carnitine acetyltransferase deficiency

Primary episodic ataxias
    Episodic ataxia type 1 (paroxysmal ataxia with myokymia)
    Episodic ataxia type 2 (acetazolamide responsive)
    Episodic ataxia types 3 and 4
    Episodic ataxia with paroxysmal dystonia

Psychogenic

[a]*Modified from Ryan MM, Engle EC. Acute ataxia in childhood. J Child Neurol. 2003;18:309–316. Reprinted with permission from Sage Publications.*

> **Box 12-3. Reported Causes of Infectious/Postinfectious Cerebellitis in Childhood[a]**
>
> Varicella-zoster
>
> Coxsackie A and B
>
> Epstein-Barr virus
>
> Scarlet fever
>
> Mumps
>
> Mycoplasma pneumoniae
>
> Bacterial meningitis (pneumococcal, meningococcal)
>
> Legionella pneumophilia
>
> Diphtheria
>
> Hepatitis A
>
> Leptospirosis
>
> Influenza A and B
>
> Herpes simplex virus I
>
> Echovirus type 6
>
> Enterovirus type 71
>
> Malaria
>
> Poliovirus type 1
>
> Japanese B encephalitis
>
> Parvovirus B19
>
> Measles
>
> ---
>
> [a]*Modified from Ryan MM, Engle EC. Acute ataxia in childhood. J Child Neurol. 2003;18:309–316.*
> *Reprinted with permission from Sage Publications.*

benzodiazepines, alcohol, and antihistamines. Less often, ataxia develops after exposure to organic chemicals and heavy metals.

Autoimmune Ataxias

Guillain-Barré syndrome is a disorder in which the body's immune system attacks part of the peripheral nervous system. Initial symptoms of this disorder include varying degrees of weakness or tingling sensations in the legs. Ataxia is present in as many as 15% of pediatric cases of Guillain-Barré syndrome.

Miller Fisher Syndrome (MFS) is a clinical variant of GBS. Neurologic symptoms commonly occur 5 to 10 days after an infectious illness (often *Campylobacter* gastroenteritis). It is defined by the triad of ataxia, areflexia, and ophthalmoplegia. This postinfectious immune-mediated phenomenon is related to antibodies to the GQ1b myelin ganglioside in more than 90% of cases.

Bickerstaff brainstem encephalitis (BBE) is a clinical syndrome characterized by ophthalmoplegia, cerebellar ataxia, disturbance of consciousness, and other CNS signs, usually associated with the presence of anti-GQ1b antibodies. Some authors argue that GBS, MFS, and BBE are all different manifestations of the same disorder. Areflexia is usually absent in BBE, whereas significant drowsiness is not present in MFS.

Multiple Sclerosis

The estimated prevalence of multiple sclerosis (MS) worldwide is 50 per 100,000 with 2.7% to 5.6% of patients presenting before the age of 15 to 16 years. Similar to the disease in adults, there is a female predominance in childhood MS, ranging from 2.1 to 3:1. Diagnosis of MS is based on clinical manifestations and biochemical, electrophysiological, and radiologic abnormalities.

Children with MS can have acute, intermittent, or chronic ataxia (Boxes 12-1, 12-2, 12-4, 12-5). Other associated symptoms include pure sensory symptoms, motor symptoms, optic neuritis, and a variety of other neurologic signs and symptoms. Cerebrospinal fluid sampling shows increases in cells and protein; however, lumbar puncture is normal in about 60% of childhood-onset MS. Visual, auditory, and somatosensory evoked potential studies may show involvement of the visual pathways, brain stem, and spinal cord, respectively. Magnetic resonance imaging (MRI) reveals asymmetrical, multifocal white matter lesions.

Treatment of MS includes disease-modifying drugs—such as corticosteroids, intravenous immunoglobulins (IVIG), immunosuppressive agents, and immunomodulators like interferon-β1—and other medications to alleviate symptoms such as fatigue, spasticity, bladder dysfunction, and depression. Rehabilitation services play an important role in maintaining function and quality of life. Neuroprotective therapies are under investigation. Very few immunomodulator trials have included children; therefore, there is no standardized treatment for childhood-onset MS.

> **Box 12-4. Chronic Nonprogressive Ataxias[a]**
>
> Head trauma
>
> Hypothyroidism
>
> Hydrocephalus
>
> Multiple sclerosis
>
> Cerebrovascular diseases
>
> Brain malformations
> > Joubert syndrome
> > Dandy-Walker malformation
> > Basilar impression
> > Cerebellar dysgenesis
> > Chiari malformations
>
> Cerebral palsy
>
> ---
>
> *[a]Modified from Berman PH. Ataxia in children. Int Pediatr. 1999;14:44–47.*

Acute Disseminated Encephalomyelitis

Acute disseminated encephalomyelitis (ADEM) and MS share similar clinical presentations, laboratory data, and neuroimaging abnormalities. Acute disseminated encephalomyelitis is usually a monophasic illness. A history of preceding infection and a presentation featuring encephalopathy or bilateral optic neuritis favor the diagnosis of ADEM. There are no specific diagnostic tests for ADEM, although MRI is regarded as the imaging modality of choice. Acute disseminated encephalomyelitis is usually treated with intravenous corticosteroids followed—or not—by oral corticosteroids and IVIG. Plasmapheresis can be considered in cases of aggressive or severe disease that has not responded to corticosteroids and IVIG.

Paraneoplastic Syndromes

Paraneoplastic neurologic disorders are autoimmune responses attacking the CNS triggered by an underlying tumor. The incidence is quite low; only 0.01% of cancer patients, predominantly adults.

Opsoclonus-myoclonus syndrome (OMS) is the most common paraneoplastic syndrome in childhood. Opsoclonus-myoclonus syndrome, also known as *Kinsbourne encephalopathy* and *dancing-eyes-dancing-feet syndrome,* is usually associated with neuroblastoma. It is an extremely rare condition, affecting only 2% to 3% of children with this form of cancer. It is

Box 12-5. Chronic Progressive Ataxias[a]

Multiple sclerosis

Hydrocephalus

Brain tumors
Medulloblastoma
Cerebellar astrocytoma
Brain stem glioma
Ependymoma

Primary hereditary ataxias
Spinal cerebellar ataxias
Friedreich ataxia
Ataxia telangiectasia
Angelman syndrome
Rett syndrome

Metabolic ataxias
Mitochondrial encephalopathies
Neurotransmitter disorders
Leukodystrophies
Urea cycle defects
Aminoacidurias
A-beta lipoproteinemia
Biotinidase deficiency
Vitamin E deficiency

[a]Modified from Berman PH. Ataxia in children. Int Pediatr. 1999;14:44–47.

thought to be caused by an immunologic reaction against cerebellum and brain stem. It is usually seen between 6 months to 3 years of age. Patients present with sudden onset of opsoclonus (rapid, chaotic, multidirectional, conjugate eye movements or jerky eyes), myoclonus, and ataxia, and there can be extreme irritability and recurrent vomiting. The underlying tumor can be detected by measurements of urinary vanillylmandelic and homo-vanillic acid levels. Chest and abdominal computerized tomography (CT) or MRI may demonstrate the tumor. If CT or MRI is negative, nuclear medicine studies using ^{131}I iobenguane may demonstrate small groups of catecholamine-producing cells. Treatment includes corticosteroids, IVIG, adrenocorticotropic hormone, monoclonal anti-B cell antibodies (ritux-imab), and plasmapheresis. Although the symptoms of OMS are typically responsive to steroids, and recovery from acute symptoms of OMS can be quite good, children often suffer lifelong neurologic sequelae that impair motor, cognitive, language, and behavioral development.

Vestibular Dysfunction

Acute labyrinthitis produces vertigo, nystagmus, and ataxia. The diagnosis is clinical, and usually it is a diagnosis of exclusion. There is commonly a concomitant viral infection. Treatment of acute labyrinthitis includes anti-histaminics (meclazine, promethazine, diphenhydramine) and sedatives (diazepam, lorazepam).

Perilymphatic fistulas may be caused by head trauma. Endolymphatic hydrops can be caused by trauma, infection, or congenital anomalies. The treatment is surgical. Antibiotics may be used if acute infection is suspected.

Meniere disease is a common cause of idiopathic endolymphatic hydrops. It features vertigo and progressive sensorineural hearing loss, and it affects adults predominantly. Children account for less than 1% of patients with Meniere disease. Treatment includes antihistamines, sedatives, and diuretics. Corticosteroids and surgery can be employed in refractory cases.

Traumatic brain injury and cerebrovascular disease are neurologic diseases that can feature acute ataxia. They are discussed elsewhere in this volume.

Episodic and Intermittent Ataxias

Several disorders can cause both acute and intermittent ataxia. Some causes of intermittent ataxia have been described above.

Migraine and Migraine Equivalents

Migraine is a paroxysmal headache disorder affecting more than 13% of the general population in the United States. *Migraine variant* or *migraine equivalent* refers to migraine manifesting itself in a form other than head pain. Basilar migraine consists of headache accompanied by dizziness, ataxia, tinnitus, nausea and vomiting, dysarthria, diplopia, syncope, and sometimes loss of consciousness. Basilar migraine is more frequent in adolescent girls and young women. Other migraine variants that can present with episodic ataxia include benign paroxysmal vertigo and benign paroxysmal torticollis of infancy. The prophylactic agents employed for the prevention of ordinary cephalgic migraine can be useful in the management of migraine variants as well, including beta-blockers, calcium channel blockers, anticonvulsants, and antidepressants.

Inherited Metabolic Disorders

Several inherited metabolic disorders can cause episodic, chronic progressive, and nonprogressive ataxia. Some metabolic disorders have their onset in childhood and therefore must be considered for any child with ataxia associated with developmental regression or other progressive neurologic findings. Common associated symptoms include mental retardation, developmental delay or regression, myopathy, peripheral neuropathy, paralysis, seizures, visual disturbances, hearing loss, and psychiatric symptoms. A list of common metabolic disorders that cause ataxia is presented in Box 12-2.

Primary Episodic Ataxias

Primary episodic ataxias (PEA) are channelopathies that manifest as attacks of imbalance and incoordination. Most PEAs are autosomal dominant. Mutations in 2 genes, *KCNA1* and *CACNA1A,* cause the best characterized ataxias and account for most identified cases of episodic ataxia. Clinical features associated with primary episodic ataxias are seizures, nystagmus, myokimia, tremor, and slurred speech. Weakness may be present in between attacks. Episodes can last from seconds to days, can be rare, or can occur several times a day. The diagnosis is mostly clinical. Currently, diagnostic genetic testing is commercially available for types 1 and 2 (EA1, EA2). Carbamazepine, valproic acid, and acetazolamide have shown to help some patients.

Psychogenic Ataxia

Conversion, malingering, and factious disorders can present with nonorganic ataxia (astasia abasia) and should be suspected in the absence of any other symptoms and in the presence of clinical inconsistencies.

Chronic Nonprogressive Ataxias

Nonprogressive ataxia is often associated with other neurological symptoms. It is a common feature of cerebral palsy (CP).

Cerebral Palsy

Cerebral palsy is a general term referring to a chronic impairment of movement caused by a non-progressive brain condition with onset before, during, or shortly after birth. Cerebral palsy is not a diagnosis, because there are many diseases that can cause it. There are 4 main clinical patterns of CP: spastic, athetoid, ataxic, and mixed type. Ataxic CP is the least common; however, ataxia is often present in other forms of CP as well. Cerebral palsy is discussed in more detail elsewhere in this volume. Other causes of chronic nonprogressive ataxias are listed in Box 12-4.

Chronic Progressive Ataxias

A list of the most frequent chronic progressive ataxias is displayed in Box 12-5.

Brain Tumors

Primary brain neoplasms occur in approximately 2,000 children in the United States each year. Forty-five percent to 60% of all childhood brain tumors arise in the posterior fossa in the brain stem or the cerebellum. Brain tumors in infants usually present with nonspecific signs of elevated intracranial pressure such as restlessness, vomiting, failure to thrive, and progressive macrocephaly, whereas older children are more likely have progressive ataxia and localizing neurologic findings. Other clinical features include headache and personality change. Recurrent bouts of headache, nausea, and vomiting with subacute, progressive ataxia are a common presentation of tumors of the posterior fossa, most frequently medulloblastoma, cerebellar astrocytoma, ependymoma of the fourth ventricle, and brain stem gliomas.

Hereditary Disorders

Hereditary ataxias are a group of genetic disorders characterized by slowly progressive incoordination of gait and often associated with poor coordination of hands, speech, and eye movements. They can be inherited in an autosomal recessive, X-linked, and sporadic pattern. Classification of hereditary ataxias is based on the pattern of inheritance or mode of genetic transmission as well as clinical presentation. The most current classification of hereditary ataxias is shown in Tables 12-1 and 12-2.

Table 12-1. Autosomal Dominant Hereditary Ataxias			
Disease	**Gene**	**Chromosome**	**Protein Name**
SCA1	ATXN1	6p23	Ataxin-1
SCA2	ATXN2	12q24	Ataxin-2
SCA3	ATXN3	14q24.3-q31	Ataxin-3
SCA4	?	6q22.1	?
SCA5	SPTBN2	11p13	Spectrin beta chain
SCA6	CACNA1A	19p13	Voltage-dependent P/Q-type calcium channel alpha-1A subunit
SCA7	ATXN7	3p21.1-p12	Ataxin-7
SCA8	ATXN80S	13q21	?
SCA10	ATXN10	22q13	Ataxin-10
SCA11	SCA11	15q14-q21.3	
SCA12	PPP2R2B	5q31-q33	Serine/threonine protein phosphatase 2A
SCA13	KCNC3	19q13.3-q13.4	Potassium voltage-gated channel subfamily C member 3
SCA14	PRKCG	19q13.4	Protein kinase C gamma type
SCA15	?	3p26.1-p25.3	?
SCA16	SCA16	3p26.2-pter	Contactin-4
SCA17	TBP	6q27	TATA-box binding protein
SCA18	SCA18	7q22-q32	?
SCA19	SCA19	1p21-q21	?
SCA20	SCA20	11p13-q11	?
SCA21	SCA21	7p21-p15.1	?
SCA22	?	1p21-q21	?
SCA23	?	20p13-p12.3	?
SCA25	SCA25	2p21-p13	?
SCA26	?	19p13.3	?
SCA27	FGF14	13q34	Fibroblast growth factor 14
SCA28	?	18p11.22-q11.2	?
DRPLA	ATN	12p13.3	Atrophin-1
EA1	KCNA1	12p13	Potassium voltage-gated channel subfamily A member 1
EA2	CACNA1A	19p13	Voltage-dependent P/Q-type calcium channel alpha-subunit
EA2	CACNB4	2q22-q23	Voltage-dependent L-type calcium beta-4 subunit
ADSA	SAX1	12p13	?

Table 12-2. Autosomal Recessive Hereditary Ataxias		
Disease	**Gene**	**Chromosome**
Friedreich ataxia	Frataxin	9q13
Ataxia-telangiectasia	ATM	11q22.3
Ataxia with vitamin E deficiency	TTPA	8q13.1-q13.3
Ataxia with oculomotor apraxia type 1	APTX	9p13.3
Ataxia with oculomotor apraxia type 2	SETX	9q34
IOSCA 1	PEO1	10q24
Marinesco-Sjögren	SIL1	5q31
AR spastic ataxia of Charlevoix-Saguenay	SACS	13q12

The autosomal dominant ataxias are also called the *spinocerebellar ataxias (SCA)*. To date, researchers have identified 28 autosomal dominant ataxia genes. Cerebellar ataxia and cerebellar degeneration are common to all types, but other signs and symptoms, as well as age of onset, differ depending on the specific gene mutation. These conditions are usually slowly progressive with gradual worsening over a period of years, although some types of SCA can progress more rapidly than others. Diagnosis can be challenging because there is an overlap of symptoms among the different types of SCA, and genetic testing is available for only about 60% of all dominant hereditary ataxias. The most common of the autosomal dominant ataxia in North America is SCA3.

Autosomal recessive cerebellar ataxias are fewer than autosomal dominant hereditary ataxias. Friedreich ataxia is an autosomal recessive disorder linked to a defect on chromosome 9. Its presentation is in the first decade of life with ataxia, pes cavus, scoliosis, and areflexia. Patients typically present between the ages of 5 and 15 with difficulty in walking or gait ataxia. Other symptoms include muscle weakness, visual impairment, hearing loss, slurred speech, scoliosis, high plantar arches, diabetes mellitus, cardiac arrhythmia, and cardiomyopathy. Diagnosis is made by careful clinical examination and gene testing. Individuals with Friedreich ataxia have identifiable mutations in the *FXN* gene. Patients should have an electrocardiogram (ECG) and an echocardiogram. Treatment of Friedreich ataxia is strictly symptomatic and includes prostheses, walking aids, and wheelchairs for mobility, speech, occupational, and physical therapy; pharmacologic agents for spasticity; orthopedic interventions for scoliosis and foot deformities; and psychological support. Surveillance includes biennial ECGs and echocardiograms, hearing assessment every 2 to 3 years, and annual measurement of fasting blood glucose to monitor for diabetes mellitus. Cardiology and endocrinology referrals may be indicated.

Ataxia telangiectasia is an autosomal recessive multisystem disorder caused by an abnormality on the long arm of chromosome 11 and is characterized by progressive truncal ataxia, oculocutaneous telangiectasias, and variable immunodeficiency with susceptibility to sinopulmonary infections, impaired organ maturation, x-ray hypersensitivity, and a predisposition to malignancy.

Ataxia with vitamin E deficiency generally manifests in late childhood or early teens with slurred speech, poor balance when walking (especially in the dark), dystonia, psychotic episodes (paranoia), pigmentary retinopathy, and intellectual decline. Most individuals become wheelchair bound between ages 11 and 50 years.

Angelman syndrome is an inherited autosomal recessive disease characterized by microcephaly, seizure disorder, global developmental delay, and ataxia. There is usually lack of speech development, excessively happy behavior, ataxia, and jerky movements. Most children have a microdeletion of 15q11.2–15q13, and confirmatory diagnosis can be achieved by gene testing.

Rett syndrome is an inherited neurodegenerative disorder that occurs almost exclusively in girls. Most cases of classic Rett syndrome are caused by mutations in the *MECP2* gene and have an estimated incidence of 1 in 10,000 to 22,000 females. Males with mutations in the *MECP2* gene often die before birth or in infancy. Babies with Rett syndrome are normal until the ages of 6 months and 18 months, when they develop progressive problems with language and communication, learning, coordination, and other brain functions. Early in childhood, affected girls lose purposeful use of their hands and begin making repeated hand wringing, washing, or clapping motions. Ataxia is a prominent feature in children with Rett syndrome. Associated symptoms include microcephaly, breathing abnormalities, seizures, and sleep disturbances.

Metabolic Ataxias

Metabolic disorders associated with intermittent or progressive ataxias in childhood include urea cycle defects, aminoacidurias, and disorders of pyruvate and lactate metabolism.

Mitochondrial Encephalomyopathies

Mitochondrial diseases are a genotypically and phenotypically complex group involving dysfunction of the cellular energy production mechanism. Mitochondrial disorders are often associated with additional clinical manifestations, such as seizures, deafness, diabetes mellitus, cardiomyopathy, retinopathy, and short stature. Some mitochondrial diseases that present with ataxia are listed in Table 12-2.

Neurotransmitter Disorders

There is a class of neurometabolic syndromes attributable to a primary disturbance of neurotransmitter metabolism or transport. They include disorders of biopterin, catecholamines, serotonin, glycine, pyridoxine, and gamma-aminobutyric acid metabolism. Patients present with progressive neurologic disturbances such as developmental delay, mental retardation, hypotonia, behavior problems, seizures, ataxia, psychiatric symptoms, and sleep disturbances. Confirmatory diagnosis requires CSF analysis. Treatment is specific for the neurotransmitter disorder in question.

Leukodystrophies

Autosomal recessive leukodystrophies must be considered in the differential diagnosis of childhood ataxia. The most common is X-linked adrenoleukodystrophy (XALD) with an incidence of 1:42,000 people in United States. The molecular basis for XALD is a defect in the *ABCD1* gene, which codes for a protein that is critical for peroxisomal degradation of long-chain fatty acids. Tissue accumulation of long-chain fatty acids is toxic to myelin and to the adrenal cortex. X-linked adrenoleukodystrophy can present as 1 of 3 syndromes: a childhood-onset cerebral syndrome, an adult-onset myeloneuropathic syndrome, and an isolated adrenocortical—so-called Addison disease only—syndrome. Strangely, all 3 syndromes can be seen in a single pedigree. Gait disturbance and ataxia can be prominent features of the childhood-onset syndrome. A distinctive clinical feature is the associated cutaneous hyperpigmentation caused by adrenocortical insufficiency. Brain imaging is usually distinctive as well, exhibiting marked symmetrical involvement of the posterior parietal and occipital white matter and the splenium of the corpus callosum.

Vanishing white-matter disease is another cause of autosomal recessive childhood ataxia that features CNS hypomyelination. It is characterized by slowly progressive cerebellar ataxia, spasticity, variable optic atrophy, and relatively preserved cognition. It follows a saltatory course with periods of stability interrupted at unpredictable intervals by declines that can be triggered by stresses such as infection or minor head injury. The MRI is characteristic, because it demonstrates a progressive disappearance over time of the affected white matter.

Evaluation and Management of Ataxias

Evaluation of a child with ataxia requires a careful history and physical examination. Intelligent selection of imaging and laboratory investigations can be informed by answers to the following questions:

- When was the onset and what has been the tempo of progression of the ataxia?
- Have there been fever, vomiting, headaches, lethargy, or other symptoms possibly attributable to elevated intracranial pressure?
- Has the child had seizures?
- Has there been a recent viral illness?
- Have there been environmental exposures: heavy metals, gases, solvents?
- Is the child taking any medications? What medications are in the household? Can there have been an ingestion?
- Has the child been depressed or have there been any other emotional or behavioral disturbances?
- Has the child's development been normal? Has there been delay or actual regression?
- Have there been chronic, progressive neurologic conditions among family members?
- Have there been premature deaths, especially in infancy or childhood?

If no cause for the ataxia is found after the initial set of imaging studies and generally available laboratory tests, then additional specific metabolic and genetic tests must be considered. The most commonly tested genetic disorders include the spinocerebellar ataxias, Friedreich ataxia, and ataxia-telangiectasia. Comprehensive evaluation of a child with ataxia is shown in Box 12-6.

There is no specific treatment for ataxia, but there are treatments for associated symptoms such as movement disorders (tremor, chorea, myoclonus), vertigo, nausea, or seizures. Patients with hydrocephalus require neurosurgical intervention. Certain metabolic disorders can be ameliorated by specific dietary modifications. Rehabilitation services play an important role in maintaining function and general quality of life.

Children with persistent ataxia are often referred to a neurologist. Referral to a cardiologist, endocrinologist, and geneticist may be necessary. Outcome of ataxias in childhood is highly dependent on the underlying disease process.

Box 12-6. Evaluation of Ataxia

Complete blood count

Electrolytes

Renal function

Liver function

Thyroid function

Toxicological screening (blood and urine)

Urine for vanillylmandelic acid/homovanillic acid if opsoclonus/myoclonus

Serum and urine organic and amino acids

Serum lactate, pyruvate, ammonia

Serum copper/ceruloplasmine

Vitamin E

Lumbar puncture

Electroencephalogram

Brain computerized tomography

Brain magnetic resonance imaging

Web Sites

National Ataxia Foundation: www.ataxia.org

Ataxia-Telangiectasia Children's Project: www.atcp.org

Friedreich's Ataxia Research Alliance (FARA): www.curefa.org

Bibliography

Albright AL, Price RA, Guthkelch AN. Brain stem gliomas of children: a clinicopathological study. *Cancer.* 1983;52:2313–2319

Berman PH. Ataxia in children. *Int Pediatr.* 1999;14:44–47

Brusse E, Maat-Kievit JA, van Swieten JC. Diagnosis and management of early- and late-onset cerebellar ataxia. *Clin Genet.* 2007;71:12–24

Dressler D, Benecke R. Diagnosis and management of acute movement disorders. *J Neurol.* 2005;252:1299–1306

Gadoth N. Multiple sclerosis in children. *Brain Dev.* 2003;25:229–232

Geller T, Loftis L, Brink DS. Cerebellar infarction in adolescent males associated with acute marijuana use. *Pediatrics.* 2004;113:e365–e370

Gieron-Korthals MA, Westberry KR, Emmanuel PJ. Acute childhood ataxia: 10-year experience. *J Child Neurol.* 1994;9:381–384

Hasan I, Wapnick S, Tenner MS, Couldwell WT. Vertebral artery dissection in children: a comprehensive review. *Pediatr Neurosurg.* 2002;37:168–177

Hayward K, Jeremy RJ, Jenkins S, et al. Long-term neurobehavioral outcomes in children with neuroblastoma and opsoclonus-myoclonus-ataxia syndrome: relationship to MR imaging findings and anti-neuronal antibodies. *J Pediatr.* 2001;139:552–559

Kazimiroff PB, Weichsel ME Jr, Grinnell V, Young RF. Acute cerebellar hemorrhage in childhood: etiology, diagnosis, and treatment. *Neurosurgery.* 1980;6:524–528

Khurana DS, Melvin JJ, Kothare SV, et al. Acute disseminated encephalomyelitis in children: discordant neurologic and neuroimaging abnormalities and response to plasmapheresis. *Pediatrics.* 2005;116:431–436

Mori M, Kuwabara S, Fukutake T, Yuki N, Hattori T. Clinical features and prognosis of Miller Fisher syndrome. *Neurology.* 2001;56:1104–1106

Odaka M, Yuki N, Yamada M, et al. Bickerstaff's brainstem encephalitis: clinical features of 62 cases and a subgroup associated with Guillain-Barre syndrome. *Brain.* 2003;126:2279–2290

Pearl PL, Capp PK, Novotny EJ, Gibson KM. Inherited disorders of neurotransmitters in children and adults. *Clin Biochem.* 2005;38:1051–1058

Pollack IF. Brain tumors in children. *N Engl J Med.* 1994;331:1500–1507

Ryan MM, Engle EC. Acute ataxia in childhood. *J Child Neurol.* 2003;18:309–316

Swift M, Morrell D, Cromartie E, Chamberlin AR, Skolnick MH, Bishop DT. The incidence and gene frequency of ataxia-telangiectasia in the United States. *Am J Hum Genet.* 1986;39:573–583

Waldman A, O'Connor E, Tennekoon G. Childhood multiple sclerosis: a review. *Ment Retard Dev Disabil Res Rev.* 2006;12:147–156

Williams CA. Neurological aspects of the Angelman syndrome. *Brain Dev.* 2005;27:88–94

Chapter 13

Neuromuscular Disorders

Sabrina W. Yum, MD
Harold G. Marks, MD

Introduction

This chapter deals with disorders involving the peripheral nervous system (PNS), including spinal cord motor neurons, spinal roots, peripheral nerves, neuromuscular junction, and muscles. In neonates and young infants, neuromuscular diseases usually present as "floppy infant" syndrome. In older children, patients frequently present with delayed motor development or a gait disorder. In general, patients with primary muscle diseases or anterior horn cell diseases have symptoms and signs of proximal limb weakness (such as waddling gait, difficulty ascending stairs or arising from the floor, inability to run, Gower sign), whereas patients with chronic neuropathies have symptoms and signs of distal weakness (such as foot deformity, toe walking, frequent falls, and inability to heel walk). Easy fatigability and fluctuating weakness is the hallmark of neuromuscular junction defects.

In some neuromuscular disorders, one sees both central nervous system (CNS) and PNS involvement (ie, myotonic dystrophy, some congenital muscular dystrophies). Some connective tissue or bone disorders (ie, Ehlers-Danlos, achondroplasia) may present with symptoms mimicking neuromuscular diseases (such as hypotonia or abnormal gait).

Investigation of children with neuromuscular disease often requires special diagnostic testing such as electromyography (EMG) and nerve conduction velocity (NCV) studies, as well as nerve or muscle biopsy. Recent development and progress in molecular genetics has made it possible to establish the diagnosis with genetic or biochemical tests in many of these patients and to provide proper genetic counseling for the family.

Disorders of the Spinal Cord Motor Neurons

Spinal Muscular Atrophy

Spinal muscular atrophy (SMA) includes a group of autosomal recessive disorders affecting the anterior horn cells, caused by abnormalities of the survival motor neuron (SMN) genes located in chromosome 5q11.2-13.3. A mutation of the telomeric SMN (SMN1) gene causes SMA. A clinical picture consistent with SMA supported by the finding of a mutation of SMN1 is diagnostic of SMA. The number of copies of the centromeric SMN (SMN2) gene modifies the severity of the disease. There are 1 to 4 copies of SMN2 in each chromosome 5q. Generally speaking, the more copies of SMN2, the milder the disease.

Spinal muscular atrophy has an incidence of 8 to 11 per 100,000 newborns. There are 3 types of SMA in children. Type I (Werdnig-Hoffman) is the most common (50%), type II (intermediate form) is seen in 30%, and type III (Kugelberg-Welander) in 20%. All children with SMA have proximal weakness involving the hip girdle more than the shoulder girdle, hyporeflexia or areflexia, and fasciculations. Fasciculations can be seen in the tongue or in the fingers (polyminimyoclonus). The Werdnig-Hoffman variant is characterized by diminished fetal movements, onset before 6 months of age, progressive respiratory problems, and death prior to age 2 years. Children with type II have onset of symptoms between 6 and 18 months of age and never walk. They are wheelchair bound. Children with Kugelberg-Welander have onset of symptoms after 18 months of age. They are usually ambulatory. Creatine kinase (CK) is normal in type I and moderately increased in type III. Clinically, children with type III may resemble limb girdle muscular dystrophy (LGMD). Electromyography demonstrates fibrillations; positive waves; and high amplitude, long duration, polyphasic motor units. Diagnosis is confirmed with DNA testing. Treatment is symptomatic and supportive. Experimental treatment presently focuses on genetic therapy aimed at increasing the amount of full-length SMN in muscle fibers.

Infectious Poliomyelitis

Poliomyelitis is an enterovirus infection that involves the motor neurons of the spinal cord and brain, causing an asymmetrical flaccid paralysis. With widespread immunization, cases have become sporadic and, in some instances, have been associated with vaccine strains. More recently, a polio-myelitis-like illness has been associated with the West Nile virus, a flavivirus transmitted by mosquitoes.

Disorders of the Peripheral Nerves

Peripheral neuropathies are disorders in which the primary pathological process affects the axons of motor or sensory neurons or both, or their myelin sheaths and associated Schwann cells. Most chronic polyneuropathies in children are genetically determined. The largest group is the family of hereditary motor and sensory neuropathies called *Charcot-Marie-Tooth disease* (CMT). Complex syndromes associated with inborn errors of metabolism or neurodegenerative disorders may have polyneuropathy as one of their features. Different from adults, the incidence of toxic neuropathy or neuropathy secondary to systemic diseases such as diabetes, cancer, and collagen vascular diseases is low. In addition to polyneuropathy, focal or compressive neuropathy such as carpal tunnel syndrome (median neuropathy at wrist), ulnar neuropathy, or peroneal neuropathy can occur, but are uncommon in children. Patients with recurrent compressive neuropathy should be evaluated for hereditary neuropathy with susceptibility to pressure palsy.

Charcot-Marie-Tooth Disease

Charcot-Marie-Tooth disease is the most common family of neuropathies in childhood, accounting for more than half of chronic neuropathies. Based on the motor NCV and pathology, CMT is commonly divided into demyelinating form with NCV less than 38 m/s (including the dominantly inherited CMT1, the X-linked CMT1X, and the recessively inherited CMT4) and axonal form with normal or slightly reduced NCV (CMT type 2, which can be inherited in both dominant and recessive fashions). Congenital hypomyelinating neuropathy or Dejerine-Sottas neuropathy (also known as *CMT3*) designates the more severe kinds of demyelinating neuropathy that are recognized in infancy or before age 3 years. About 50 loci and 30 genes have been identified (www.molgen.ua.ac.be/CMTMutations); some cause both demyelinating and axonal phenotypes. Peripheral myelin protein 22 duplications are by far the most common cause for CMT, and about one-fourth of CMT2 cases have dominant mutations in MFN2, which encodes mitochondrial fusion protein mitofusin 2.

Onset of disease is usually within the first decade, although very early onset during the neonatal period or later onset of disease in the second decade can occur. Gait disturbance and foot deformity are the usual presenting symptoms. Patients frequently have toe walking, difficulty running, and frequent falls due to distal weakness and gait instability. Symmetrical atrophy and weakness of distal intrinsic foot, peroneal and, later, leg muscles are evident, and the weakness and atrophy are progressive in a length-dependent pattern to involve eventually the lower thigh and hand muscles in some patients, resulting in poor handwriting and difficulty with tieing shoes and buttoning. Deep tendon reflexes, especially the ankle jerks, are often absent, although they may be present and even brisk in the axonal form of CMT. In patients with a longstanding disease, high-arched feet, some with hammer toes and pes cavus, are frequently found (Figure 13-1). The severity of symptoms can vary greatly from patient to patient, and even within the family. Some patients may have no noticeable symptoms but are found to have CMT on examination; therefore, examination of both parents is necessary. Progression of disease is usually slow, and most patients remain active and ambulatory, although some may eventually become wheelchair bound.

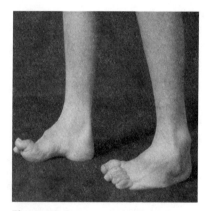

Figure 13-1.
Teenage boy with Charcot-Marie-Tooth type 1 neuropathy and typical deformities of his feet. Note cavus feet, clawing of toes, varus heel, and forefoot adduction.

Diagnosis is based on the mode of inheritance and clinical and electrophysiological features. Selection of genetic testing based on these features greatly increases the yield of identifying specific mutations. Nerve biopsy is rarely performed, except in unusual cases.

Medical interventions have improved the quality of life for many of these patients. These interventions focus on enhancing physical mobility and social interactions, and preventing complications and contractures. Physical therapy, braces, and heel cord and foot joint surgery are used to correct foot deformities and contractures and, therefore, to improve the quality of gait and prolong walking. Scoliosis surgery is performed in patients with serious spinal curvature.

Neuropathies as Part of a Complex Syndrome or a Metabolic Disease

Neuropathy may be a component of many other genetic or inherited metabolic conditions discussed elsewhere in this volume, in which case it may be overshadowed by involvement of the CNS. Demyelination or dysmyelination of peripheral axons is frequently found in patients with Krabbe disease (galactosylceramide lipidosis or globoid cell leukodystrophy), metachromatic leukodystrophy, Cockayne syndrome, and Refsum disease. Axonal neuropathy can be seen in porphyria, X-linked adrenoleukodystrophy, mitochondrial cytopathy (especially neuropathy, ataxia, retinitis pigmentosa [NARP] and mitochondrial myopathy, encephalopathy, lactic acidosis, stroke [MELAS]), neuraxonal dystrophy, some types of hereditary spastic paraparesis, and spinocerebellar ataxia and is a feature of Friedrich ataxia and giant axonal neuropathy.

Acquired Generalized Neuropathies

Guillain-Barré Syndrome

Guillain-Barré syndrome (GBS) is a monophasic inflammatory disorder of peripheral nerves and nerve roots. The incidence of GBS in children younger than 15 years is near 1.1 per 100,000 children, making it the most common cause of acute generalized paralysis in this age group. About two-thirds of patients have a history of an antecedent respiratory or diarrheal illness. Immune-mediated mechanisms involving both cellular and humoral responses have been postulated in GBS.

Clinical Characteristics

Guillain-Barré syndrome is characterized by ascending symmetrical weakness progressing over hours to days. Weakness usually affects legs first, causing gait instability, difficulty standing, ascending stairs, or ambulation. The illness may begin with numbness and tingling in fingers, toes, or trunk. In some individuals, the facial nerves are disproportionately affected at onset. Approximately 50% of patients reach their nadir by 2 weeks.

The key features on examination include symmetrical, proximal more than distal weakness and diffuse hyporeflexia or areflexia. Up to 50% of patients have facial weakness and as many as 30% have ophthalmoparesis. Signs of autonomic involvement include sinus tachycardia, hypertension, and orthostatic hypotension. About 15% to 25% of patients develop respiratory failure, with loss of airway protective reflexes or neurogenic hypoventilation, or both.

Diagnostic Evaluation

Cerebrospinal fluid (CSF) examination and electrophysiological studies should be performed in most cases to establish the diagnosis of GBS. The CSF protein level is elevated (especially in those with symptoms for at least 1 week), and there are fewer than 10 mononuclear leukocytes/mm^3 (so-called albumino-cytologic dissociation). The finding of CSF pleocytosis greater than 50 white blood cells/mm^3 casts doubt on the diagnosis of GBS. Electrophysiological studies reveal signs of segmental demyelination by the third week of illness in 80% of patients. Suspected associated infections should prompt serologic or microbiologic testing, particularly if the suspected pathogens require antibiotic treatment (eg, *Campylobacter, Mycoplasma, Borrelia*) or threaten serious illness in their own right (eg, hepatitis, HIV).

Guillain-Barré syndrome in its typical form is unlikely to cause diagnostic confusion. Rarely, the Miller Fisher syndrome variant of GBS, characterized by ophthalmoplegia, ataxia, and areflexia without weakness of the extremities, occurs in children. About 20% of children (especially infants and young children) may present with decreased activity, pain, and irritability, leading to a misdiagnosis of viral syndrome or toxic encephalopathy. Among conditions that may mimic GBS, acute spinal cord lesions (transverse myelitis, tumor, and trauma) are the most important etiologies to be considered as flaccid paraparesis or quadriparesis with areflexia may occur during the early stage of a spinal cord injury (spinal shock). A sensory level or bowel and bladder dysfunction may point to a spinal process. An imaging study of the spine may be necessary in uncertain cases. Patients with poliomyelitis usually have fever and meningism. Asymmetrical weakness, and marked CSF pleocytosis also distinguish polio from GBS. The advent of widespread immunizations has made both polio and diphtheria (another acute neuromuscular disorder of childhood) rare in many parts of the world.

Management

Patients with suspected GBS should be hospitalized for observation because of concern of potential respiratory compromise and autonomic dysfunction. Respiratory function, blood pressure, cardiac rhythm, bulbar function, and urinary function should be monitored. Forced vital capacity (FVC) should be checked at least every 4 to 6 hours, or even hourly if necessary. Signs of impending respiratory failure include deterioration in FVC, rapid and shallow breathing, or decreased alertness. A fall in FVC below 15 mL/kg, arterial partial pressure of oxygen below 70 mm Hg in room air, or signs of respiratory fatigue or impaired airway protective reflexes should prompt consideration of intubation. Patients with cardiac arrhythmia or marked fluctuation of blood pressure should have continuous eletrocardiographic and blood pressure monitoring in an intensive care setting.

Pain may require treatment with analgesics, including acetaminophen, and nonsteroidal anti-inflammatory agents. Neurontin or amitriptyline may alleviate neuropathic pain.

Physical therapy, including passive range of motion exercises and splinting of wrists and ankles, prevents joint contracture and deep vein thrombosis in paralyzed patients. A graduated program of active rehabilitation should be implemented once the acute phase of GBS has passed.

Immunomodulatory Therapy

Children with mild cases of GBS who remain ambulatory can be managed without immunomodulatory therapy. For children with gait instability, rapid progression of symptoms, impending respiratory failure, or bulbar insufficiency, either plasmapheresis (PE) or immune globulin intravenous (human) (IGIV) should be instituted. Corticosteroids are not effective in the treatment of GBS, and oral prednisone has been shown to delay recovery.

Plasmapheresis. Plasmapheresis has proven unequivocally beneficial in 3 large, randomized trials conducted primarily among adults with GBS. The time of initial improvement, time to regaining ambulation, and duration of mechanical ventilation were each significantly reduced. Neurologic status was significantly better at 6- and 12-month follow-up visits in the treated groups compared with control subjects. Plasmapheresis is reported to be effective in children with GBS; however, no controlled therapeutic trial has been conducted. Prompt initiation of this therapy probably improves its effectiveness. A total of 5 treatments over approximately 10 days, with net plasma exchange of 200 to 250 mL/kg of body weight is the protocol commonly used in the author's institution. Potential complications of PE include hypotension, transfusion reaction, infection, hypocalcemia, and arrhythmia.

Immune globulin intravenous. A large controlled study in adults comparing IGIV with PE indicated that IGIV was at least as effective. A recent randomized clinical trial demonstrated that IGIV did hasten motor recovery sooner in children, although the severity and long-term outcome were not significantly different between treated and untreated subjects with mild disease. At the authors' institution, IGIV (400 mg/kg/d) is infused over 6 to 8 hours for 5 consecutive days. A 2-day high-dose IGIV regimen showed no clear benefit over a more protracted 5-day regimen in terms of disease recovery, but had an increased likelihood of potential secondary deterioration. Serious anaphylactic reactions can occur in patients with immunoglobulin A (IgA) deficiency. Concurrent administration of diphenhydramine may reduce the chance of adverse events that occur in about 15% of patients receiving IGIV therapy. These include hypotension, headache, aseptic meningitis, congestive heart failure, renal failure, and infection with hepatitis B virus, although solvent detergent treatment or pasteurization of IGIV substantially decreases the possibility of hepatitis or other virus transmission. Because PE frequently requires central venous access in children, IGIV has substantial advantages in young children or infants.

Prognosis
Special effort must be taken to convey the nature and prognosis of GBS. Reassurance and communication, especially for patients who require mechanical ventilation, can play an important role in recovery. The overall prognosis for GBS is good in childhood. Although GBS in adults carries a mortality of 2% to 3%, and as many as 15% of patients experience long-term disability, children seem to fare better than adults with this condition. Recovery of function usually begins 2 to 4 weeks after the progression stops. Early improvement decreases the likelihood of long-term residue deficits. Only small numbers of patients experience relapse of symptoms.

Chronic Inflammatory Demyelinating Polyneuropathy

Chronic inflammatory demyelinating polyneuropathy (CIDP) is an autoimmune, acquired, chronic, sensory and motor, multifocal demyelinating polyneuropathy. Unlike patients with GBS, those with CIDP rarely have a history of an antecedent event, such as a viral or bacterial infection, or a vaccination.

Clinical Characteristics

Pediatric presentations range from hypotonia in infants to gait disturbance in adolescents. Occasionally, patients may present with floridly progressive quadriparesis and respiratory insufficiency. Subsequent relapse or persistent signs of inflammation on nerve biopsy or CSF examination ultimately distinguish these cases from GBS. More often, CIDP is insidious in its onset, with a chronic-progressive or relapsing-remitting course. In many patients, peak impairment may occur a year or longer after the initial symptoms.

Physical examination may reveal distal contractures and dystrophic changes of skin. Cranial nerve dysfunction is uncommon. Symmetrical distal weakness and sensory abnormalities are characteristic findings. Proximal weakness may simulate a myopathic pattern of weakness (in contrast to hereditary neuropathy, in which proximal weakness appears late in the course of the disorder). Muscle wasting indicates that the disease has been active for at least a month. Patients with CIDP uniformly have hyporeflexia or areflexia. Proprioceptive deficits commonly cause sensory ataxia. Patchy small-fiber sensory (pain and temperature) loss may be asymptomatic.

Diagnostic Evaluation

The diagnosis of CIDP is confirmed by electrophysiological studies, CSF examination, and nerve biopsy. Slowed nerve conduction velocities or conduction block corroborates the diagnosis. The CSF usually demonstrates an elevated protein level, with or without a low-grade lymphocytic pleocytosis (albumino-cytologic dissociation). Sural nerve biopsy shows multifocal demyelination and remyelination, onion bulb formation, edema, and lymphocytic infiltration. Because of the uneven distribution of pathological changes, a normal sural nerve biopsy cannot exclude the diagnosis of CIDP.

Management

Proven therapies for CIDP, including prednisone, PE, and IGIV therapy, have similar efficacy. The therapeutic options in CIDP require that the physician, child, and family consider the cost, availability, and potential side effects for each individual patient.

Prednisone is convenient, cheap, and effective, and is the mainstay of therapy for CIDP. Most patients respond to corticosteroid therapy within 2 months, and the response is often greater in proximal muscles. Initial dose is usually 1 to 2 mg/kg/d (but not more than 80 mg/d), and slow taper of the dose over the next 4 to 8 weeks may be followed, decreasing no more than 20% of the previous dose every 4 weeks, and given on alternate days to minimize potential side effects. Once symptoms recur or worsen during the taper, a relative large prednisone increase of 10 to 20 mg/d may be required to restore the previous function, and many of those who relapse seem to have an attenuated response to the intensification of therapy. Continuation of low-dose prednisone over several years may decrease the frequency of exacerbation, but may result in well-known and sometimes serious side effects. Patients should be followed closely for their weight and growth, hypertension, glucosuria, cataracts, and osteoporosis. Ophthalmologic screening should be carried out yearly, and serial bone density (DEXA) scans may help to monitor bone density changes.

Because IGIV is easier to deliver than PE and has fewer side effects than prednisone, it has become the treatment of choice for many patients with CIDP. The authors have followed a protocol calling for an initial dose of 400 mg/kg/d for 5 days, with maintenance infusions 6 to 8 weeks apart at 1 g/kg/d for 2 days. Side effects include rare anaphylaxis, of particular concern in individuals with IgA deficiency. Some patients experience transient but severe headache. Mild pleocytosis and severe headache may be seen with aseptic meningitis.

Plasmapheresis was demonstrated to be helpful in a small, sham-controlled, double-blind clinical trial in adults. Patients with rapid deterioration in motor function and compromised respiratory status should usually be treated with PE initially, although IGIV may also be useful in this setting. Plasmapheresis should also be considered in patients with slowly progressive symptoms who are either refractory or intolerant to prednisone therapy.

Unlike GBS, CIDP is a chronic condition that requires the involvement of occupational therapists, physical therapists, psychological counselors, orthopedists, and neuromuscular specialists as appropriate. Orthoses for the hands and feet prevent contractures. The outlook for pediatric CIDP may be more favorable than that for adults with this condition.

Primary Muscle Diseases

The Muscular Dystrophies

The muscular dystrophies (MDs) are a group of genetic myopathies in which the muscle is dystrophic (Figure 13-2). They can be subdivided into

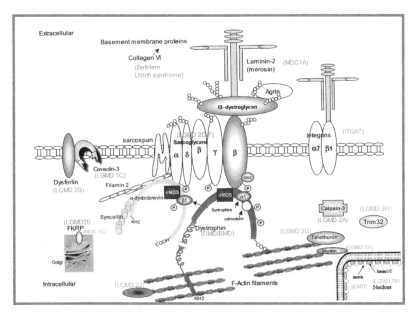

Figure 13-2.

Diagram of the muscle membrane, illustrating association of dystrophin-glycoprotein complex linkage to contractile proteins, extracellular matrix proteins with signaling properties (syntrophins, Grb2). It also illustrates the multiple phosphorylation sites at the 3-prime ends of dystrophin, dystrobrevin, and dystroglycan. Diseases associated with defect in individuals proteins are also listed in parenthesis. Abbreviations: BMD, Becker muscular dystrophy; DMD, Duchenne muscular dystrophy; ITGA7, integrin α7; LGMD, limb-girdle-muscular dystrophy; MDC1a, merosin-negative congenital muscular dystrophy; MDCqC, merosin-positive congenital muscular dystrophy; nNOS, neuronal nitric oxide synthase. (From Escolar DM, Leshner RT. Muscular dystrophies. In: Swaiman KF, Ashwal S, Ferriero DM, ed. *Pediatric Neurology. Principles & Practice.* Philadelphia, PA: Mosby Elsevier; 2006:1970, with permission from Elsevier.)

5 groups: the dystrophinopathies, which include Duchenne and Becker MD; congenital MD; limb girdle MD (LGMD) and can be subdivided into autosomal dominant (LGMD1) and autosomal recessive (LGMD2) forms; facioscapulohumeral MD; and others, including Emery-Dreifuss, ocular pharyngeal MD, etc (Table 13-1).

Dystrophinopathies

The dystrophinopathies are the most common MD. They can be subdivided into Duchenne MD (DMD), Becker MD (BMD), X-linked cardiomyopathy, and X-linked myalgia syndrome. By definition, in DMD there is an absence of dystrophin (<3%), and in BMD there is a dystrophin of abnormal molecular weight or of decreased quantity or both.

Duchenne MD is the most common MD in children and the most common X-linked disorder in humans. It has an incidence of 1 per 3,500 male births. Onset is usually before 3 years of age, but it is usually not diagnosed until 5 or 6 years of age. Children with DMD present with an abnormal, waddling gait; frequent falls; or difficulty going up stairs. They may have toe walking or flat feet. On examination, they have proximal greater than distal weakness that involves the legs more than the arms. At an early age, deep tendon reflexes are absent or depressed in the arms and patella, but they may persist at the ankles into the teen years. Muscle hypertrophy usually occurs in the calves, but may affect other muscles or be generalized (Figure 13-3). Weakness is rapidly progressive, and children will stop walking between 7 and 12 years of age (mean age: 10 years). Death usually occurs before 20 years of age (mean survival: 19.25 years). In children treated with nocturnal ventilation, mean survival improves to 25.3 years. The causes of death are pulmonary (75%) and cardiac (25%).

Although only 15 % of children younger than 16 years with DMD have symptomatic cardiomyopathy, electrocardiogram (ECG) abnormalities are often seen in the early stages of the disease. Gastrointestinal abnormalities include constipation and delayed gastric emptying. Thirty percent of children with DMD have mental retardation with a specific impairment of verbal rather than performance IQs. Prior to treatment with steroids, more than 90% of patients developed scoliosis. Corticosteroid treatment has resulted in fewer boys with scoliosis (30%) and milder curves.

Table 13-1. Classification and Genetics of the Muscular Dystrophies[a]

Disease	Gene locus	Gene product	Inheritance
Limb-girdle muscular dystrophy (LGMD) Caused by Sarcolemma or Cytosolic Protein Defects			
Duchenne/Becker MD	Xp21	Dystrophin	XR
LGMD1A	5q22	Myotilin	AD
LGMD1B	1q11-q21	Lamin A/C	AD
LGMD1C	3p25	Caveolin-3	AD
LGMD1D	6q23	Not identified	AD
LGMD1E	7q	Not identified	AD
LGMD1F	2q	Not identified	AD
LGMD2A	15q15	Calpain-3	AR
LGMD2B/Myoshi myopathy	2p13	Dysferlin	AR
LGMD2C	13q12	γ-Sarcoglycan	AR
LGMD2D	17q112	α-Sarcoglycan	AR
LGMD2E	4q12	β-Sarcoglycan	AR
LGMD2F	5q23	δ-Sarcoglycan	AR
LGMD2G	17q11	TCAP	AR
LGMD2H	9q31	TRIM32	AR
LGMD2I	13q13	FKRP	AR
LGMD2J/Tibial MD	2q31	Titin	AR/AD
Congenital Muscular Dystrophies (CMDs) Secondary to Glycosylation Disorder			
Fukuyama MD	9q31-q33	Fukutin	AR
Muscle-eye-brain disease	1p3	POMGnT1 Glycosyltransferase	AR
Walker-Warburg syndrome	9q34	POMT1	AR
MDC1A	6q22	Laminin-2 (merosin)	AR
MDC1B	1q42	Not identified	AR
MDC1C	19q13	FKRP	AR
MDC1D	22q12	LARGE	AR
Other Congenital Muscular Dystrophies			
CMD with early rigid spine	1p36	Selenoprotein 1	AR
CMD with ITGA7 mutations	12q	Integrin α7	AR
Ullrich syndrome	21q22.3 (A1, A2)	Collagen 6 A1, A2, A3	AD
Bethlem myopathy	2q37 (A3)		

Table 13-1. Classification and Genetics of the Muscular Dystrophies,[a] continued

Disease	Gene locus	Gene product	Inheritance
Muscular Dystrophies Secondary to Nuclear Envelope Defects ("Nuclear Envelopathies")			
Emery-Dreifuss MD (EDMDX)	Xq28	Emerin	XR
Emery-Dreifuss MD (EDMD1)	1q11-q23	Lamin A/C	AD/sporadic
Muscular Dystrophies Secondary to RNA Metabolism Defect			
Myotonic dystrophy 1 (DM1)	19q13	DM	AD
Myotonic dystrophy 2 (DM2)	3q21	ZFN9	AD
Muscular Dystrophies of Unknown Mechanism			
Faciosapulohumeral MD	4q35	Not identified	AD
Oculopharyngeal MD	14q11.2-q13	PABp2	AD

Abbreviations: MD, muscular dystrophy; AD, autosomal dominant; AR, autosomal recessive; MDC, merosin-negative congenital muscular dystrophy; XR, X-linked recessive.

[a]From Escolar DM, Leshner RT. Muscular dystrophies. In: Swaiman KF, Ashwal S, Ferriero DM, ed. *Peditric Neurology. Principles & Practice*. Philadelphia, PA: Mosby Elsevier; 2006:1971, with permission from Elsevier.

Initial evaluation should include CK and ECG. Creatine kinase is usually 50 to 100 times normal. A child who demonstrates signs and symptoms of DMD and elevation of CK should have DNA analysis. Initial DNA analysis is directed at common deletions or duplications. This test is abnormal in 60% to 70% of children with DMD. Direct sequencing of all exons increases the yield to 90% or 95% but is very expensive. Insurance often does not pay for this test. In the 5% or 10% of children with clinical features of DMD but normal DNA analysis, muscle biopsy for dystrophin analysis (by immunostain or immunoblot) may be necessary.

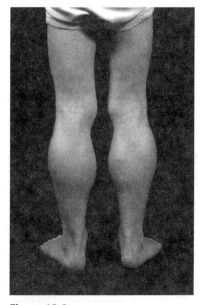

Figure 13-3.
Boy with Duchenne muscular dystrophy and marked pseudohypertrophy of his calves.

Treatment is symptomatic. It should include timely evaluation and treatment of pulmonary, cardiac, orthopedic, and educational problems. Prednisone has been shown to improve strength and function mildly, to prolong ambulation for up to 3 years, and to decrease the risk of scoliosis. Unfortunately, it has many side effects (weight gain and osteoporosis are the most significant). It is usually started between 5 and 7 years of age. There is significant practice variation in dosing. The dose supported by the greatest number of studies is 0.75 mg/kg/d, given daily.

Thirty percent of children with DMD have new mutations. Appropriate genetic counseling should be given to all female relatives of children with DMD.

Becker MD has a more variable presentation. Clinical findings are similar to DMD but they usually have later onset (mean age of onset: 12 years) and slower progression. Mean age at loss of ambulation is the mid 30s and at death is 42 years (range: 23–89 years).

Facioscapulohumeral Muscular Dystrophy

Facioscapulohumeral MD is the second most common form of MD. Its prevalence is 1 per 20,000. Onset is in late childhood and adolescence. This disorder is slowly progressive and initially affects the face, upper arms (sparing the deltoids), and scapula (Figure 13-4). Later it affects the abdominal and lower extremity muscles. Weakness is often asymmetrical. Two-thirds of these children have high-frequency hearing loss. By fluorescent angiography, two-thirds have a vascular retinopathy (Coat disease), but less than 1% are symptomatic.

Facioscapulohumeral MD is an autosomal dominant disorder with variable penetrance. Ten percent to 30% are new mutations. Creatine kinase is mildly elevated (1–5 times normal). In 95% of children, diagnosis is made by DNA analysis. There

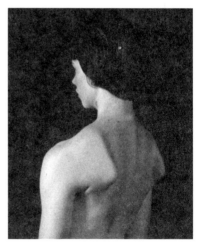

Figure 13-4.
Teenage girl with facioscapulohumeral muscular dystrophy showing winging of her scapula.

is contraction of a tandem repeat (D4Z4 repeat) located at 4q35. Treatment is symptomatic. Life expectancy is normal.

Limb Girdle Muscular Dystrophy

Children with LGMD have weakness of the hip/shoulder girdle. There are 13 forms of LGMD2 and 7 forms of LGMD1 (Table 1). Children with a DMD-like phenotype and normal dystrophin should be suspected of having LGMD2C-F (sarcoglycanopathies) or LGMD2I (Fukutin-related protein deficiency). Children with LGMD usually have normal intelligence.

Congenital Muscular Dystrophy

Children with congenital MD (CMD) present in the newborn period with hypotonia, weakness, and possibly contractures. They have variably elevated or normal CK. The inheritance is autosomal recessive (Table 13-1). The CMDs can be subdivided into those that have mental retardation and CNS structural anomalies and those that have normal intelligence. The most common forms of CMD with CNS structural anomalies are Fukuyama CMD, Walker-Warburg CMD, and muscle-eye-brain disease. In the United States, these conditions are rare. The 2 most common forms of CMD with normal intelligence are merosin deficiency and the Ullrich form. Both present at birth with hypotonia and weakness, which are very slowly progressive or static. The latter is caused by collagen 6 abnormalities and is characterized by proximal contractures and distal hypotonia and hypermobility. In the former, magnetic resonance imaging (MRI) shows white matter hyperintensity.

Other Muscular Dystrophies

Of the other MDs, the one that presents in older children and is most important to recognize is Emery-Dreifuss MD (Table 13-1). These children have early contractures of the elbows, Achilles tendons, and posterior cervical muscles and slowly progressive weakness and atrophy, which begin in a scapulohumeral distribution. Early recognition is important because these children will develop a cardiomyopathy that begins with conduction defects and culminates in complete heart block and atrial paralysis. There is a sex-linked form caused by abnormalities of the emerin protein (*STA* gene) and an autosomal dominant form caused by abnormalities of lamin A and C (*LMNA* gene).

Benign Congenital Myopathies

The benign congenital myopathies are a group of genetic myopathies that usually present at birth with hypotonia, hyporeflexia, and weakness. They usually have a slowly progressive or nonprogressive course. On muscle biopsy they show structural abnormalities of the muscle fiber. Although in most of them genetic defects have been identified, the tests are usually not commercially available, and diagnosis is based on muscle biopsy with histochemistry and EMG. The CK may be normal or mildly elevated, and EMG may be myopathic, normal, or even neurogenic.

Myotonic Syndromes

Myotonia is characterized clinically by delayed relaxation or sustained contraction of skeletal muscle. Myotonic syndromes can be subdivided into dystrophic and non-dystrophic. Non-dystrophic myotonic syndromes are rare and include myotonia congenita (chloride channel myotonias) and paramyotonia congenita (sodium channel myotonia).

Myotonic Dystrophy

Two types of myotonic dystrophy (DM) are now known (Table 13-1). Both are autosomal dominant. Type 1 has an estimated prevalence of 1 per 20,000. Type 1 may have a congenital or childhood onset, and type 2 (also called *proximal myotonic myopathy*) may present in the second decade. The childhood presentations of types 1 and 2 are similar. The congenital form of type 1 will be discussed in more detail.

Congenital myotonic dystrophy presents at birth with proximal greater than distal weakness, hypotonia, facial weakness (ptosis and tent-shaped mouth) (Figure 13-5), feeding difficulties (50%–60%), talipes equinovarus (50%), and respiratory problems (50%). Respiratory problems

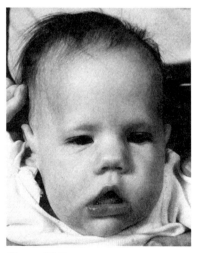

Figure 13-5.
Infant girl with congenital myotonic dystrophy. She has facial weakness: notice ptosis and tent-shaped mouth.

are secondary to weakness, pulmonary immaturity, aspiration pneumonia, and diaphragmatic paralysis. Infants do not have clinical or EMG myotonia. Although they may be quite severe initially, hypotonia and weakness improve, and almost all children who survive will be weaned off the respirator and walk. Sixty percent to 70% will have mental retardation, which is usually mild to moderate. Ninety-five percent of children inherit the disease from their mothers. Diagnosis is suspected after examining the mother, and it is confirmed with DNA analysis. Children with congenital DM have greatly expanded cytosine-thymidine-guanosine (CTG) repeats (730–4,300 repeats) at the 3-prime end of the myotonin kinase gene. Creatine kinase is normal or mildly elevated.

Inflammatory Myopathies

The inflammatory myopathies are a heterogeneous group of disorders that have infectious, genetic, and autoimmune causes. Excluding the viral myositides, polymyositis and dermatomyositis are the most common. In children, dermatomyositis is more common. Its incidence is about 2 to 3 cases per million children per year and it is more common in girls (2:1).

Dermatomyositis

Most cases of dermatomyositis present between 4 and 11.5 years of age with insidious weakness and rash, and possibly with systemic symptoms. In one study of 79 children, all had weakness and rash. Sixty-five percent had fever, 73% muscle pain, 44% dysphagia, 35% arthritis, and 10% melena. Heliotrope eyelid rash and Grotton papules are seen in about 80% of children. A papulosqamous rash is often seen over the extensor surfaces.

Weakness is generalized (more proximal than distal) and symmetrical and starts in the legs. Muscle calcifications (calcinosis) and knee joint contractures may be present. Ulceration of the gastrointestinal mucosa and pulmonary fibrosis are known systemic complications. The course of the disease is variable. About 37% have a monophasic course and the rest have a chronic or relapsing-remitting illness.

Laboratory tests show CK to be normal or mildly elevated, sedimentation rate and C-reactive protein (CRP) are also normal or elevated. Electromyography shows myopathic action potentials with or without fibrillations or stimulation-induced repetitive high-frequency discharges. Abnormal muscles on MRI show increased signal in T2-weighted images. Muscle biopsy shows endomysial, perivascular, and perimysial inflammation and perifascicular atrophy. Diagnosis is based on clinical findings supplemented by appropriate supporting laboratory data.

Initial treatment includes prednisone (1–2 mg/kg/d) or IGIV, or both. If symptoms are not controlled, immunosuppressive therapy, including methotrexate, azathioprine, or cytoxan, is indicated.

Disorders of the Neuromuscular Junction

Myasthenia Gravis

Myasthenia gravis (MG) is characterized by fluctuating skeletal muscle weakness that worsens after repeated or sustained muscle activity and improves with rest, due to a neuromuscular junction transmission defect. Three forms of MG occur in childhood: transient neonatal myasthenia in the infant born to a myasthenic mother, congenital myasthenia in the child of a non-myasthenic mother (CMGs), and the immune-mediated form of MG (also known as *juvenile MG*).

Juvenile Myasthenia Gravis

Clinical Characteristics

Juvenile MG is not different from the adult form of MG. First symptoms occur after age 10 years in 75% of patients, but may appear as early as infancy. Unilateral or bilateral ptosis, which is often asymmetrical, is the most common presenting symptom. Signs of fatigability of the eyelid include increased drooping on sustained up gaze (Simpson test) and an upward overshoot of the eyelid with several twitches followed by repositioning of the lid to the original ptotic state after looking down for 10 to 15 seconds (Cogan lid twitch sign). Diplopia secondary to extraocular muscle involvement may occur separately or accompany ptosis. Specific ocular muscles affected may change from examination to examination. The "peek" sign occurs when the palpebral fissure widens after a period of voluntary eye closure and is an indication of weakness and fatigability of the orbicularis oculi muscle. Individual patients can have very different patterns and severity of weakness. Weakness may remain in the ocular muscles (ocular MG) or spread to the facial and bulbar (bulbar MG) or also involve the limbs and respiratory muscles (generalized MG). Hypophonia, difficulty chewing, and dysphagia indicate bulbar involvement, and choking and respiratory failure can be life-threatening. Difficulty in raising the arms to wash, brush hair, or shave, and difficulty ascending stairs or getting up from the floor indicate proximal limb weakness. Fatigability of the arms can be demonstrated by timing the patient's ability to hold the arms forward in extension. Weakness classically worsens over the course of the day or with repetition or exertion and improves with rest or with the use of acetylcholinesterase inhibitors.

Diagnostic Evaluation

Patients should be referred to a specialist for evaluation. A transient response to edrophonium (Tensilon test), elevated acetylcholine receptor (AChR) antibody levels, significant decremental responses to repetitive nerve stimulation, excessive "jitter" with single-fiber EMG, and response to therapy provide a total clinical picture that is the basis of diagnosis.

Tensilon is fast acting (usually within 30–60 seconds), with short duration of action of about 10 minutes. Overall, it is a relatively safe test, but serious side effects such as hypotension, bradycardia, cardiac arrest, and respiratory distress may occur, and it should be performed only if appropriate resuscitation equipment is available. The ice-pack test can be a safe and simple alternative test. The ice-pack is applied to the eyelid for about 2 minutes and the eyelid is observed to see if the drooping improves. However, this is a nonspecific test for MG and can be misleading as improvement has been seen in other conditions such as mitochondrial diseases and myopathy. Negative Tensilon tests or ice-pack tests do not exclude the diagnosis of MG however.

If AChR antibody levels are elevated, the diagnosis of autoimmune MG is certain. Acetylcholine receptor antibody levels, however, are not elevated in all patients (seronegative). Indeed, the highest proportion of seronegative patients is among the youngest patients: 36% to 50% of prepubertal patients are seronegative, compared with 25% to 32% of peripubertal patients and 0% to 9% of postpubertal adolescent patients. Differentiation between seronegative juvenile MG and CMGs is therefore most difficult in these youngest patients. Repeated AChR antibody measurements over years may identify a conversion from seronegative to seropositive in some of these patients, supporting the diagnosis of juvenile MG. Small numbers of the seronegative patients may have an evaluated anti-muscle specific tyrosine kinase (anti-MuSK) antibody. Where clinically indicated (eg, severe weakness), a therapeutic response to steroid, PE, or IGIV would support a diagnosis of juvenile MG.

Other differential diagnosis includes congenital myopathy and mitochondrial cytopathy. Serologic tests for thyroid disease should be ordered because dysthyroidism may coexist with MG in up to 9% of males and 18% of females. All patients suspected of having MG also need a computed tomography scan of the chest and anterior mediastinum for evaluation for thymoma.

Management

Treatment options include cholinesterase inhibitors, steroids and other immunosuppressants, PE, IGIV, and thymectomy. The goal of treatment for patients with MG should be to induce and maintain maximum clinical remission with minimal adverse effects. It is important to avoid those common drugs that exacerbate MG, as shown in Box 13-1.

Pyridostigmine or mestinon, a cholinesterase inhibitor, is often the first line of therapy. The initial dose is 0.5 to 1 mg/kg/dose every 3 to 6 hours.

Box 13-1. Drugs to Be Avoided or Used With Caution in Patients With Myasthenia Gravis

Antibiotics
  Aminoglycosides, ciprofloxacin, erythromycin, telithromycin

Beta-adrenergic receptor blockers
  Propranolol, timolol, oxprenolol

Neuromuscular junction blocker
  Curare, non-depolarizing (vecuronium), botulinum toxin

Antirheumatic drugs
  Chloroquine, high-dose prednisone

Calcium channel blockers
  Verapamil

Anticholinergics
  Trihexyphenidyl

Others
  D-penicillamine, α-interferon, quinidine, procainamide, procaine, lithium, magnesium

Comparison of strength and activity 1 hour after a dose and immediately before the next dose facilitates individualized tailoring of the dosage schedule. The main side effects are nausea, vomiting, abdominal pain, diarrhea, sweating, and (potentially) cholinergic crisis (ie, exacerbated weakness due to excess cholinesterase inhibition).

For patients with bulbar and generalized MG, immunomodulatory agents and thymectomy are the mainstays of therapy. Corticosteroids, specifically prednisone, provide the core immunosuppressive treatment, although few randomized controlled trials have been done. The initial dosage is usually 1 mg/kg/d, but caution must be taken as prednisone may exacerbate symptoms of MG at introduction, sometimes to the point of marked respiratory muscle weakness requiring mechanical ventilation. Improvement usually begins within 2 weeks, but may take as long as 2 months. A very slow tapering every 4 weeks (no more than 20% of the previous dose) can then be attempted, although many patients require a low-maintenance dose for a prolonged period. Azathioprine is commonly used as a steroid-sparing agent in MG, but the onset of action may be delayed until after 12 months. In addition, within the first few weeks of treatment, about 10% of the patients develop an idiosyncratic reaction. Other immunosuppressive agents, such as methotrexate, cyclosporine, and CellCept, have been reported to be effective and are used as second-line adjunctive therapy in MG. Cyclophosphamide (pulsed intravenously) was used in 8 patients with severe refractory MG.

Plasmapheresis should be used in myasthenic crisis. Controlled clinical trials have shown that IGIV is effective in acute worsening of symptoms, to prepare for thymectomy, or as an adjuvant to other immunosuppressive therapies. For long-standing fixed deficits, prisms, and ptosis or strabismus, surgery can be helpful.

Congenital Myasthenia Syndromes

Congenital myasthenia syndromes (CMSs) are a heterogeneous group of inherited disorders involving neuromuscular junction transmission, and are classified according to their target as presynaptic, synaptic basal lamina-associated, or post-synaptic.

Myasthenic symptoms are usually recognized at birth or shortly thereafter in infants who are not born to myasthenic mothers, although it may also present later in life. Most patients have reached maximum disease severity within 2 years of onset. Spontaneous remissions may occur over many years. The presentation is similar to myasthenia acquired in the first 2 years of life. Patients with the slow-channel CMS typically show selective severe weakness of cervical, wrist, and finger extensors. Cranial muscles are usually spared. Measurement of the AChR antibodies is necessary to establish the proper diagnosis, because these antibodies are often present in juvenile autoimmune myasthenia but absent in congenital myasthenia gravis.

Congenital myasthenia syndromes often improve with mestinon treatment. The dosage is the same as that recommended for acquired autoimmune myasthenia gravis. Occasionally, the addition of ephedrine provides additional benefit. However, mestinon and 3,4-diaminopyridine may lead to worsening in patients with slow-channel syndrome and end-plate acetylcholinesterase deficiency. Immunomodulatory therapy is not effective.

Infant Botulism

Infant botulism is the most common form of human botulism in the United States, with between 80 and 110 cases recognized annually and the highest incidences found in Utah, Pennsylvania, and California. It results from the ingestion of spores of *Clostridium botulinum* (or rarely, neurotoxigenic *Clostridium butyricum* or *Clostridium baratii*), which germinate and temporarily colonize the lumen of the large intestine and produce botulinum neurotoxin. These spore-forming bacteria are known to produce 8 different toxin types, but more than 90% of US cases of infant botulism are due to toxin types A or B, with rare cases due to toxin type E (from *C butyricum*) and type F (from *C baratii*). Botulinum toxin binds irreversibly to presynaptic nerve terminals and inhibits the release of acetylcholine, thereby causing muscle paralysis.

Clinical Characteristics

Infant botulism usually occurs between 2 weeks and 1 year of age, with a median age of 10 weeks, although one infant with confirmed botulism was only 54 hours old at the onset of symptoms. Symptoms range from mild hypotonia to severe paralysis and fulminant respiratory failure. Paralysis is flaccid and symmetrical, always progressing in a descending pattern from muscles innervated by cranial nerves; to upper then lower extremities proximally; to trunk, distal extremities, and diaphragm. Constipation is often one of the early but frequently overlooked symptoms, and most infants have some combination of poor feeding and weak suck, weak cry, ptosis, facial weakness, decreased gag reflex, floppiness with poor head control, weakness and decreased spontaneous movement, and autonomic dysfunction during the course of illness. More than 50% will show sluggishly reactive pupils and ophthalmoplegia. Deep tendon reflexes can be normal or diminished. Infants with severe symptoms may require lengthy hospital stays, admission to the intensive care unit, and mechanical ventilation. Fever is usually absent. Generally, the disease progresses for about 1 to 2 weeks, followed by gradual improvement over the next few weeks.

Diagnostic Evaluation

The diagnosis of infant botulism can be confirmed by detecting botulinum toxin via the biologic mouse toxin assay (using a specimen of filtered stool) or by isolating toxigenic clostridia in fecal material, but results may take a few days. Electrophysiology is usually the quickest way to make a diagnosis of botulism, but is rarely indicated in classical cases. Typically, compound motor action potentials are small, a finding that may be misinterpreted as indicative of a motor neuropathy or a neuronopathy. Rapid (30–50 Hz) repetitive nerve stimulation causes abnormal incremental responses, whereas slow (2–3 Hz) repetitive nerve stimulation may cause abnormal decremental responses. Septicemia and meningitis are the most frequent misdiagnosis. Other differential diagnoses include uncommon diseases such as Guillain-Barré syndrome, tick paralysis, metabolic disorders, hypothyroidism, anterior horn cell disease, MG, myopathy, poliomyelitis, and organophosphate poisoning.

Management

Urgent treatment with BabyBIG, botulism immune globulin intravenous (human) (BIG-IV), is the current standard of treatment, and it must not be delayed for confirmatory testing. Botulism immune globulin intravenous is derived from pooled plasma of immunized adult volunteers; it neutralizes free toxin. BabyBIG is available only through the California Department of Healthcare Services (CDHS) Botulism Treatment and Prevention Program (510/231-7600; www.infantbotulism.org). To be most effective, BabyBIG should be administered as early as possible during the course of illness. A 5-year placebo controlled, randomized clinical trial showed that a single intravenous dose of human-derived botulinum immunoglobulin decreased the duration of hospital stay from 5.5 weeks to 2.6 weeks, and the rate of intubation by two-thirds. Antibiotics should be avoided, especially aminoglycosides, which can exacerbate neuromuscular junction blockade. In addition, measures must be taken to prevent serious, mainly avoidable, complications. Acute otitis media, aspiration pneumonia, and urinary tract infection are the most common infectious complications. Hospital-associated *Clostridium difficile* can cause toxic megacolon and necrotizing enterocolitis.

Prognosis

The prognosis for full recovery is excellent if appropriate nutritional and respiratory supportive cares are provided; the case-fatality rate is less than 2%.

Web Sites

Charcot-Marie-Tooth Association: www.charcot-marie-tooth.org

Guillain-Barré Syndrome Foundation International: www.gbsfi.com

Muscular Dystrophy Association: www.mdusa.org

Muscular Dystrophy Family Foundation Inc.: www.mdff.org

Muscular Dystrophy Canada: www.muscle.ca

FSH Society, Inc.: www.fshsociety.org

Myotubular Myopathy Resource Group: www.mtmrg.org

Myasthenia Gravis Foundation of America, Inc.: www.myasthenia.org

Bibliography

Agrawal S, Peake D, Whitehouse WP. Management of children with Guillain-Barré syndrome. *Arch Dis Child Educ Pract Ed.* 2007;92:161–168

Andrews PI. Autoimmune myasthenia gravis in childhood. *Semin Neurol.* 2004;24:101–110

Angelini C. The role of corticosteroids in muscular dystrophy: a critical appraisal. *Muscle Nerve.* 2007;36:424–435

Arnon SS, Schechter R, Maslanka SE, Jewell NP, Hatheway CL. Human botulism immune globulin for the treatment of infant botulism. *N Engl J Med.* 2006;354:462–471

Barisic N, Claeys KG, Sirotković-Skerlev M, Löfgren A, Nelis E, De Jonghe P, Timmerman V. Charcot-Marie-Tooth disease: a clinico-genetic confrontation. *Ann Hum Genet.* 2008;72(pt 3):416–441

Beals TC, Nickisch F. Charcot-Marie-Tooth disease and the cavovarus foot. *Foot Ankle Clin.* 2008;13:259–274

Bertoni C. Clinical approaches in the treatment of Duchenne muscular dystrophy (DMD) using oligonucleotides. *Front Biosci.* 2008;1:517–527

Bhagavati S. Stem cell based therapy for skeletal muscle diseases. *Curr Stem Cell Res Ther.* 2008;3:219–228

Bradley WG, Jones MZ, Mussini JM, Fawcett PRW. Becker-type muscular dystrophy. *Muscle Nerve.* 1978;1:111–132

Braun S. Muscular gene transfer using nonviral vectors. *Curr Gene Ther.* 2008;8:391–405

Bressolin N, Castelli E, Comi GP, et al. Cognitive impairment in Duchenne muscular dystrophy. *Neuromusc Disord.* 1994;4:359–369

Compeyrot-Lacassagne S, Feldman BM. Inflammatory myopathies in children. *Pediatr Clin N Am.* 2005;52:493–520

Cossu G, Sampaolesi M. New therapies for Duchenne muscular dystrophy: challenges, prospects and clinical trials. *Trends Mol Med.* 2007;13:520–526

Darabi R, Santos FN, Perlingeiro RC. The therapeutic potential of embryonic and adult stem cells for skeletal muscle regeneration. *Stem Cell Rev.* 2008;4:217–225

Domingo RM, Haller JS, Gruenthal M. Infant botulism: two recent cases and literature review. *J Child Neurol.* 2008;23:1336–1346

Driscoll SW, Skinner J. Musculoskeletal complications of neuromuscular disease in children. *Phys Med Rehabil Clin N Am.* 2008;19:163–194

Eagle M, Baudouin SV, Chandler C, Giddings DR, Bullock R, Bushby K. Survival in Duchenne muscular dystrophy: improvements in life expectancy since 1967 and the impact of home nocturnal ventilation. *Neuromuscul Disord.* 2002;12:926–929

Eagle M, Bourke J, Bullock R, et al. Managing Duchenne muscular dystrophy—the additive effect of spinal surgery and home nocturnal ventilation in improving survival. *Neuromuscul Disord.* 2007;17:470–475

Engel AG. The therapy of congenital myasthenic syndromes. *Neurotherapeutics.* 2007;4:252–257

Escolar DM, Leshner RT. Muscular dystrophies. In: Swaiman KF, Ashwal S, Ferriero DM, ed. *Pediatric Neurology. Principles & Practice.* Philadelphia, PA: Mosby Elsevier; 2006:1969–2013

Evoli A, Bianchi MR, Riso R, et al. Response to therapy in myasthenia gravis with anti-MuSK antibodies. *Ann NY Acad Sci.* 2008;1132:76–83

Fabbro F, Marini A, Felisari G, et al. Language disturbances in a group of participants suffering from Duchenne muscular dystrophy: a pilot study. *Percept Motor Skills.* 2007;104:663–676

Guglieri M, Straub V, Bushby K, Lochmüller H. Limb-girdle muscular dystrophies. *Curr Opin Neurol.* 2008;21:576–584

Harper PS. *Myotonic Dystrophy.* Philadelphia, PA: W.B. Saunders Company; 1979

Herrmann DN. Experimental therapeutics in hereditary neuropathies: the past, the present, and the future. *Neurotherapeutics.* 2008;5:507–515

Hetherington KA, Losek JD. Myasthenia gravis: myasthenia vs. cholinergic crisis. *Pediatr Emerg Care.* 2005;21:546–548

Hughes RA, Raphaël JC, Swan AV, van Doorn PA. intravenous immunoglobulin for Gullain-Barré syndrome. *Cochrane Database Syst Rev.* Jan 25;(1)CD002063

Hughes RA, Swan AV, Raphaël JC, Annane D, van Koningsveld R, van Doorn PA. Immunotherapy for Guillain-Barré syndrome: a systematic review. *Brain.* 2007;130(pt 9):2245–2257

Jani-Acsadi A, Krajewski K, Shy ME. Charcot-Marie-Tooth neuropathies: diagnosis and management. *Semin Neurol.* 2008;28:185–194

Kabzinska D, Hausmanowa-Petrusewicz I, Kochanski A. Charcot-Marie-Tooth disorders with an autosomal recessive mode of inheritance. *Clin Neuropathol.* 2008;27:1–12

King WM, Ruttencutter R, Nagaraja HN, et al. Orthopedic outcomes of long-term daily corticosteroid treatment in Duchenne muscular dystrophy. *Neurology.* 2007;68:1607–1613

Kirschner J, Bonnemann CG. The congenital and limb girdle muscular dystrophies. *Arch Neurol.* 2004;61:189–199

Koepke R, Sobel J, Arnon SS. Global occurrence of infant botulism, 1976–2006. *Pediatrics.* 2008;122:e73–e82

Kupersmith MJ, Ying G. Ocular motor dysfunction and ptosis in ocular myasthenia gravis: effects of treatment. *Br J Ophthalmol.* 2005;89:1330–1334

Long SS. Infant botulism and treatment with BIG-IV (BabyBIG®). *Pediatr Infect Dis J.* 2007;26:261–262

Maddison P, Newsom-Davis J. Treatment for Lambert-Eaton myasthenic syndrome. *Cochrane Database Syst Rev.* 2005 Apr 18;(2):CD003279

Maggi L, Andreetta F, Antozzi C, et al. Two cases of thymoma-associated myasthenia gravis without antibodies to the acetylcholine receptor. *Neuromuscul Disord.* 2008;18:678–680

Manzur AY, Kuntzer T, Pike M, Swan A. Glucocorticoid corticosteroids for Duchenne muscular dystrophy. *Cochrane Database Syst Rev.* 2008 Jan 23;(1):CD003725.

McCreery KM, Hussein MA, Lee AG, Paysse EA, Chandran R, Coats DK. Major review: the clinical spectrum of pediatric myasthenia gravis: blepharoptosis, ophthalmoplegia and strabismus. A report of 14 cases. *Binocul Vis Strabismus Q.* 2002;17:181–186

Meregalli M, Farini A, Torrente Y. Combining stem cells and exon skipping strategy to treat muscular dystrophy. *Expert Opin Biol Ther.* 2008;8:1051–1061

Muntoni F, Brockington M, Godfrey C, et al. Muscular dystrophies due to defective glycosylation of dystroglycan. *Acta Myol.* 2007;26:129–135

Muntoni F, Wells D. Genetic treatments in muscular dystrophies. *Curr Opin Neurol.* 2007;20:590–594

Ortiz S, Borchert M. Long-term outcomes of pediatric ocular myasthenia gravis. *Ophthalmology.* 2008;115:1245–1248

Palmieri B, Sblendorio V, Ferrari A, Pietrobelli A. Duchenne muscle activity evaluation and muscle function preservation: is it possible a prophylactic strategy? *Obes Rev.* 2008;9:121–139

Pillen S, Arts IM, Zwarts MJ. Muscle ultrasound in neuromuscular disorders. *Muscle Nerve.* 2008;37:679–693

Pitt M. Neurophysiological strategies for the diagnosis of disorders of the neuromuscular junction in children. *Dev Med Child Neurol.* 2008;50:328–333

Poysky J, Behavior in DMD Study Group. Behavior patterns in Duchenne muscular dystrophy: report on the Parent Project Muscular Dystrophy Behavior Workshop 8-9 of December 2006, Philadelphia, USA. *Neuromuscul Disord.* 2007;17:986–994

Ryan MM. Guillain-Barré syndrome in childhood. *J Paediatr Child Health.* 2005;41:237–241

Sackley C, Disler PB, Turner-Stokes L, Wade DT. Rehabilitation interventions for foot drop in neuromuscular disease. *Cochrane Database Syst Rev.* 2007 Apr 18;(2):CD003908

Scherer SS. Finding the causes of inherited neuropathies. *Arch Neurol.* 2006;63:812–816

Scimè A, Rudnicki MA. Molecular-targeted therapy for Duchenne muscular dystrophy: progress and potential. *Mol Diagn Ther.* 2008;12:99–108

Seguier-Lipszyc E, Bonnard A, et al. Left thoracoscopic thymectomy in children. *Surg Endosc.* 2005;19:140–142

Sewry CA, Jimenez-Mallebrera C, Muntoni F. Congenital myopathies. *Curr Opin Neurol.* 2008;21:569–575

Sladky JT. Guillain-Barré syndrome in children. *J Child Neurol.* 2004;19:191–200

Tarnopolsky MA. Clinical use of creatine in neuromuscular and neurometabolic disorders. *Subcell Biochem.* 2007;46:183–204

Tawil R. Facioscapulohumeral muscular dystrophy. *Neurotherapeutics.* 2008;5:601–606

Toussaint M, Chatwin M, Soudon P. Mechanical ventilation in Duchenne patients with chronic respiratory insufficiency: clinical implications of 20 years published experience. *Chron Respir Dis.* 2007;4:167–177

Wagner AJ, Cortes RA, Strober J, et al. Long-term follow-up after thymectomy for myasthenia gravis: thoracoscopic vs open. *J Pediatr Surg.* 2006 Jan;41:50–54

Young P, De Jonghe P, Stögbauer F, Butterfass-Bahloul T. Treatment for Charcot-Marie-Tooth disease. *Cochrane Database Syst Rev.* 2008 Jan 23:CD006052

Chapter 14

Sleep Disorders of Childhood and Adolescence

Chandra Matadeen-Ali, MD
Navasuma Havaligi, MD, MPH
Sanjeev V. Kothare, MD

Introduction

Sleep problems in early childhood and development are a cause for great parental concern and anxiety. Sleep is the primary activity of the brain during early development; during childhood and adolescence it accounts for about 40% of an average day. Consequently, approximately 25% of all children experience some type of sleep problem at some point during childhood. Sleeplessness in childhood is a major contributor to mood, behavior, intellectual, and general health problems.

Childhood sleep problems are common, chronic, treatable, and preventable. Sleep is necessary for a child's optimal functioning, because it affects every aspect of his or her physical, emotional, cognitive, and social development. The clinical symptoms of any primary medical or psychiatric disorder are likely to be worsened by comorbid sleep problems. Childhood sleep disorders may also extend their impact by causing increased stress for parents, adding to marital disruption, and resulting in negative effects on parental sleep and daytime function. Inadequate recognition and treatment may have significant repercussions not only for the individual child, but also for the family as a whole. It is also a public health issue. It has been estimated that there is a 226% increase in health care utilization in children with obstructive sleep apnea and is consequently a huge financial burden. This reinforces the need for pediatricians and primary care health providers to screen for and recognize symptoms of sleep disorders in children.

In a survey of community-based and academic pediatricians, the percentage of pediatricians rating the impact on children of sleep problems in a variety of domains as important ranged from 50% (non-intentional injuries) to 93% (academic performance). However, only 46% of the surveyed physicians felt confident or very confident about their own ability to screen for sleep problems. Another study investigating pediatricians' training and practices regarding sleep disorders in children showed that 50% of them believed that the symptoms would subside by themselves.

Questionnaires such as the BEARS algorithm (Table 14-1) for information about sleep in general, Pediatric Daytime Sleepiness Scale to assess daytime sleepiness (Box 14-1), and other questionnaires to screen for obstructive sleep apnea and movement disorders in sleep have been developed to help pediatricians screen for sleep disorders of childhood.

Normal Sleep Structure From Birth to Adolescence

Changes in sleep architecture occur across the entire lifespan, but the most significant ones happen throughout early childhood.

Newborns (0–3 Months)
The normal newborn sleeps 16 to 20 hours per day. Sleep generally occurs in 1- to 4-hour periods, followed by 1- to 2-hour wake periods. Classic electroencephalogram (EEG) patterns are not present in the first months of life, and sleep staging is divided equally into active sleep and quiet sleep.

Infants (3–12 Months)
Non–rapid eye movement (NREM) sleep stages 1 through 4 can be identified, and sleep is entered through one of these stages. The proportion of REM sleep begins to decline around 3 months of age (Figures 14-1 and 14-2, Table 14-2). Throughout the first 12 months of life, total sleep time decreases to about 14 hours per day. Sleep consolidation into a 6- to 8-hour nighttime period occurs in about 75% by age 9 months and in nearly all children by 12 months. Naps persist about twice a day in 2- to 4-hour blocks.

Toddlers (1–3 Years)
Total sleep time decreases to about 12 hours per day with one nap daily, but the duration of the nap decreases to 1 to 3 hours. Up to 25% of toddlers have sleep problems with bedtime resistance and frequent night awakenings. Behavioral insomnia of childhood is the primary sleep disorder in this age group.

Table 14-1. BEARS: Sleep Screening Algorithm[a,b]		
	Toddler/preschool (2–5 yrs)	**School-aged (6–12 y)**	**Adolescent (13–18 y)**
Bedtime problems	Does your child have any problems • Going to bed? • Falling asleep?	Does your child have any problems at bedtime? (P) Do you have any problems going to bed? (C)	Do you have any problems falling asleep at bedtime? (C)
Excessive daytime sleepiness	Does your child seem overtired or sleep a lot during the day? Does she still take naps?	Does your child have difficulty waking in the morning, seem sleepy during the day, or take naps? (P) Do you feel tired a lot? (C)	Do you feel sleepy a lot during the day? In school? While driving? (C)
Awakenings during the night	Does your child wake up a lot at night?	Does your child seem to wake up a lot at night? Any sleepwalking or nightmares? (P) Do you wake up a lot at night? Have trouble getting back to sleep? (C)	Do you wake up a lot at night? Have trouble getting back to sleep? (C)
Regularity and duration of sleep	Does your child have a regular bedtime and wake time? What are they?	What time does your child go to bed and get up on school days? Weekends? Do you think he/she is getting enough sleep? (P)	What time do you usually go to bed on school nights? Weekends? How much sleep do you usually get? (C)
Snoring	Does your child snore a lot or have difficulty breathing at night?	Does your child have loud or nightly snoring or any breathing difficulties at night? (P)	Does your teenager snore loudly or nightly? (P)

Abbreviations: P, parent-directed question; C, child-directed question.

[a]The BEARS instrument is divided into five major sleep domains, providing a comprehensive screen for the major sleep disorders affecting children in the 2- to 18-year-old range.

[b]From Owens JA, Dalzell V. Use of the 'BEARS' sleep screening tool in a pediatric residents' continuity clinic: a pilot study. *Sleep Med.* 2005;6:63–69, with permission from Elsevier.

Box 14-1. Pediatric Daytime Sleepiness Scale (PDSS)[a,b]

Please answer the following questions as honestly as you can by circling one answer only:

1. **How often do you fall asleep or get drowsy during class periods?**
   Always   Frequently   Sometimes   Seldom   Never

2. **How often do you get sleepy or drowsy while doing your homework?**
   Always   Frequently   Sometimes   Seldom   Never

[c]3. **Are you usually alert most of the day?**
   Always   Frequently   Sometimes   Seldom   Never

4. **How often are you ever tired and grumpy during the day?**
   Always   Frequently   Sometimes   Seldom   Never

5. **How often do you have trouble getting out of bed in the morning?**
   Always   Frequently   Sometimes   Seldom   Never

6. **How often do you fall back to sleep after being awakened in the morning?**
   Always   Frequently   Sometimes   .   Seldom   Never

7. **How often do you need someone to awaken you in the morning?**
   Always   Frequently   Sometimes   Seldom   Never

8. **How often do you think that you need more sleep?**
   Always   Frequently   Sometimes   Seldom   Never

[a]From Drake C, Nickel C, Burduvali E, Roth T, Jefferson C, Badia P. The pediatric daytime sleepiness scale (PDSS): sleep habits and school outcomes in middle-school children. Sleep. 2003;26:455–458. Reprinted by permission of the American Academy of Sleep Medicine.

[b]Scoring: 4 3 2 1 0; scores above 20 indicate hypersomnia

[c]Reverse score this item

Preschoolers (3–6 Years)

Total sleep time may decrease slightly and generally is 11 to 12 hours per day. Most children stop taking naps by age 5 years. Bedtime resistance, nightmares, and nighttime fears are common in this age group. Obstructive sleep apnea syndrome (OSAS) and arousal parasomnias peak during this stage.

School-aged Children (6–12 Years)

Children still require 10 to 11 hours of sleep, with rare naps. Sleep problems in this age group include insufficient sleep, bedtime resistance, OSAS, and poor sleep hygiene. Sleep restriction has been related to cognitive and behavior problems.

Adolescents (13–18 Years)

Sleep requirements are 8 to 9 hours (Figure 14-3); however, most adolescents are sleep deprived due to social and school activities. Delayed sleep phase syndrome, OSAS, insufficient sleep, insomnia, restless legs syndrome (RLS), periodic limb movements in sleep (PLMS), and narcolepsy are seen in this age group.

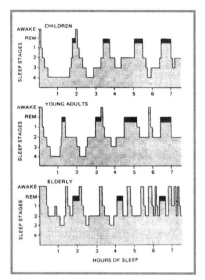

Figure 14-1.
Non–rapid eye movement/rapid eye movement sleep cycles through ages. (From Mindell JA, Owens JA. *A Clinical Guide to Pediatric Sleep. Diagnosis and Management of Sleep Problems.* Philadelphia, PA: Lippincott Williams & Wilkins; 2003. Reprinted by permission.)

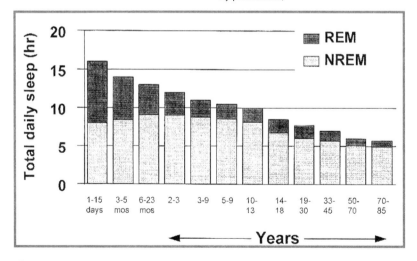

Figure 14-2.
Total sleep time and rapid eye movement/non–rapid eye movement distribution over ages. (From Roffwarg HP, Muzio JN, Dement WC. Ontogenetic development of the human sleep-dream cycle. *Science.* 1966;152:604–619. Reprinted with permission from AAAS.)

Table 14-2. Developmental Changes in Sleep Architecture		
	Newborn	**Adult**
% REM/NREM	50/50	20/80
REM/NREM cycles	50–60 min	90–100 min
Sleep onset stage	REM	NREM

Abbreviations: REM, rapid eye movement; NREM, non–rapid eye movement.

Evaluation of Sleep Disorders in Children

Assessment of sleep disorders should include

- *Sleep history:* Difficulty going to bed or initiating or maintaining sleep, excessive daytime sleepiness, nocturnal awakenings, unusual behaviors at night, snoring, and difficulty breathing
- *Medical and psychiatric history:* Asthma, allergies, gastroesophageal reflux disease (GERD), chronic lung disease, sickle cell disease, neurologic problems such as epilepsy, headaches, cerebral palsy, developmental delay, attention-deficit/hyperactivity disorder (ADHD), autism, depression, bipolar disorder, and anxiety
- *Family history:* sleep-disordered breathing (SDB), narcolepsy, and PLMS
- *Developmental screen:* Assessment of school functioning and behavior
- *Physical examination:* Special attention should be paid to
  - *Growth parameters:* Height, weight, and body mass index
  - *Ear, nose, throat examination:* Looking for deviated septum, adenotonsillar hypertrophy, adenoid facies, and oropharyngeal crowding
  - *Neurologic examination:* Especially in children with excessive sleepiness and seizures

Further evaluation may include sleep diaries, polysomnography (PSG), and multiple sleep latency test (MSLT).

Polysomnography and Multiple Sleep Latency Test

A PSG is a continuous recording of multiple physiological parameters during sleep, including EEG, electrocardiogram, electro-oculogram, respiratory effort using chest and abdominal belts, airflow, gas exchange using pulse oximetry and end tidal carbon dioxide, electromyography for legs and chin activity, snore microphone, and pH probe.

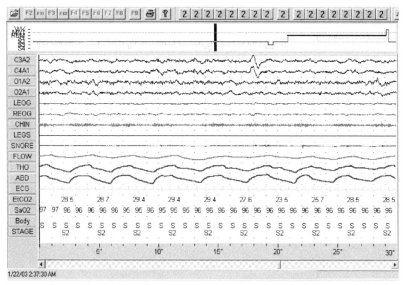

Figure 14-3.

Normal polysomnogram. (C3A2, C4A1, O1A2, O2A1: electroencephalogram electrodes; LEOG and REOG: left and right extraocular movement; tho: thoracic movements; abd: abdominal movements; EtCO₂: end-tidal carbon dioxide; SaO₂: oxygen saturation; stage: sleep stage.)

A PSG is warranted to investigate

- Sleep-related causes of excessive daytime sleepiness such as SDB
- Sleep fragmentation due to frequent nocturnal arousals from PLMS, bruxism, GERD, etc
- The etiology of episodic nocturnal phenomena (ie, parasomnias vs nocturnal seizures)

A PSG must be performed prior to MSLT to ensure at least 6 to 7 hours of sleep on the previous night. The contents of the PSG report and the normative values for pediatric PSGs are shown in Boxes 14-2 through 14-4. Figure 14-4 shows a graphic representation of a PSG epoch on digital recording.

The MSLT is a validated objective measure of the ability or tendency to fall asleep. It is indicated as part of the evaluation of patients with suspected narcolepsy and idiopathic hypersomnia. This test involves 5 daytime naps lasting 20 minutes each, with each nap being separated by 2 hours. The sleep onset for each nap is determined as sleep latency. Onset of REM sleep within 15 minutes of sleep onset constitutes a SOREMP (sleep onset REM period).

Box 14-2. Polysomnogram Report Parameters

Total sleep time

Sleep efficiency = total sleep time divided by time in bed

Sleep latency = time to fall asleep

REM latency = time taken to go into REM sleep after sleep onset

Sleep architecture = percentage of stages 1, 2, 3, 4 NREM and REM sleep

Arousal index = number of arousals per hour

Apnea hypopnea index = number of apneas and hypopneas per hour

Movement index = number of leg movements per hour

Movement arousal index = number of leg movements with arousals per hour

Pulse oximetry

End tidal carbon dioxide value

Other: pH probe with pH values simultaneously recorded

Abbreviations: REM, rapid eye movement; NREM, non–rapid eye movement.

Box 14-3. Polysomnogram Normative Values[a]

Central apneas lasting <20 s without
  -SpO_2 drop <89% or
  -SpO_2 drop >4% from baseline

A central apnea index of ≤1.0

An obstructive apnea index of ≤1.0

SpO_2 nadir >92%

Partial pressure of CO2 level >45 mm Hg for <10% of total sleep time

PLM index <5/hour

Sleep efficiency >85%

Abbreviations: SpO_2, saturation of peripheral oxygen; CO_2, carbon dioxide; PLM, periodic limb movement.

[a]Adapted from Marcus CL Omlin KJ, Basinki DJ, et al. Normal polysomnographic values for children and adolescents. Am Rev Respir Dis. 1992;146:1235–1239.

Box 14-4. Polysomnogram Empiric Norms for Apneas and Desaturations in Normal Children[a]

Obstructive apnea: Absence of airflow with continued chest wall and abdominal movement for at least 2 breaths (≥2 respiratory cycles).

Hypopnea: A decrease in nasal airflow of ≥50% with a corresponding decrease in SpO_2 ≥4% and/ or with an associated arousal.

Central apnea: An absence of flow and effort not immediately preceded by an arousal or awakening and lasting ≥20s; or any duration associated with an SpO_2 fall of ≥3%.

Abbreviations: SpO_2, saturation of peripheral oxygen.

[a]From Montgomery-Downs HE, O'Brien LM, Gulliver TE, Gozal D. Polysomnographic characteristics in normal preschool and early school-aged children. Pediatrics. 2006; 117:741–753 and Marcus CL, Omlin KJ, Basinki DJ, et al. Normal polysomnographic values for children and adolescents. Am Rev Respir Dis. 1992;146:1235–1239.

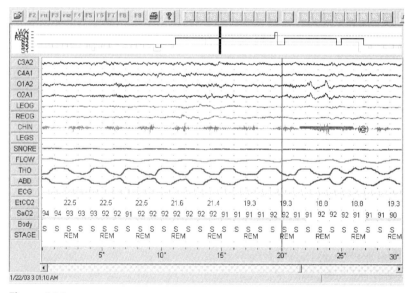

Figure 14-4.
Obstructive sleep apnea syndrome polysomnogram showing paradoxing, obstruction, and desaturation.

A mean sleep latency of less than 10 minutes and presence of 2 or more SOREMPs on an MSLT is abnormal and diagnostic of narcolepsy.

Behavioral Insomnia of Childhood

The essential feature of behavioral insomnia of childhood is difficulty in falling asleep, staying asleep, or both, which is related to an identified behavioral etiology. Two types are described (Box 14-5). Limit-setting type is characterized by bedtime stalling or refusal that is the result of inadequate limit setting by a caregiver. Sleep-onset association type is characterized by the child's dependency on specific stimulation, objects, or settings for initiating sleep or returning to sleep following an awakening. In the absence of these conditions, sleep onset is significantly delayed. They can have night awakenings with associated fearful or resistive behaviors.

Night awakenings are actually the norm in early childhood. They occur in association with the normal sleep cycle, so that brief awakenings occur every 90 to 120 minutes. The response to this waking is variable. Children, who are able to go back to sleep without parental intervention are referred to as *self-soothers*. Children who alert their parents with crying or getting out of bed are referred to as *signalers*. The signalers typically develop this pattern as a result of reinforcement by the caregiver. Self-soothers, on the other hand, are put to bed drowsy but awake and tend to develop associations with sleep onset that do not involve interaction with the caregiver. Other causes of night awakenings are shown in Box 14-6. In our experience, insomnia in infants or toddlers may be an initial manifestation of autism.

Good sleep hygiene is the key to promotion of self-soothing. Caregivers are advised to set regular bedtimes and naptimes, use positive reinforcement to increase appropriate behaviors and avoid punishment to decrease inappropriate behaviors. A consistent bedtime routine and putting the child to bed drowsy but awake is also advised. Either complete or gradual extinction may be used when reinforcement is not possible or practical.

Recent studies have related the lack of enough sleep with metabolic complications like obesity and diabetes.

Box 14-5. Behavioral Insomnia of Childhood[a]

A. A child's symptoms meet the criteria for insomnia based upon reports of parents or other adult caregivers.

B. The child shows a pattern consistent with either the sleep-onset association or limit-setting type of insomnia described below.

I. Sleep-onset association type includes each of the following:

  1. Falling asleep is an extended process that requires special conditions.

  2. Sleep-onset associations are highly problematic or demanding.

  3. In the absence of the associated conditions, sleep onset is significantly delayed or sleep is otherwise disrupted.

  4. Nighttime awakenings require caregiver intervention for the child to return to sleep.

II. Limit-setting type includes each of the following:

  1. The individual has difficulty initiating or maintaining sleep.

  2. The individual stalls or refuses to go to bed at an appropriate time or refuses to return to bed following a nighttime awakening.

  3. The caregiver demonstrates insufficient or inappropriate limit setting to establish appropriate sleeping behavior in the child.

C. The sleep disturbance is not better explained by another sleep disorder, medical or neurologic disorder, or medication use.

---

[a]From *American Academy of Sleep Medicine.* The International Classification of Sleep Disorders Diagnostic and Coding Manual. *2nd ed. Westchester, IL: American Academy of Sleep Medicine; 2005. Reprinted by permission.*

Pediatric Parasomnias

According to the *International Classification of Sleep Disorders Diagnostic and Coding Manual, 2nd Edition,* parasomnias are "undesirable physical events or experiences that occur during entry into sleep or during arousals from sleep." Parasomnias are classified as (1) disorders of arousal from NREM sleep, (2) parasomnias usually associated with REM sleep, and (3) other parasomnias.

A brief mention must be made of normal NREM sleep phenomena, including hypnic jerks (sleep starts) and hypnagogic imagery. These are experienced by most people during the transition from wake to sleep. Hypnic jerks are sudden jerks of all or part of the body, occasionally waking the individual or bed partner. Hypnagogic imagery is a dream-like mentation occurring at sleep onset in light NREM sleep. They do not necessarily imply REM onset sleep and should not be used as a clinical marker of narcolepsy.

Box 14-6. Causes of Nighttime Awakenings

Inadequate sleep hygiene
Inappropriate napping
Inconsistent sleep schedule
Excessive caffeine
Environmental factors

Child behavior/parent-child interaction
Sleep onset association disorder
Limit-setting sleep disorder
Nighttime fears
Primary insomnia

Fragmented sleep secondary to arousals
OSAS
PLMS
Narcolepsy
Bruxism

Parasomnias
NREM parasomnias
Confusional arousals
Sleep walking
Sleep terrors

REM parasomnias
REM behavior disorder
Nightmares

Other
Nocturnal seizures

Medical or psychiatric conditions
Anxiety
Depression
Substance abuse
Psychoses
Epilepsy
Headaches
Asthma
GERD
Pain
Medications

Abbreviations: OSAS, obstructive sleep apnea syndrome; PLMS, periodic limb movements in sleep; NREM, non–rapid eye movement; REM, rapid eye movement; GERD, gastroesophageal reflux disease.

Disorders of Arousal From NREM Sleep

These tend to occur in the first half of the night, when slow-wave sleep (SWS) is most prominent. Sleep walking, confusional arousals, and sleep terrors are included here. Prevalence estimates in childhood for sleep terrors range from 1% to 6%, for sleep walking up to 17% with a peak at 8 to 12 years, and for confusional arousals up to 17%. They are so common that they are often considered normal by most pediatricians. In these disorders, the transition from SWS to lighter sleep, just prior to REM sleep onset, is abnormal. The patient is neither awake nor fully asleep. The EEG demonstrates a combination of mixed frequencies.

Sleepwalking in children shares features with sleepwalking in adults. Children are usually calm and may walk into different parts of the house. They are at risk for injury from falls, lacerations from broken windows, and even hypothermia from exposure.

Confusional arousals occur mainly in infants and toddlers. A typical episode begins with moaning and evolves to confused and agitated behavior with crying and thrashing. The child cannot be fully aroused. Reassurance and comforting is not helpful. It may take 5 to 15 minutes before the child returns back to sleep.

Sleep terrors are dramatic partial arousals from SWS. The child may sit up suddenly and scream, with an intense blood-curdling "battle cry." Autonomic activation occurs with diaphoresis, mydriasis, and tachycardia. Sleep terrors are more prevalent in childhood with a peak between 5 and 7 years, and resolution typically before adolescence. There is usually no recollection of these events on the following day. They have to be differentiated from nightmares, nocturnal panic attacks, epileptic events, and cluster headaches.

Sleep deprivation is associated with more frequent and severe parasomnias. Other factors that influence arousal parasomnias include medications (neuroleptics, sedative hypnotics, stimulants, antihistamines), noisy environment, fever, stress, GERD, and intrinsic sleep disorders (ie, OSAS and PLMS). An overnight PSG is indicated when there is concern for another intrinsic sleep disorder and to rule out nocturnal seizures. Table 14-3 describes the differences between parasomnias and nocturnal seizures.

Evaluation of parasomnias should address questions regarding what events typically look like, how soon after sleep onset these events are noted, and whether they happen during nap or wakefulness as well as at night. A

Table 14-3. Comparison of Pediatric Parasomnias and Nocturnal Seizures[a]

Characteristic	Sleep-walking	Confusional arousals	Sleep terrors	Nightmares	Seizures
Timing during sleep	First third	First third	First third	Second half	Any
Sleep stage at start	SWS	SWS	SWS	REM	Any, especially stage 2
Duration	2–30 min	5–40 min	1–10 min	3–20 min	2–15 min
Agitation	None/mild	Moderate	Marked	Mild	Variable
Autonomic arousal	None/mild	Moderate	Severe	Mild	Variable
EEG abnormalities	No	No	No	No	Yes
Amnesia	Yes	Yes	Yes	No	Yes
Post-event confusion	Usual	Usual	Usual	Very rare	Usual
Family history/genetic	Yes	Yes	Yes	No	Rare
Episodes in wakefulness	No	No	No	No	Possible
Structural CNS lesion	No	No	No	No	Possible

Abbreviations: SWS, slow-wave sleep; REM, rapid eye movement; EEG, electroencephalogram; CNS, central nervous system.

[a]From Mason TBA, Pack A. Pediatric parasomnias. *Sleep.* 200; 30:141–151. Reprinted by permission of the American Academy of Sleep Medicine.

detailed history, along with a sleep log/diary, and in occasional cases simultaneous video-EEG monitoring, will help to differentiate these disorders from epilepsy.

Treatment of parasomnias includes reassuring parents that they are common in childhood. Safety measures should be instituted where appropriate. Maintenance of a sleep diary to reinforce the principle of minimizing sleep deprivation, avoiding stimulants, and evaluation for other intrinsic sleep disorders should be advised. Parents should also be told not to try to restrain or awaken the child during the episode. When arousal disorders occur consistently at a particular time, scheduled or anticipatory awakenings several minutes before hand may help; scheduled awakenings may be ineffective in children who do not have arousal parasomnias frequently and at a predictable time. Medications are preserved for rare protracted cases with no associated sleep disorder, with frequent parasomnias, and a threat of injury to self/others. Low-dose clonazepam and tricyclic antidepressants have been used with some success.

Disorders of Arousal From REM Sleep

Nightmares are the most common type of these arousals in children. They are noted at least occasionally in 30% to 90% of children between the ages of 3 and 6 years. Nightmares are vivid dreams with intense feelings of terror or dread that typically awaken a patient from sleep. Children may be anxious after awakening and can usually give a detailed description of the dream imagery. While infrequent nightmares likely do not require further evaluation, the presence of frequent ones have been associated with an increased prevalence of psychiatric disorders, such as schizophrenia, generalized anxiety disorder, and separation anxiety. It may also be a marker for sexual abuse.

Rapid eye movement sleep behavior disorder is very uncommon in children. Instead of REM sleep atonia, patients with this disorder have dreams associated with complex movements that can be vigorous and violent. It may occur in the setting of narcolepsy and other neurologic disorders such as brain stem tumors, juvenile Parkinson disease, and olivopontocerebellar degeneration.

Sleep paralysis is a fleeting inability to speak or move the trunk, head, and extremities that occurs during the transition from sleep to wakefulness, causing significant distress to the patient. It occurs as part of the narcolepsy tetrad, or as an isolated form in otherwise healthy children. Factors such as sleep deprivation, fatigue, and stress predispose to sleep paralysis.

Other Parasomnias

Nocturnal Enuresis

This is common in children. It is defined as enuresis in a child meeting the following criteria: (1) a chronological age of at least 5 years with a mental age of 4 years; (2) 2 or more incontinent events in a month between the age 5 and 6 years, or one or more events after age 6 years; and (3) absence of a physical disorder associated with incontinence, such as diabetes, urinary tract infection, or seizure disorder.

Sleep enuresis is primary if a child has never had a prolonged period of nocturnal continence and secondary if wetting recurs after 1 year of continence. It is quite common, affecting 25% of boys and 15% of girls at age 6. With each advancing year, the percentage of children with sleep enuresis decreases by about 15%. Enuresis typically occurs in NREM sleep. There is generally a family history of nocturnal enuresis. Sleep-disordered breathing has been identified as a potential cause of sleep enuresis.

Evaluation should include emotional and psychological assessment, physical examination for masses in the abdomen, motor/sensory disturbances associated with spina bifida and laboratory testing with urinalysis for assessment of infection, proteinuria, and glycosuria.

Treatment is directed at the underlying cause, then at development of skills and behaviors to promote dryness including alarms, retention control training, waking, and responsibility training. Imipramine and desmopressin have been used for short-term management.

Sleep-related dissociative disorder, exploding head syndrome, sleep-related eating disorder, and catathrenia (nocturnal groaning) are some other rare parasomnias.

Sleep-Related Movement Disorders

Sleep-Related Rhythmic Movement Disorder
Rhythm movement disorder is characterized by repetitive, stereotyped, and rhythmic motor behaviors that occur predominantly during drowsiness or sleep and involve large muscle groups. Head banging and body rocking are very common in late infancy and early toddlers. This behavior is seen in about 67% of 9-month-old infants, declining to 10% of 4-year-olds. It is commonly believed to be a means of soothing in the transition to sleep. There is little need for intervention, as behaviors do not cause harm to the infant.

Bruxism (Teeth Grinding)
This is another movement disorder that is very prevalent in childhood, approximately 14% to 17%, and then decreases over the lifespan.

Sleep-related bruxism without clear cause is termed *primary,* whereas *secondary* sleep-related bruxism may be associated with the use of psychoactive medications, recreational drugs, or a variety of medical disorders. It can lead to abnormal wear of teeth, jaw muscle pain, or temporal headache. Dental examination and oral appliances may be indicated.

Restless Legs Syndrome and Periodic Limb Movements in Sleep

Restless legs syndrome does occur in children. Prevalence is not well defined. The same essential criteria apply as in adult RLS: (1) urge to move or unpleasant sensation of the legs, (2) sensation worsens with inactivity, (3) sensation improves with activity, and (4) occurs predominantly at night. Current diagnostic guidelines for definite RLS in children are displayed in Box 14-7. While RLS is mainly a clinical diagnosis, PLMS is a polysomnographic diagnosis characterized by leg movements detected on PSG.

Primary RLS is idiopathic in nature. It has been postulated that it has a genetic basis with an autosomal dominant pattern of inheritance. Secondary RLS can occur in relation to a number of different medical conditions, including iron deficiency anemia, renal disease, pregnancy, and certain drugs. RLS and PLMS often occur concomitantly, and both result in sleep disruption. In adults, studies indicate that 70% of those with RLS also have

---

Box 14-7. Diagnosis of Restless Leg Syndrome in Pediatric Patients (Age 2-12 y)[a]

A. The child meets all four essential adult criteria for RLS and relates a description, in his or her own words, that is consistent with leg discomfort.

OR

B. The child meets all four essential adult criteria, but does not relate a description in his/her own words that is consistent with leg discomfort.

AND

C. The child had at least two of the following three findings:

I.   A sleep disturbance for age

II. A biological parent or sibling with definite RLS

III. A polysomnographically documented periodic limb movement index of five or more per hour of sleep

---

[a]From *American Academy of Sleep Medicine.* The International Classification of Sleep Disorders Diagnostic and Coding Manual. *2nd ed. Westchester, IL: American Academy of Sleep Medicine; 2005. Reprinted by permission.*

PLMS; whereas only 20% of patients with PLMS have RLS. Similar studies have not been conducted in children. Attention-deficit/hyperactivity disorder has shown associations with RLS and PLMS among small samples of referred children. Whether RLS and PLMS are a cause or effect of ADHD remains to be determined.

Management of RLS and PLMS includes replacing iron if deficient, sleep hygiene, avoiding caffeine, antihistamines, cold/sinus preparations, and antiemetics. Medications used in treatment include benzodiazepines and dopamine agonists, starting at the lowest possible dose and titrating upward. Data on their use in children are scant.

Excessive Daytime Sleepiness

Excessive daytime sleepiness is generally considered uncommon in early and middle childhood. Its prevalence in adolescence, however, compares with or exceeds the adult prevalence. As in adults, the most important cause of this disorder is inadequate quantity and quality of sleep. It is important to note that sleepiness in children may not be recognizable as drowsiness or other manifestations of sleepiness that occur in adults. Instead, it takes the form of moodiness, behavioral problems such as hyperactivity and poor impulse control, and neurocognitive dysfunction. Sleep need is on the order of 8 to 9 hours for most adolescents. Actual sleep time, however, is less than 7 hours for a significant number of adolescents. Frequently cited reasons for restricted sleep are evening activity levels (sports, homework, television, etc) and early school start time.

Other causes of excessive daytime sleepiness in children include delayed sleep phase syndrome and other sleep disorders such as SDB and RLS (Box 14-8). Uncommon causes of hypersomnolence that must be considered after other secondary causes have been ruled out include narcolepsy, idiopathic hypersomnolence, and recurrent hypersomnias (Kleine-Levin syndrome).

Circadian Rhythm Sleep Disorder

Prolonged periods of sleep deprivation or persistent irregularities in sleep hygiene inevitably lead to delayed sleep phase syndrome (DSPS), which is predominantly seen in adolescents. Adolescents begin to stay up later and later, sleeping only 6 to 7 hours per weeknight. In an attempt to recover lost sleep, they tend to sleep longer on weekends. However, over time, the short

---

Box 14-8. Causes of Excessive Daytime Sleepiness in the Pediatric Population

Insufficient sleep
Sleep deprivation/sleep restriction

Fragmented sleep
Obstructive sleep apnea/sleep-disordered breathing
Obesity hypoventilation syndrome
PLMS
Bruxism

Circadian rhythm disorders
DSPS

Primary disorders of EDS
Narcolepsy
Idiopathic hypersomnia
Recurrent hypersomnia

Sleep disorders associated with mental or medical conditions
Anxiety
Depression
Substance abuse
Psychoses
Epilepsy
Headaches
Asthma
GERD
Pain
Medications

Abbreviations: PLMS, periodic limb movements in sleep; DSPS, delayed sleep phase syndrome; EDS, excessive daytime sleepiness ; GERD, gastroesophageal reflux disease.

---

sleep periods followed by irregular long sleep periods disrupts the biological clock and leads to DSPS.

Patients with DSPS display an inability to fall asleep at the customary bedtime and an inability to rise at the usual time in the morning. There is no difficulty maintaining sleep once asleep, but there is great difficulty arousing at an appropriate hour in the morning. Total sleep time is greatly reduced during the week and prolonged on weekends. Once the circadian rhythm is disrupted, DSPS persists on vacations. It is often resistant to treatment with hypnotics. Treatment requires behavior management and chronotherapy (gradually shifting the time of sleep onset over 1 week). Light therapy (use of a light box with a 10,000 lux source of light used for 20 minutes in the morning) is often used in conjunction with chronotherapy.

Narcolepsy

Narcolepsy is a neurologically based disorder characterized by uncontrollable and overwhelming daytime sleepiness. Other symptoms that constitute the tetrad of symptoms are cataplexy, hypnagogic hallucinations, and sleep paralysis. Although it is a relatively rare sleep disorder in adolescents, it is important to recognize it early. Retrospectively, most adults with narcolepsy report that their symptoms started in childhood.

Narcolepsy with cataplexy can be observed at any age, but is rarely diagnosed before 5 years of age. It is very tightly associated with human leukocyte antigen subtypes DR2/DRB1*1501 and DQB1*0602. Current evidence suggests that most cases of narcolepsy with cataplexy are associated with loss of hypothalamic neurons containing the neuropeptide hypocretin. The lack of this peptide can be assessed by measuring cerebrospinal fluid levels of hypocretin-1. Diagnostic guidelines for narcolepsy with and without cataplexy are shown in Box 14-9.

Treatment of narcolepsy in adolescents is similar to that in adults. Providing education and supportive counseling to the adolescent and his or her family and teachers is the most important element of therapy. Stimulant medications, usually methyphenidate or modafinil, are also important to improve daytime alertness. γ-hydroxybutyrate (Xyrem) has been used in the treatment of narcolepsy with cataplexy. Selective serotonin reuptake inhibitors and tricyclic inhibitors have been found to be useful in controlling symptoms of cataplexy. Early identification and treatment will result in improved quality of life for children and their families.

Recurrent Hypersomnias

These are extremely rare. Kleine-Levin syndrome is the best representative example. It is characterized by recurrent episodes of hypersomnia often associated with other behaviors, such as overeating and sexual disinhibition, that typically occur weeks or months apart. The patient has normal alertness and behavior between episodes.

Box 14-9. Diagnostic Criteria for Narcolepsy With Cataplexy[a]

A. The patient has a complaint of excessive daytime sleepiness occurring almost daily for at least three months.

B. A definite history of cataplexy, defined as sudden and transient episodes of loss of muscle tone triggered by emotions, is present.

C. The diagnosis of narcolepsy with cataplexy should, whenever possible, be confirmed by nocturnal polysomnography followed by an MSLT; the mean sleep latency on the MSLT is less than or equal to eight minutes and two or more SOREMPs are observed following sufficient nocturnal sleep (minimum six hours) during the night prior to the test. Alternatively, hypocretin-1 levels in the CSF are less than or equal to 110 pg/ml or one third of mean normal control values.

D. The hypersomnia is not better explained by another sleep disorder, medical or neurological disorder, mental disorder, medication use, or substance use disorder.

Abbreviations: MSLT, multiple sleep latency test; SOREMP, sleep onset rapid eye movement period; CSF, cerebrospinal fluid.

[a]From *American Academy of Sleep Medicine*. The International Classification of Sleep Disorders Diagnostic and Coding Manual. 2nd ed. Westchester, IL: American Academy of Sleep Medicine; 2005. Reprinted by permission.

Recurrent episodes of sleepiness that occur in association with the menstrual cycle may be indicative of the menstrual-related hypersomnia.

Sleep Disorders Associated With Medical and Psychiatric Conditions

Primary sleep disorders should be differentiated from sleep disorders that accompany medical and psychiatric conditions (Box 14-10). Clinicians who evaluate and treat children with behavior disorders need to be aware that primary sleep disorders may present as behavior disorders; and treatment of behavior disorders may require treatment of the concomitant sleep disorders.

Seizures and Sleep

Benign rolandic epilepsy is the most common idiopathic epilepsy of childhood, occurring predominantly in sleep. Age of onset is typically 5 to 10 years. Seizures are usually infrequent, occurring less than 3 to 4 times a year.

Box 14-10. Sleep Disorders Associated With Mental Disorders or Medical Conditions[a]

Associated with mental disorders
Psychoses
Mood disorders
Anxiety/panic disorders
Substance abuse disorders

Associated with neurologic disorders
Sleep-related epilepsy
Sleep-related headaches
Degenerative disorders

Associated with other medical disorders
Sleep-related asthma
Gastroesophageal reflux

---

[a]*From Anders TF, Eiben LA. Pediatric sleep disorders: A review of the past 10 years.* J Am Acad Child Adolesc Psychiatry. *1997;36:9–20. Reprinted by permission of Lippincott Williams & Wilkins.*

Attacks begin with a somatosensory aura, usually referred to the *tongue and cheek,* followed by speech arrest, excessive salivation, and tonic-clonic movement involving the face. Prognosis is excellent, with most children responding to antiepileptic medications. Most patients stop having seizures in their teens.

Frontal lobe epilepsy can mimic parasomnias. Seizures tend to be primarily nocturnal, frequently repetitive with complex motor activity, of brief duration, and with only a brief or no postictal period.

Electrical status epilepticus of SWS and Landau-Kleffner syndrome are epileptic encephalopathies characterized by behavioral abnormalities and regression of language, with infrequent nocturnal seizures. The EEG shows continuous spike-wave discharges during NREM sleep and normal activity in REM sleep and wakefulness.

Obstructive Sleep Apnea Syndrome and Sleep-Disordered Breathing

Definition

Sleep-disordered breathing in children encompasses a continuum of upper airway obstruction during sleep ranging from primary snoring to obstructive sleep apnea syndrome.

Obstructive sleep apnea syndrome is a disorder of breathing during sleep characterized by prolonged partial upper airway obstruction and/or intermittent complete obstruction (obstructive apnea) that disrupts normal ventilation during sleep and normal sleep patterns. Multiple arousals resulting from these obstructive events lead to sleep fragmentation and frequent sleep stage transitions and, consequently, to symptoms of daytime sleepiness that often are neurobehavioral.

Epidemiology

Obstructive sleep apnea syndrome occurs in children of all ages, from neonates to adolescents; however, it is most common in preschool-aged children. The prevalence of habitual snoring in children ranges from 3.2% to 12.1%. Obstructive sleep apnea syndrome however has traditionally been considered to have a prevalence of 1% to 3% in children of preschool age, though more recent studies including older, more obese children indicate prevalence as high as 5%.

Epidemiological studies indicate several factors that influence the development of SDB in children.

Age. Obstructive sleep apnea syndrome occurs in all ages but peaks between the ages of 2 and 6 years. This coincides with the peak age of lymphoid hyperplasia and adenotonsillar hypertrophy. A second peak occurs in adolescence and it is most likely secondary to obesity.

Race. A clear racial predilection has been noted, with higher prevalence among African American and Asian children than among white children.

Gender. Gender appears to play no significant role in pediatric SDB.

Family history. A family history of SDB (among parents or siblings) is common among children with SDB.

Etiology and Pathogenesis

A number of risk factors for pediatric SDB have been identified. Adenotonsillar hypertrophy is the predominant underlying mechanism in non-adolescent children. Adenotonsillar hypertrophy is most prominent in children up to about age 6 to 8 years, when natural regression of this tissue begins to occur. Obstructive sleep apnea syndrome is usually due to a combination of upper airway obstruction, decreased upper airway diameter, and muscle tone.

Specific factors related to these underlying mechanisms are shown in Box 14-11.

Down syndrome is perhaps the most prevalent of the pediatric conditions leading to risk for OSAS. Children with Down syndrome may have any or all of the predisposing factors for OSAS, including macroglossia, midface hypoplasia, micrognathia, and muscular hypotonia.

Central ventilatory drive may be reduced in some patients (eg, brain stem injury or masses, Arnold Chiari malformation type 2, and myelomeningocele), resulting in ventilatory control instability and hence leading to central sleep apnea.

Box 14-11. American Thoracic Society's Indications for Cardiopulmonary Sleep Studies in Children[a]

Differentiate benign snoring from snoring associated with sleep-disordered breathing.

Assess severity of OSAS.

Clarify diagnosis when symptoms and risk factors are discordant.

Screen children at high risk for OSAS (eg, trisomy 21, achondroplasia).

Delineate severity of OSAS in children at risk for perioperative and postoperative symptoms.

Titrate CPAP in children with diagnosed OSAS.

Abbreviations: OSAS, obstructive sleep apnea syndrome; CPAP, continuous positive airway pressure.

[a]Adapted from American Thoracic Society, Standards and indication for cardiopulmonary sleep studies in children. Am J Respir Crit Care Med. 1996;153:866–876.

Clinical Manifestations

The clinical manifestations of SDB in children are fairly broad. The classic presentation of OSAS in children involves obstructive hypoventilation without marked daytime somnolence, which is somewhat different from that seen in the classic adult form of the disease. A comparison of the clinical features of pediatrics and adult OSAS is provided in Table 14-4. In reality, however, pediatric SDB exists as a continuum under which individuals can be categorized in 1 of 4 clinical variants or phenotypes translated into increased clinical severity. These include the following:

- Chronic, habitual snoring that results in sleep disruption without associated blood gas abnormalities
- Upper airway resistance, similar to that seen in adults, including snoring without identifiable airflow obstruction and increasingly negative esophageal pressure swings and arousals
- Obstructive hypoventilation, which consists of long periods of persistent, partial, upper airway obstruction associated with hypercarbia with or without arterial oxygen desaturation (classic pattern)
- Cyclic episodes of obstructive apnea, similar to that of adults with OSAS

The relative prevalence of each of these patterns is not well studied. Among all variants, the most commonly encountered presenting symptom is snoring.

Table 14-4. Comparison of Pediatric and Adult OSAS		
Factor	**Children**	**Adults**
Estimated prevalence	Variable depending on phenotype	Up to 5%
	1% to 3% in young children	
Peak age	2 to 6 years for classic phenotype	30 to 60 yrs
Gender	M=F	M>F
Weight	Commonly normal, but can be underweight or overweight	Most obese
Snoring	Often continuous	Usually alternating with pauses
Excessive daytime sleepiness	Uncommon	Very common
Major cause	Adenotonsillar hypertrophy	Obesity

Abbreviations: OSAS, obstructive sleep apnea syndrome; M, male; F, female.

Common presenting symptoms of OSAS in childhood are listed in Box 14-12.

Complications

Major complications of childhood OSAS include failure to thrive, developmental delay, cor pulmonale, systemic hypertension, and death. More common, however, are the cognitive and behavioral complications of SDB (Table 14-5).

Box 14-12. Diagnostic Criteria for Pediatric OSAS[a]

A. Caregiver reports snoring, labored or obstructed breathing, or both snoring and labored or obstructed breathing during sleep.

B. Caregiver reports observing at least one of the following:
   I. Paradoxical, inward rib cage motion during inspiration
   II. Movement arousals
   III. Diaphoresis
   IV. Neck hyperextension during sleep
   V. Excessive daytime sleepiness, hyperactivity, or aggressive behavior
   VI. Slow rate of growth
   VII. Morning headaches
   VIII. Secondary enuresis

C. PSG recording demonstrates one or more scoreable respiratory events per hour (ie, apnea or hypopnea of at least 2 respiratory cycles in duration).[b]

D. PSG recording demonstrates either I or II (below):
   I. At least one of the following is observed:
      a. Frequent arousals from sleep associated with increased respiratory effort
      b. Arterial oxygen desaturation in association with the apneic episodes
      c. Hypercapnia during sleep
      d. Markedly negative esophageal pressure swings
   II. Periods of hypercapnia, desaturation, or hypercapnia and desaturation during sleep, associated with the following: snoring; paradoxical, inward rib cage motion during inspiration; and at least one of the following:
      a. Frequent arousals from sleep
      b. Markedly negative esophageal pressure swings

E. The disorder is not better explained by another current sleep disorder, medical or neurologic disorder, medication use, or substance use disorder.

---

[a]Adapted from American Academy of Sleep Medicine. The International Classification of Sleep Disorders Diagnostic and Coding Manual. 2nd ed. Westchester, IL: American Academy of Sleep Medicine; 2005. Reprinted by permission.

[b]Very few normative data are available for hypopneas, and the data that are available have been obtained using a variety of methodologies. These criteria may be modified in the future, once more comprehensive data become available.

Table 14-5. Complications of Childhood OSAS[a]	
Body System	**Complications**
Growth	Failure-to-thrive
	Short stature
	Impaired growth hormone release
Cardiovascular	Cor pulmonale/pulmonary hypertension
	Polycythemia
	Hypertension
Gastrointestinal	Feeding difficulties
	Gastroesophageal reflux
Pulmonary	Chronic aspiration
	Pulmonary edema (postoperative)
	Pectus excavatum
Behavioral	Developmental delay
	Behavioral problems
	School problems
Neurologic	Enuresis
	Increased intracranial pressure
	Lethargy/ dull affect
	"Hypoxia headache"
Surgical	Death (intraoperative, RVH/RVD)
	Death (postoperative)
	Postoperative respiratory compromise

Abbreviations: OSAS, obstructive sleep apnea syndrome; RVH, right ventricular hypertrophy; RVD, right ventricular dilation.

[a]Adapted from Sheldon SH, Kryger NH, Ferber R. Principles and Practice of Pediatric Sleep Medicine. Philadelphia, PA: WB Saunders and Co; 2005.

The incidence of death as a result of SDB is unknown. There is an association of OSAS and sudden infant death syndrome (SIDS) in patients with a family history of this condition. While it is unlikely that SIDS represents a pure form of OSAS, some characteristics of this disorder may lead to death in some infants. Overall, however, death as a complication of SDB is likely limited to the extreme cases of OSAS when it is associated with other medical or surgical conditions.

Assessment and Diagnosis

History and Physical Examination

A sleep history screening for snoring and other symptoms of OSAS should be part of routine health care visits. In children, OSAS is very unlikely in the absence of habitual snoring. Findings on physical examination during the wake state are often normal. There may be nonspecific findings related to adenotonsillar hypertrophy. Evidence of complications of OSAS may be present, including systemic hypertension, pulmonary hypertension, and poor growth, although some children with OSAS are obese. Although the history and physical examination are important in diagnosing OSAS, no combination of symptoms and physical findings has been found to reliably distinguish OSAS from habitual snoring. Therefore, overnight PSG performed in a sleep laboratory remains the diagnostic gold standard for OSAS, and there are currently no satisfactory alternatives.

Polysomnography

A PSG should be performed in every child with risk factors for OSAS. A PSG can differentiate habitual snoring from OSAS, delineate severity of OSAS in children at risk for perioperative and postoperative symptoms, and is also an important baseline measure for children with OSAS who may need additional PSG after treatment.

Presently there are no universally accepted PSG parameters for diagnosing OSAS in children; however, there are commonly accepted criteria. On the basis of normative data, an obstructive apnea index of 1 is often chosen as the cutoff for normality. However, while an apnea index of 1 is statistically significant (ie, at the 97.5th percentile for an asymptomatic, normative population), it is not known what level is clinically significant (Figure 14-4, Box 14-3, Box 14-4, Box 14-13, Box 14-14).

Treatment

The treatment of SDB in children may encompass a broad spectrum of therapy from surgery to device therapy, as well as medical therapy.

Adenotonsillectomy

Adenotonsillectomy provides curative therapy in most patients (75%–100%), including those who are obese. Children with OSAS clearly seem to be at high risk of postoperative respiratory compromise, and increased vigilance in postoperative monitoring is warranted, particularly in those with a high preoperative apnea-hypopnea index. Identified risk factors for respiratory complications are shown in Box 14-15.

Postoperative laryngeal edema may take up to 6 to 8 weeks to completely resolve and, therefore, OSAS may still be present during this period. Risk

Box 14-13. Risk Factors for Postoperative Respiratory Compromise in Children With OSAS Undergoing Adenotonsillectomy[a]

Age <3 years

Severe OSAS on polysomnography

Cardiac complication of OSAS (eg, right ventricular hypertrophy)

Failure to thrive

Obesity

Prematurity

Recent respiratory infection

Craniofacial anomalies

Neuromuscular disorders

Abbreviation: OSAS, obstructive sleep apnea syndrome.

[a]Adapted from McColley SA, April MM, Carroll JL, Nacleria RM, Loughlin GM. Respiratory compromise after adenotonsillectomy in children with obstructive sleep apnea. Arch Otolaryngol Head Neck Surg. *1992;118:940–943.*

Box 14-14. Factors Related to Pediatric Sleep-Disordered Breathing

Upper airway obstruction
- Adenotonsillar hypertrophy results from multiple etiologies (the most common are recurrent upper respiratory infection and allergic irritants)
- Chronic nasal obstruction from allergies
- Pharyngeal edema from GERD
- Velopharyngeal flap cleft palate repair

Upper airway size and muscle tone
- Obesity is the most common contributor to decreased airway size in adults and, with the increasing prevalence of obesity in children, it will likely play a larger role in OSAS in children.
- Airway size is also decreased in many syndromes, such as Prader-Willi, achondroplasia, mucopolysaccharidoses, Pierre Robin, Treacher Collins, Apert, Down, and many others.
- Decreased upper airway tone results from brain stem lesions (such as tumors and malformations).
- Neuromuscular diseases and diseases affecting overall neuromuscular tone (ie, hypotonic cerebral palsy).

Box 14-15. Common Presenting Symptoms of OSAS in Childhood

Nocturnal symptoms
- Loud continuous snoring
- Apneic pauses, choking, gasping, dyspnea
- Paradoxical breathing
- Excessive sweating
- Restless sleep
- Enuresis
- Abnormal sleeping position (ie, hyperextended neck)
- Nocturnal awakening
- Behavioral sleep problems (ie, bedtime resistance)
- Increase in partial arousal parasomnia (ie, sleepwalking, sleep terrors, etc)

Daytime symptoms
- Mouth breathing
- Chronic nasal congestion
- Hyponasal speech
- Difficulty swallowing
- Morning headaches
- Frequent infections (eg, otitis media and sinusitis)
- Poor appetite
- Excessive daytime sleepiness (rare)

Behavioral and cognitive dysfunction
- Hyperactivity/aggression and inattention (ADHD-like symptoms)
- Mood changes
- Academic difficulties

Others
- Increase in seizure frequency in predisposed children

---

factors for persistent OSAS after adenotonsillectomy include continued snoring, and a high apnea-hypopnea index on the preoperative PSG. All patients should be reevaluated postoperatively to determine whether additional treatment is required.

Other surgical options are available for patients not responding to the usual treatment. They include uvulopharyngoplasty, maxillofacial surgery, and tracheotomy; however, they are rarely performed in children but may be indicated in select cases.

Continuous Positive Airway Pressure

Certain patients may not derive full benefit from adenotonsillectomy. In a recent population-based study of children from 1 to 18 years, 6% of them snored nightly post-adenoidectomy with or without tonsillectomy. Continuous positive airway pressure (CPAP), the standard of care in adults with OSAS, is also effective in children. Continuous positive airway pressure is a noninvasive therapy of providing positive pressure to maintain upper airway patency and improve functional residual capacity in the lungs.

Indications for CPAP include

- Post-adenotonsillectomy with residual symptoms
- Prior to surgery in patients with severe OSAS
- Contraindications to adenotonsillectomy

Medical Treatment

Treatment has been limited to those agents that reduce upper airway tissue burden. Two studies have demonstrated efficacy of nasal steroids in pediatric SBD. One preliminary study has shown efficacy of the leukotriene-modifying agent montelukast in mild SDB. Other agents, such as nasal decongestants, may be helpful for intermittent snoring associated with intercurrent illness, but these agents should not be considered for long-term management.

Weight Management and Lifestyle Changes

In obese patients, weight management is likely to be of benefit. It should include comprehensive nutritional, exercise, and behavioral counseling for both the patient and the family. When appropriate, smoking cessation counseling should be offered to parents and caregivers.

Oral Appliances

Oral appliances such as mandibular advancing devices and tongue retainers may be used in adolescents when facial bone growth is complete. Referral to an orthodontist specializing in these devices should be recommended.

Guidelines

The American Academy of Pediatrics has published clinical guidelines for the evaluation and management of children with uncomplicated OSAS (Box 14-16).

> **Box 14-16. Summary of Recommendations for the Diagnosis and Management of Uncomplicated Childhood OSAS[a]**
>
> 1. All children should be screened for snoring.
> 2. Complex, high-risk patients should be referred to a specialist.
> 3. Patients with cardiorespiratory failure cannot await elective evaluation.
> 4. Diagnostic evaluation is useful in discriminating between primary snoring and OSAS; the gold standard is PSG.
> 5. Adenotonsillectomy is the first line of treatment for most children, and CPAP is an option for those who are not candidates for surgery or do not respond to surgery.
> 6. High-risk patients should be monitored as inpatients postoperatively.
> 7. Patients should be reevaluated postoperatively to determine whether additional treatment is required.
>
> ---
>
> *Abbreviations: OSAS, obstructive sleep apnea syndrome; PSG, polysomnography; CPAP, continuous positive airway pressure.*
>
> *[a]From American Academy of Pediatrics Section of Pulmonology, Subcommittee on Obstructive Sleep Apnea. Clinical practice guideline: diagnosis and management of childhood obstructive sleep apnea syndrome. Pediatrics. 2002;109:704–712.*

Web Sites

The National Sleep Foundation: www.sleepfoundation.org

The National Institutes of Health National Center on Sleep Disorders Research: www.nhlbi.nih.gov/about/ncsdr/

American Sleep Apnea Association: www.sleepapnea.org

The Restless Legs Syndrome Foundation: www.rls.org

Web MD Sleep Disorders Center: www.webmd.com/sleep-disorders

Information on Sleep Disorders: www.sleepnet.com

Information on Sleep Disorders: http://sleepdisorders.about.com

Bibliography

Alexopoulos EI, Kaditis AG, Kalampouka E, et al. Nasal corticosteroids for children with snoring. *Pediatr Pulmonol.* 2004;38:161–167

American Academy of Pediatrics Section on Pediatric Pulmonology, Subcommitee on Obstructive Sleep Apnea Syndrome. Clinical practice guideline: diagnosis and management of childhood obstructive sleep apnea syndrome. *Pediatrics.* 2002;109:704–712

American Academy of Sleep Medicine. *The International Classification of Sleep Disorders Diagnostic and Coding Manual.* 2nd ed. Westchester, IL: American Academy of Sleep Medicine; 2005

American Thoracic Society. Cardiorespiratory sleep studies in children. Establishment of normative data and polysomnographic predictors of morbidity. *Am J Respir Crit Care Med.* 1999;160:1381–1387

Amin RS, Carroll JL, Jeffries JL, et al. Twenty-four-hour ambulatory blood pressure in children with sleep disordered breathing. *Am J Respir Crit Care Med.* 2004;169:950–956

Anders TF, Eiben LA. Pediatric sleep disorders: a review of the past 10 years. *J Am Acad Child Adolesc Psychiatry.* 1997;36:9–20

Anstead M. Pediatric sleep disorders: new developments and evolving understanding. *Curr Opin Pulm Med.* 2000;6:501–506

Bokkala S, Napalinga K, Pinninti N, et al. Correlates of periodic limb movements of sleep in the pediatric population. *Pediatr Neurol.* 2008;39:33–39

Brouillette RT, Manoukian JJ, Ducharme FM, et al. Efficacy of fluticasone nasal spray for pediatric obstructive sleep apnea. *J Pediatr.* 2001;138:838–844

Chervin RD, Archbold KH, Dillon JE, et al. Inattention, hyperactivity, and symptoms of sleep-disordered breathing. *Pediatrics.* 2002;109:449–456

Chervin RD, Dillon JE, Archbold KH, Ruzicka DL. Conduct problems and symptoms of sleep disorders in children. *J Am Acad Child Adolesc Psychiatry.* 2003;42:201–208

Gaylor EE, Goodlin-Jones BL, Anders TF. Classification of young children's sleep problems: a pilot study. *J Am Acad Child Adolesc Psychiatry.* 2001;40:61–67

Goldbart AD, Goldman JL, Veling MC, Gozal D. Leukotriene modifier therapy for mild sleep-disordered breathing in children. *Am J Respir Crit Care Med.* 2005;172:364–370

Gottlieb DJ, Chase C, Vezina RM, et al. Sleep-disordered breathing symptoms are associated with poorer cognitive function in 5-year-old children. *J Pediatr.* 2004;145:458–464

Gozal D. Obstructive sleep apnea in children: implications for the developing central nervous system. *Semin Pediatr Neurol.* 2008;15:100–106

Gozal D. Sleep-disordered breathing and school performance in children. *Pediatrics.* 1998;102:616–620

Guilleminault C, Li K, Quo S, Inouye RN. A prospective study on the surgical outcomes of children with sleep-disordered breathing. *Sleep.* 2004;27:95–100

Kaditis AG, Finder J, Alexopoulos EI, et al. Sleep-disordered breathing in 3,680 Greek children. *Pediatr Pulmonol.* 2004;37:499–509

Knutson KL, Van Cauter E. Associations between sleep loss and increased risk of obesity and diabetes. *Ann N Y Acad Sci.* 2008;1129:287–304

Kothare SV, Kaleyias J. The clinical and laboratory assessment of the sleepy child. *Semin Pediatr Neurol.* 2008;15:61–69

Kryger MH, Roth T, Dement WC, eds. *Principles and Practice of Sleep Medicine.* Philadelphia, PA: WB Saunders; 2005

Marcus CL, Omlin KJ, Basinki DJ, et al. Normal polysomnographic values for children and adolescents. *Am Rev Respir Dis.* 1992;146:1235–1239

Marcus CL. Sleep-disordered breathing in children. *Am J Respir Crit Care Med.* 2001;164:16–30

Marcus CL, Rosen G, Ward SL, et al. Adherence to and effectiveness of positive airway pressure therapy in children with obstructive sleep apnea. *Pediatrics.* 2006;117:e442–e451

Mason TB II, Pack AI. Pediatric parasomnias. *Sleep.* 2007;30:141–151

McColley SA, April MM, Carroll JL, Naclerio RM, Loughlin GM. Respiratory compromise after adenotonsillectomy in children with obstructive sleep apnea. *Arch Otolaryngol Head Neck Surg.* 1992;118:940–943

Mindell JA, Moline ML, Zendell SM, Brown LW, Fry JM. Pediatricians and sleep disorders: training and practice. *Pediatrics.* 1994;94:194–200

Mindell JA, Owens JA. *A Clinical Guide to Pediatric Sleep. Diagnosis and Management of Sleep Problems.* Philadelphia, PA: Lippincott Williams and Wilkins; 2003

Mitchell RB. Sleep-disordered breathing in children. *Mo Med.* 2008;105:267–269

Montgomery-Downs HE, O'Brien LM, Gulliver TE, Gozal D. Polysomnographic characteristics in normal preschool and early school-aged children. *Pediatrics.* 2006;117:741–753

Owens JA. The practice of pediatric sleep medicine: results of a community survey. *Pediatrics.* 2001;108:e51

Owens JA. Dalzell V. Use of the 'BEARS' sleep screening tool in a pediatric residents' continuity clinic: a pilot study. *Sleep Med.* 2005;6:63–69

Picchietti DL, Underwood DJ, Farris WA, et al. Further studies on periodic limb movement disorder and restless legs syndrome in children with attention-deficit hyperactivity disorder. *Mov Disord.* 1999;14(6):1000–1007

Picchietti MA, Picchietti DL. Restless legs syndrome and periodic limb movement disorder in children and adolescents. *Semin Pediatr Neurol.* 2008;15:91–99

Redline S, Tishler PV, Schluchter M, Aylor J, Clark K, Graham G. Risk factors for sleep disordered breathing in children. Associations with obesity, race, and respiratory problems. *Am J Respir Crit Care Med.* 1999;159:1527–1532

Salzarulo P, Chevalier A. Sleep problems in children and their relationship with early disturbances of the waking-sleeping rhythms. *Sleep.* 1983;6:47–51

Sheldon SH, Kryger NH, Ferber R. *Principles and Practice of Pediatric Sleep Medicine.* WB Saunders and Co; 2005

Tishler PV, Redline S, Ferrette V, Hans MG, Altose MD. The association of sudden unexpected infant death with obstructive sleep apnea. *Am J Respir Crit Care Med.* 1996;153:1857–1863

Zaremba EK, Barkey ME, Mesa C, Sanniti K, Rosen CL. Making polysomnography more "child friendly": a family-centered care approach. *J Clin Sleep Med.* 2005;1:189–198

Chapter 15

Brain Tumors

Duncan Stearns, MD
Joseph H. Piatt Jr, MD

Introduction

Cancer remains the leading cause of non-traumatic mortality in children. Neoplasms of the central nervous system (CNS), while quite heterogeneous in biology and clinical presentation, represent the most common solid tumor of childhood and are a significant cause of death and disability. While the treatment of children with CNS tumors is best served at institutions with multidisciplinary neuro-oncology teams, the general pediatrician can play an important role in the diagnosis of patients, in counseling and supporting the family, and in the management of late treatment effects.

Brain tumors in children are different from tumors that arise in later years. Infratentorial tumors are much more common in the pediatric population, representing half of all brain tumors in children compared with 20% of tumors in adults. This distinction leads to differences in presenting symptomatology. Tumor types are also somewhat age specific. Medulloblastoma, for example, accounts for a large fraction of brain tumors among school-aged children but is a very uncommon diagnosis among adults, and CNS lymphoma is rarely seen in children. In addition to these inherent differences in tumor biology, the effects of treatment on the developing nervous system are unique to pediatrics. Children who are cured of their initial disease often experience late neurocognitive effects. For these and many other reasons, supervision of treatment and long-term follow-up by a pediatric neuro-oncologist are critical components of optimal care.

This chapter will outline the identification of patients, appropriate initial evaluations, and general principles of multimodality therapy. Tumor predisposition syndromes will be reviewed, along with guidelines for monitoring. Specific tumor types will be described briefly, along with current treatment approaches and expected outcomes. Interested readers will be directed to more complete references.

Epidemiology

In the United States, more than 3,000 patients younger than 20 years receive the diagnosis of primary brain tumor each year. This represents a wide variety of histopathological subtypes with differing age peaks and gender predilections. There is little evidence to support significant differences in tumor incidence between racial groups. Tumors can be low grade (benign) or malignant. The most common class of tumor is low-grade astrocytoma, followed by medulloblastoma, high-grade glioma, ependymoma, and a large group of relatively rare miscellaneous tumor types. There has been some concern that the incidence of childhood brain tumors is rising; however, many researchers feel that this has been due to increased use of magnetic resonance imaging (MRI) and improved detection.

Cancer is a genetic disease, but for most patients, the causes of their brain tumors are unknown. A very small subset of pediatric brain tumors is related to genetic tumor predisposition syndromes such as neurofibromatosis, Li-Fraumeni syndrome, Gorlin or basal cell nevus syndrome, and Turcot syndrome. With the exception of neurofibromatosis, these syndromes are very rare, but they have provided indispensable windows onto molecular mechanisms critical to the development of more common cancers. Environmental factors have been studied with interest; however, only exposure to ionizing radiation has been shown definitively to increase the risk of developing a CNS neoplasm. Diet, exposure to pesticides or electromagnetic fields, head trauma, viral infections, and medication use have been examined, but no consistent link to increased risk has been identified. It is likely that the somatic mutations or the epigenetic events that result in tumor formation in most patients are multistep, multifactorial processes, possibly involving host genetics, host immune response, and environmental factors. One implication of the negative epidemiological investigations and the rarity of pediatric cancer is that tumor prevention strategies are not likely to be of significant impact.

Presentations

The presenting symptoms of a child with a brain tumor vary with tumor location and are often nonspecific. Consequently, the initial evaluation of patients can be problematic because typical complaints of headache, vomiting, and dizziness are also typical of much more common childhood illnesses. Headache, specifically, can be a difficult symptom to address. In infants and young children unable to verbalize, headache can be expressed as a variety of behaviors including irritability, head holding, and head banging. Headaches that awaken a child from sleep deserve investigation, as do headaches of subacute onset and progressive frequency and intensity. Conversely, headaches of duration greater than 6 months are almost never symptoms of a brain tumor. Often there are other clues that can enhance the practitioner's suspicion and lead to appropriate diagnostic imaging. A complete and thorough neurologic examination is essential, including assessment of head growth and funduscopic examination, as is review of school performance, personality, and behavior in older children.

For posterior fossa tumors, that is, tumors located in the brain stem, fourth ventricle, or cerebellum, the presenting complaints are often related to cerebrospinal fluid (CSF) outflow obstruction leading to increased intracranial pressure and hydrocephalus. For infants, hydrocephalus can cause accelerated head growth, bulging fontanel, split calvarial sutures, and forced down-gaze, so-called sun setting. Papilledema is not always detected in infants due to the increased cranial capacity from unclosed sutures, but it is a sign that warrants immediate evaluation if found at any age. Cerebellar dysfunction can be determined by the presence of ataxia, more easily seen in children who are walking, but can be detected as truncal instability in infants. Nystagmus may also be found. Brain stem lesions often produce cranial nerve dysfunction, commonly resulting in complaints of diplopia and the finding of strabismus. Head tilt or torticollis may reflect an adaptive behavior to suppress diplopia, or it may reflect asymmetrical cerebellar herniation at the foramen magnum. Although there are other causes besides brain tumor, acquired torticollis lasting more than a few days requires investigation.

Supratentorial neoplasms can present with signs and symptoms of hydrocephalus related to obstruction of the aqueduct of Sylvius or the foramina of Monroe, but more often, they present with seizures or localizing neurologic findings such as weakness, speech disturbance, or visual field abnormalities (Figure 15-1). Optic pathway gliomas can cause decreased visual acuity and strabismus. Other suprasellar tumors, such as craniopharyngiomas, germ cell tumors, and chiasmatic/hypothalamic gliomas, typically cause some combination of symptoms of elevated intracranial pressure from hydrocephalus, visual impairment, and hypopituitarism. The presence of diabetes insipidus at the time of presentation is fairly specific for suprasellar germ cell tumors or for the hypothalamic involvement of Langerhans cell histiocytosis. Diffuse bilateral involvement of the thalamus and hypothalamus by infiltrative astrocytic tumors in early childhood causes a rare but distinctive clinical picture of failure to thrive with preserved development and social responsiveness, sometimes referred to as the *diencephalic syndrome of Russell.* Affected children seem happy and active, but they are virtually bereft of subcutaneous adipose tissue. Pineal region tumors commonly present with hydrocephalus due to obstruction of the nearby aqueduct,

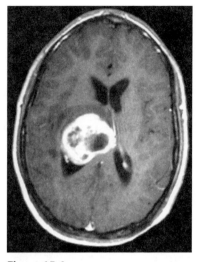

Figure 15-1.
An axial, T1-weighted magnetic resonance imaging of the brain with contrast enhancement shows a tumor arising in the right thalamus filling the trigone of the lateral ventricle. There is peripheral contrast enhancement with central areas of low signal intensity signifying necrosis. The patient came to attention with headaches from hydrocephalus and a mild left hemiparesis. The histopathological diagnosis was glioblastoma multiforme.

but they can cause a distinctive disturbance of ocular motility: the Parinaud syndrome. The most consistent feature of the Parinaud syndrome is paralysis of up-gaze, but the fully elaborated syndrome includes light-near dissociation and nystagmus retractorius. Light-near dissociation refers to suppression of pupillary reactivity to light with preservation of reactivity to accommodation. Nystagmus retractorius is an exaggerated form of gaze-paretic nystagmus. When the patient with paralysis of up-gaze attempts to look upward, all of the extraocular muscles begin firing synchronously causing the globes to retract into the orbits in a rhythmic fashion. Addition of the clinical feature of precocious puberty to a presentation with hydrocephalus and paralysis of up-gaze in a school-aged male is almost pathognomonic for a germ cell tumor of the pineal region.

Primary spinal cord tumors are rare in children, but metastatic disease spreading to the spinal cord or the spinal leptomeninges can cause back or radicular pain, bowel or bladder dysfunction, or long tract signs distinct from the primary tumor. Spinal cord involvement also becomes an issue in patients with refractory disease and a difficult challenge in palliative care.

Investigations

Neuroimaging is the primary means of initial evaluation for patients with suspected CNS tumors. Currently, computed tomography (CT) is usually the first test to consider because of its ready availability and its quickness, which obviates the need for sedation in young children. Computed tomography without contrast will provide information regarding ventricular size, will identify intracranial calcification, and may detect tumors from their mass effect or edema. The addition of contrast does improve detection in some cases, but for most patients, MRI of the brain with and without the administration of a gadolinium contrast agent is far superior. The sensitivity and improved anatomical detail of the MRI make it the modality of choice in most cases, even though the scanning time is longer and the need for immobility sometimes requires the use of anesthesia. Magnetic resonance imaging is also the modality of choice to evaluate the spinal cord. Newer imaging techniques such as MR spectroscopy, MR diffusion tensor imaging, MR perfusion imaging, and positron emission tomography are being examined for their ability to evaluate physiological aspects of a tumor as well as to improve the mapping of the tumor-normal tissue interface.

Tumor staging may require additional investigations for some patients. In recent years MRI of the spine with contrast has rendered lumbar puncture for CSF cytology unnecessary in many cases in the evaluation of tumors with a propensity for leptomeningeal dissemination, such as medulloblastoma, but CSF sampling is still critical for patients with CNS leukemia and the very rare child with CNS lymphoma. Key decisions in the management of children with germ cell tumors may turn on the presence or absence of tumor markers in blood and CSF: beta-human chorionic gonadotropin (βHCG) and alpha-fetoprotein (αFP).

Differential Diagnosis

Brain imaging is usually definitive in the diagnosis of a CNS tumor; however, there are infectious and inflammatory processes that can mimic both the presenting symptomatology and imaging characteristics of neoplasms. Brain abscesses can present as mass lesions with enhancement and surrounding vasogenic edema. Neurocystercercosis, formerly an affliction of developing nations but now encountered on a regular basis in this country, can present as a mass lesion with various degrees of calcification and may cause seizures. Likewise, vascular malformations sometimes exhibit mass effect, but they can usually be distinguished by the presence of vessel flow voids and hemosiderin in typical patterns. Metabolic and inflammatory conditions, such as acute necrotizing encephalopathy and tumefactive demyelinating disease, can masquerade as brain tumors. With few exceptions to be discussed below, treatment of childhood brain tumors is never undertaken without tissue diagnosis.

Treatment

Surgery

Treatment of childhood brain tumors begins with surgery. The tasks of the neurosurgeon are to relieve symptoms of elevated intracranial pressure due to mass effect or hydrocephalus, obtain tissue for diagnosis, and begin definitive therapy by partial or complete excision of the tumor. Children who come to attention with seizures due to small, benign-appearing lesions and the occasional patient with an incidentally discovered asymptomatic lesion can be managed electively, but symptoms attributable to mass effect or to elevated intracranial pressure are indications for urgent admission to a neurosurgical service. Such symptoms can often be ameliorated by dexamethasone while preoperative diagnostic investigations are conducted before surgery can be scheduled. Its usefulness has been recognized for decades, but only recently have MRI investigations shown that dexamethasone reduces peritumoral cerebral blood volume in addition to restoring the impermeability of the blood-brain barrier. For many cases, particularly for posterior fossa lesions, hydrocephalus can be eliminated by excision of the tumor, but if tumor surgery cannot be undertaken immediately, temporary external ventricular drainage may be necessary. Treatment of persisting hydrocephalus may be undertaken either by CSF shunt insertion or by endoscopic third ventriculostomy, as discussed elsewhere in this volume. Historically there has been concern about dissemination of malignant childhood brain tumors by drainage of CSF to the peritoneal cavity, but contemporary management of all such cases with adjuvant chemotherapy has suppressed this phenomenon.

Regions of the brain that are critical for basic neurologic functions, such as vision, voluntary movement, speech, and comprehension of language, are sometimes referred to as *eloquent*. That there are parts of the brain considered by neurosurgeons to be "non-eloquent" may be counter-intuitive but, in fact, surgical procedures in the prefrontal cortex, selected regions of the parietal lobes, and the cerebellum carry very low risk of lasting functional disability. The safety of surgery adjacent to or within regions of eloquent cerebral cortex has been greatly enhanced by recent refinements in clinical neurophysiology and advances in anatomical and functional imaging and related computer systems. Critical functions can be localized by recording of evoked potentials, by brain stimulation, and by functional MRI (fMRI). Among adults, recording and stimulation on the surface of the brain can often be performed intraoperatively in the awake patient under local anesthesia. The issue of cooperation by children can usually be finessed by a 2-stage process entailing craniotomy for implantation of subdural electrode grids under general anesthesia, stimulation and recording in the comfortable and awake patient in the electrophysiology laboratory, and a return to the operating room for the definitive surgical resection once again under general anesthesia. Safety is further enhanced by image-guided, computer-assisted surgical navigation systems, which permit precise correlation of imaging anatomy and patient anatomy in the operating room. Functional data from fMRI can be imported into such systems as well. Employment of these technologies has been motivated by accumulating clinical data suggesting that complete—or more nearly complete—removal of a variety of benign and malignant brain tumors improves prospects for survival, especially among children.

Surgical issues affecting prospects for cure and quality of survival will be addressed in the discussions of individual tumor types that follow.

Radiation Therapy

For most brain tumors, external beam radiation therapy is, next to surgery, the most effective therapeutic modality. The doses and target volumes depend on tumor type and location, but many children require radiation even after a complete surgical resection and often require treatment to areas quite distant from the original tumor. Due to the sensitivity of the child's developing nervous system, all efforts are made to use minimal doses and spare uninvolved tissue. Radiation is usually delivered in daily fractions of 1.8 Gy for 4 to 8 weeks to achieve total doses of 18 to 54 Gy. Immobilization is important, and many younger children require sedation. Preoperative scans are used for treatment planning and target dosimetry. Advances in computation and robotics have lead to vast improvements in treatment planning and have created a bewildering menu of technological options. Computed tomography– and MRI-based conformal therapy and intensity modulated radiation therapy techniques permit fractionated treatment of very complex tumor geometries while minimizing exposure of adjacent structures—a factor of crucial importance for the developing brain. High-dose, low-fraction, tightly collimated, stereotactically targeted radiation therapy, referred to as *radiosurgery,* has a limited track record in pediatric neuro-oncology, but it may be useful for selected small, recurrent tumors. The preceding techniques employ x-ray energy photons. The physics of proton beam radiotherapy create a potential for reduced dose to surrounding tissue compared with photon therapy, but this technology is available only at select centers. Its theoretical advantages have yet to be confirmed with properly controlled clinical evidence, but it has become a consideration in the management of certain rare lesions, such as clivus chordoma. Brachytherapy likewise has a limited role in pediatric neuro-oncology.

Acute effects of radiotherapy include skin breakdown; subacute effects include somnolence syndrome (4–8 weeks after therapy) and radionecrosis (6 months and beyond). Radionecrosis may be tumefactive and is often virtually impossible to distinguish by brain imaging from recurrent tumor. Surgery may be necessary for diagnosis and for management of mass effect. The definition of brain radiation tolerance limits the risk of this complication to less than 5%. Late effects are significant but variable. They can range from asymptomatic white matter changes to a progressive decline in general neurocognitive function. Central endocrine effects tend to be limited to growth hormone failure, but regular screening for all hormonal axes should be done for patients who have received cranial radiation. Patients are also at increased risk for secondary neoplasms and cerebrovascular disease.

Chemotherapy

Because of the propensity of many childhood brain tumors to disseminate in the CSF, radiation therapy often must include the entire cranium and the spine as far inferior as the termination of the thecal sack. Doses of craniospinal radiation that can be tolerated by older children and adults cause impaired axial growth and disabling encephalopathy in toddlers and infants. Such devastating side effects—to say nothing of the generally unacceptable cure rates from surgery and radiation alone—have motivated many groups to investigate chemotherapeutic approaches to the treatment of brain tumors. For some tumor types, chemotherapy has been successful in improving outcomes and reducing morbidity from radiation. In medulloblastoma, the use of chemotherapy allows for dose reduction in the craniospinal radiation without any trade-off in survival. The side effects of chemotherapy are usually acute and self-limiting, but chemotherapy is best undertaken at centers with experience in pediatric oncology ideally as part of a clinical trial. The agents used are commonly administered intravenously at regular intervals (vincristine, cisplatin, cyclophosphamide, etoposide), but some newer ones are oral (temozolomide). The limitations of chemotherapy are thought to be due to a combination of incomplete penetrance through the blood-brain barrier, resulting in reduced tissue penetration as well as intrinsic tumor resistance. Several approaches are under investigation to improve results. Chemotherapy is used for some diseases as a radiosensitizer. High-dose, bone marrow ablating chemotherapy with autologous stem cell rescue has been used successfully for both newly diagnosed and relapsed patients. Novel agents designed to target pathways important for tumor cell survival, migration, and blood vessel formation are also under active study.

Acute effects of chemotherapy include nausea and bone marrow and immune suppression, but these are usually not limiting. Late effects from chemotherapy include ototoxicity from cisplatin therapy, especially when combined with radiation to the posterior fossa. Exposure to etoposide or other epipodophyllotoxins can result in secondary leukemia. Fertility with standard dosing of agents is rarely an issue, but may be threatened by high-dose regimens.

Specific Tumor Types

Pediatric brain tumors can be classified by microscopic appearance or location, but the usefulness of classification is to predict ultimate tumor behavior and response to therapy. Histopathological criteria are constantly being updated and refined, so no classification scheme can be viewed as an eternal truth. Furthermore, explosive advances in molecular diagnostics and bioinformatics soon may displace histopathology as the primary guide to treatment and prognosis.

Gliomas

Tumors arising from glia, that is, from astrocytes, oligodendroglial cells, or ependymal cells, comprise more than 50% of all childhood brain tumors and are graded customarily from lower (grade I and II) to higher (grade III and IV). Low-grade astrocytomas are categorized either as pilocytic (grade I) or fibrillary (grade II). Pilocytic tumors have discrete borders and displace normal brain as they expand. Fibrillary tumors are infiltrative. Higher-grade tumors are likewise fibrillary and infiltrative but are distinguished successively by the presence of cytoplasmic and nuclear atypia (anaplastic astrocytoma, grade III) and by necrosis (glioblastoma multiforme, grade IV).

Pilocytic astrocytoma is predominantly a disease of childhood, although it can be seen in patients of all ages. Common locations include the cerebellum, the optic pathways and the adjacent hypothalamus, the white matter of the cerebrum, and the spinal cord. Pilocytic astrocytomas are often cystic, and the solid portions of the tumor enhance homogeneously on CT scanning or MRI (Figure 15-2). From anatomically favorable sites, particularly the cerebellum, non-eloquent sectors of the cerebrum, the spinal cord, and the optic nerve, pilocytic astrocytomas can often be resected for cure. Deep tumors involving the optic chiasm and hypothalamus require additional therapy after biopsy or subtotal resection. For older children, radiation is usually the therapy of choice. For younger patients, carboplatin-based chemotherapy has been associated with stable disease for prolonged periods. From a strategic standpoint, the management of the unresectable pilocytic astrocytoma is characterized by long periods of clinical and imaging stability punctuated by periods of generally slow disease progression that can often by arrested by careful selection among a variety of therapeutic options. If morbidity attributable to the treatment itself can be minimized, long-term survival with excellent quality of life is a realistic expectation in many cases. Malignant transformation of low-grade tumors has been reported, but it is exceptional, unlike the eventual degeneration of low-grade gliomas among adults into glioblastoma, which is the rule.

Because of its infiltrative biology, the prospects for surgical cure of the grade 2 fibrillary astrocytoma are not as good as for pilocytic astrocytoma, but in favorable anatomical locations such as non-eloquent regions of the cerebrum, total surgical extirpation may be a possibility nevertheless. In view of its expected indolent behavior, the overall approach to the management of the fibrillary astrocytoma follows the same principles as the management of unresectable pilocytic tumors, likewise for other low-grade neuroglial diagnoses, such as ganglioglioma, oligodendroglioma, and supratentorial ependymoma.

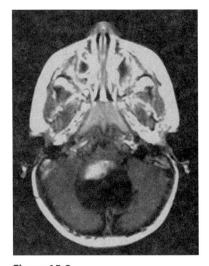

Figure 15-2.
A cystic tumor fills the fourth ventricle in this axial, T1-weighted magnetic resonance imaging of the brain with contrast enhancement. In the wall of the cyst is a solid nodule of enhancing tumor tissue. The tumor obstructed flow of cerebrospinal fluid through the fourth ventricle and caused hydrocephalus that led to headaches and gait instability in this preschool-aged child. The imaging appearance of this lesion is typical of juvenile pilocytic astrocytoma of the cerebellum.

With infrequent exceptions, high-grade gliomas are not curable, although affected children have much longer survivals than adults with the same histologic diagnoses. In a landmark multicenter trial conducted by the Children's Cancer Group, 5-year progression-free survivals ranged between 22% and 44% for anaplastic astrocytoma and between 4% and 26% for glioblastoma depending on extent of resection. Because of aggressive growth, they present more commonly with headache and subacute, progressive neurologic deficit rather than with seizures. Imaging characteristics are highly variable, but the lesions are often heterogeneous with significant peritumoral edema. Treatment is usually maximal surgical resection followed by radiotherapy in doses of 55 to 60 Gy to the tumor bed and a surrounding margin. Craniospinal radiation is not indicated. Evidence from studies of the Children's Cancer Group and its successor organization, the Children's Oncology Group, support the use of adjuvant chemotherapy, but there is an active search for more effective agents. High-dose bone marrow-ablative chemotherapy has not been shown to improve outcome, but it is still under investigation. Eventual macroscopic tumor recurrence in the bed of the original tumor is the norm, but autopsy invariably demonstrates widespread microscopic infiltration of surrounding and even remote regions of the brain.

Ependymal tumors are most commonly found in the posterior fossa arising in the fourth ventricle; however, they can occur in the cerebrum and the spinal cord. They are thought to arise from the ependymal lining of the ventricular system, although macroscopic continuity with the wall of a ventricular cavity may not be readily apparent. Signal intensities and enhancement characteristics may vary, but the growth pattern of the common fourth ventricle ependymoma is often distinctive. These lesions typically arise on the floor of the fourth ventricle and emerge out the foramina of Luschka and Magendie to coat the dorsal surface of the cervical spinal cord and to envelope the cranial nerves of the posterior fossa cisterns. Ependymomas are generally low-grade lesions, but anaplastic ependymomas do occur and may have poorer prognosis. There is a significant risk of CSF dissemination, so patients are generally staged with spinal MRI and CSF analysis. Gross total resection seems to be necessary, but not sufficient, to preserve a chance for cure. Unfortunately, these tumors are locally invasive and quite adherent to important neural and vascular structures, so a complete resection is not always possible, particularly for the more common posterior fossa lesions. Postsurgical focal radiation for patients with posterior fossa tumors has been shown to improve outcomes. Chemotherapy has not improved outcomes, but some degree of tumor response can be seen. Current clinical trials use chemotherapy prior to radiation for patients with initially unresectable tumors. Prognosis is variable, but rates of long-term disease-free survival range between 50% and 75% for patients who have undergone complete resections.

Two other glial tumor classes are defined by location and imaging characteristics and often are not biopsied. Optic pathway gliomas are tumors that can occur anywhere along the optic tract from the optic nerve to post-chiasmatic radiations. These tumors are strongly associated with neurofibromatosis type 1 (NF1) and are almost always pilocytic astrocytomas. Magnetic resonance imaging typically shows thickening of the optic nerves, chiasm, and tracts with preservation of recognizable anatomical structure; biopsy is seldom necessary. Approaches to therapy are aimed at preserving vision where possible, so frequent ophthalmologic evaluations are crucial along with regular imaging. The natural history of the optic pathway glioma is erratic, so treatment is usually indicated for symptomatic patients with clearly progressive disease. Surgery and radiation both have roles; however, carboplatin-based chemotherapy has been an effective approach at inducing tumor regression or stabilization. As would be expected given the unpredictable growth pattern, the study of clinical outcomes and responses to treatment is difficult. Long-term survival is expected for most patients; however, visual loss is common as are neuroendocrine sequelae from tumor involvement of the hypothalamus or as side effects of treatment.

Brain stem tumors are almost entirely glial, although primitive neuroectodermal tumors have been described. Magnetic resonance imaging has delineated a variety of different tumor patterns associated with vastly different patient outcomes. The tectal glioma is an infiltrative but extremely indolent glial tumor arising in the tectum of the midbrain and presenting invariably with hydrocephalus due to aqueductal obstruction. It is usually managed by endoscopic third ventriculostomy for diversion of CSF around the site of obstruction of ventricular drainage. Biopsy and treatment of the tumor itself is undertaken only in the event of progression. The dorsally exophytic pontine tumor arises on the floor of the fourth ventricle and fills it to cause hydrocephalus, but as a pilocytic astrocytoma, it characteristically refrains from invading the brain stem itself. It can be managed often by surgery alone. The classic diffuse intrinsic pontine glioma typically afflicts children in the early school years. They present with a combination of headache, cranial nerve signs such as abnormal ocular motility and facial palsy, and corticospinal signs such as asymmetrical reflexes or hemiparesis. Magnetic resonance imaging is characterized by diffuse expansion of the pons, hypointense on T1-weighted MR images with limited contrast enhancement and hyperintense on T2-weighted images (Figure 15-3). Sadly, the imaging diagnosis is sufficiently reliable that no tissue diagnosis is necessary

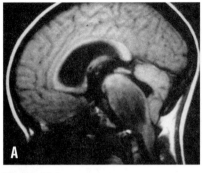

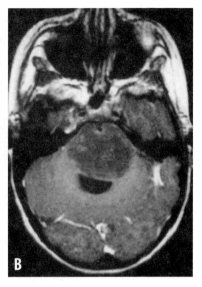

Figure 15-3.
Sagittal (Figure 3A) and axial (Figure 3B)
T1-weighted magnetic resonance imaging
shows diffuse expansion of the pons by a
mass with indistinct borders and low signal
intensity. The clinical diagnosis was diffuse
pontine glioma; no biopsy was performed.

for unequivocal counseling of parents about the dreadful prognosis of this
condition. Radiation therapy effects a transient improvement in symptoms
for most patients, but clinical and radiographic progression usually occurs
within 9 to 12 months following diagnosis. Chemotherapy has not been
helpful. Survival at 2 years is only 5% to 10%.

Medulloblastoma and the Primitive Neuroectodermal Tumors

Medulloblastoma is the most common malignant brain tumor of childhood. It is a high-grade tumor arising in the posterior fossa, most commonly
from the cerebellar vermis. It is believed to derive from an early neuroglial
precursor, and the range of its cytological phenotypes includes cells with
either neuronal or glial features in addition to completely undifferentiated
elements—hence the alternative term *cerebellar primitive neuroectodermal
tumor.* The peak age of incidence is 5 years, and there is a male predominance. Patients generally present with symptoms of increased intracranial
pressure due to hydrocephalus, cerebellar dysfunction, or symptoms of
metastatic disease. Imaging characteristics of the tumor itself are variable,
but some degree of enhancement on MRI is common. Up to one-third of all
patients will present with metastatic disease, so spine imaging and analysis

of CSF cytology are imperative. Medulloblastoma is the most likely of all CNS malignancies to exhibit extraneural spread, with metastasis to bone, bone marrow, lymph nodes, and liver described. Early diagnosis likely has resulted in the decrease in incidence of patients with extraneural disease at diagnosis; however, it is always a consideration in the relapse setting. Therapy for most patients begins with surgical attack on the fourth ventricle tumor to achieve tissue diagnosis, treat associated hydrocephalus, and maximize the likelihood of long-term survival, as long as the tumor can be reduced to a residual less than 1.5 mL in volume. Craniospinal radiation and adjuvant chemotherapy follow. For patients younger than 3 years, chemotherapy alone is commonly recommended, and radiation is withheld because of abhorrence of the catastrophic encephalopathy exhibited by survivors of whole-brain radiation therapy in infancy. Current treatment approaches have focused on efforts to reduce radiation exposure for patients without evidence of metastatic disease and on maximizing therapy for high-risk patients. Long-term disease-free survival rates approaching 80% to 90% for standard-risk patients have been reported. For patients with metastatic disease prognosis is not as good, but recent trials have shown short-term (3–5 year) survival rates approaching 60% to 70%.

The supratentorial primitive neuroectodermal tumor (sPNET) of childhood is a relatively rare high-grade tumor of the cerebrum occurring primarily in the first decade of life. There remains some controversy about a link between these tumors and medulloblastoma, but it is subsiding, and most neuropathologists consider them distinct diseases. (Additional nosological confusion can arise in relation to the *peripheral* primitive neuroectodermal tumor, which falls within the Ewing sarcoma family of tumors and possesses a chromosomal translocation, t(11;22)(q24;q12), that distinguishes it from its CNS namesake.) The sPNET is generally more radioresistant and chemoresistant than medulloblastoma, but it is often included in clinical trials for high-risk medulloblastoma. Local and distant recurrences are common, and survival rates of only 40% to 50% are seen. Pineoblastoma is also an sPNET, but it is more treatment responsive, so survival rates are higher. Pineoblastoma is also notable for a rare but curious association with retinoblastoma, so-called trilateral retinoblastoma.

Atypical Teratoid/Rhabdoid Tumor

This highly malignant tumor commonly presents in infancy. It has been encountered throughout the CNS, but it has a predilection for the posterior fossa, at which site historically it has been confused with medulloblastoma. The entity of atypical teratoid/rhabdoid tumor has been carved out of medulloblastoma only in recent years on the basis of the recognition of typical cytogenetic abnormalities: monosomy 22, 22q11 deletions, or mutation of the *INI1* tumor suppressor gene. It is a consistently and rapidly lethal tumor, and survival after aggressive therapy has been reported only infrequently.

Germ Cell Tumors

Germ cell tumors of the CNS are indistinguishable histologically from germ cell tumors arising in the gonads or other sites. The germ cell tumor family includes germinoma, choriocarcinoma, endodermal sinus tumor (or yolk sack tumor), embryonal carcinoma, and teratomas of the mature, immature, and malignant varieties. Mixed histologies are common. These tumors are found in the pineal region and the suprasellar region, occasionally appearing either synchronously or metachronously at both sites. Germinomas are extremely radiosensitive, and cure rates of 80% to 90% are reported. Non-germinomatous germ cell tumors (NGGCTs) are much more resistant to treatment and carry a guarded prognosis. They secrete one or both of the tumor markers βHCG and αFP, and under some circumstances, the detection of a marker in the blood or CSF can obviate the need for tissue diagnosis. These markers can be assayed to assess response to treatment as well. Mature teratoma is a surgical condition, but immature and malignant teratomas are managed like NGGCTs (Figure 15-4).

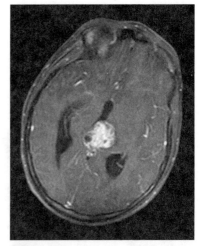

Figure 15-4.
An axial, T1-weighted magnetic resonance imaging of the brain with contrast enhancement shows a tumor of the pineal region invading the left thalamus, filling the posterior portion of the third ventricle, and causing obstructive hydrocephalus. Alpha fetoprotein was present in the cerebrospinal fluid. The histopathological diagnosis was malignant teratoma.

Despite their rarity, NGGCTs are the subject of several current multicenter research protocols featuring various combinations and sequences of radiation, carboplatin-based chemotherapy, and second-look surgery. Such aggressive treatment seems to have improved the outlook for long-term survival, which has risen from nil to 30% to 50% in contemporary reports.

Craniopharyngioma

Craniopharyngioma is a histologically benign tumor related developmentally to the epithelium of the pharyngeal pouch from which the anterior pituitary arises. It can be situated in the sella or in the suprasellar region in relation to the infundibulum, or more commonly it occupies both sites. Larger lesions can fill the third ventricle to cause hydrocephalus and expand laterally into a Sylvian fissure or posteriorly down the clivus. The tumor tends to be adherent to critical adjacent structures such as the hypothalamus, the optic chiasm, and the internal carotid arteries, so although in theory surgical extirpation is curative, in practice it can be very difficult and morbid. At a minimum, complete excision of craniopharyngiomas can be expected to cause panhypopituitarism in all but the most favorable cases. Surgical attack on lesions that are adherent to the walls of the third ventricle carries a risk of cognitive disabilities and behavioral disturbances, most notably a very difficult to manage syndrome of hyperphagia and morbid obesity. The alternative to surgical extirpation is radiotherapy, which historically has been associated in long-term follow-up with a similar pattern of morbidity from radiation injury to the same structures jeopardized by surgery. Recent technological developments have made possible the execution of very tightly focused radiation treatment plans that spare these structures, and the current trend in the management of craniopharyngiomas is toward more limited surgery combined with postoperative, conformal radiation therapy, although wide variation in tumor volume and anatomical relationships requires highly individualized therapy. Its cystic components can expand suddenly, but the tumor itself grows very slowly. The course of craniopharyngioma typically runs decades, and very delayed recurrences are not uncommon. Alternative treatment strategies are therefore very difficult to compare in a controlled fashion and, because long-term survival is expected in every case, there is a not yet resolved tension between the goals of cure and quality of life.

Choroid Plexus Tumors

Choroid plexus papillomas and carcinomas are tumors of the first 2 years of life. They arise in the bed of the choroid plexus of the lateral and third ventricles, and they come to attention because of hydrocephalus. Not only do these lesions obstruct the drainage of the ventricular system, but they also secrete excessive quantities of CSF. The imaging features are characteristic and vivid. The tumors possess a cauliflower- or frond-like morphology, they can be calcified to varying degrees, and they enhance brightly and homogeneously with intravenous contrast (Figure 15-5). Treatment is surgical, and the technical challenges are control of intraoperative hemorrhage from these highly vascular lesions and management of the postoperative disproportion between the volume of the brain and the volume of the cranial cavity, which is often grossly enlarged by long-standing, preoperative hydrocephalus. Choroid plexus carcinoma requires postoperative adjuvant chemotherapy, but if the tumor has not disseminated at the time of presentation, and if the surgical excision has been complete, the prospects for cure are good.

Hematologic Neoplasms of the Central Nervous System

The central nervous system is a common site of both presentation and relapse in children with acute lymphoblastic leukemia. Manifestations of CNS leukemia range from microscopic recognition of asymptomatic leukemic blasts in the CSF to headache to cranial neuropathy. Aggressive intrathecal chemotherapy has improved outcomes and reduced the need for prophylactic CNS irradiation. Radiation is very effective at treating patients with CNS leukemic relapse.

Langerhans cell histiocytosis is a non-neoplastic condition that commonly comes to attention because of symptoms and signs related to the head. The most common presentation is the subacute development of a painful skull mass. The radiographic appearance of a lytic lesion with eroded, indistinct margins is usually diagnostic (Figure 15-6). Central nervous system involvement is much less common. The favored site is the hypothalamus, infundibulum, and pituitary. Diabetes insipidus is a common complication, and from clinical, imaging, and even histologic perspectives, histiocytosis can be difficult to distinguish from germinoma. Even without treatment, oligoostotic disease in school-aged children usually follows a monophasic course with eventual disappearance of the granuloma and

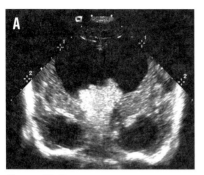
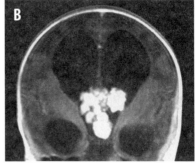

Figure 15-5.
An infant underwent transfontanel head ultrasound examination because of accelerated head growth. This coronal ultrasound image shows an echogenic, cauliflower-like tumor filling the third ventricle and erupting through the foramina of Monroe into the frontal horns of both lateral ventricles (Figure 5A). A coronal, T1-weighted magnetic resonance imaging in roughly the same plane demonstrates intense contrast enhancement. The histopathological diagnosis was choroid plexus papilloma.

healing of the bone. Curettage is sometimes performed for diagnosis or symptomatic relief. The prognosis of CNS involvement is less predictable, and the outlook for infants, who commonly present with systemic disease, is guarded. Treatment options include radiation therapy and chemotherapy with vinblastine and etoposide.

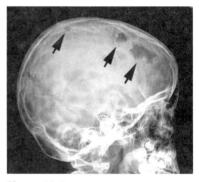

Figure 15-6.
A lateral radiograph of the skull of a school-aged child with a tender bump shows several lytic lesions with irregular, eroded borders (black arrowheads). The tender lesion was curetted for symptom relief, and the pathology was Langerhans cell histiocytosis. The remaining lesions healed without treatment over the following year.

Neurofibromatosis

While most tumor predisposition syndromes are rare, NF1 is not. Affecting 1 in 3,500, it is caused by an autosomal dominant mutation in the neurofibromin gene on the short arm of chromosome 17. It is heralded by the presence of café-au-lait spots; axillary or inguinal freckling; Lisch nodules, which are raised, pigmented, hamartomatous growths on the iris; and the predilection for peripheral and CNS tumor formation. While family history is significant in making the diagnosis, up to 50% of patients will not have any relatives with NF1, their disease presumably arising from a new mutation. Although patients with NF1 exhibit a predisposition for glial and meningeal tumors in general, the signature CNS tumor occurring in patients with NF1 is the optic pathway glioma, which is found in up to 20% of all patients. The biological behavior of optic pathway gliomas is a function of patient age. In infancy, optic gliomas often pursue an aggressive course, but among older children with NF1, they can be extremely indolent, remaining static from a clinical and imaging standpoint for years and decades. Because of the high prevalence of these lesions, all patients with NF1 should undergo regular ophthalmologic evaluation. The role of screening neuroimaging is controversial; however, regular MRI surveillance for patients with recognized optic pathway lesions is customary.

Neurofibromatosis type 1 is by far the most common of the neurocutaneous syndromes, so called because of the association of distinctive congenital or developmental skin lesions with brain tumors. The other most frequently encountered neurocutaneous syndromes are tuberous sclerosis, von Hippel-Lindau disease, and neurofibromatosis type 2. These conditions are discussed in more detail elsewhere in this volume.

Additional Considerations

Late Effects

Survivors often experience significant neurologic, cognitive, and neuroendocrine sequelae from their therapy. Multidisciplinary approaches should include physical, occupational, and speech therapy; audiology; neuropsychiatry; neurology; endocrinology; and social work involvement. Many patients will need the services of specialized occupational placement or training groups to achieve post-educational goals. Some patients will not be able to live independently. The primary care provider must be prepared to coordinate the input from multiple services in support of the patient and his or her family.

Relapse

For children with recurrence or progression of low-grade tumors, there often remain reasonable options with regard to subsequent therapy, whether it is additional surgical intervention, radiation, or chemotherapy. For patients with recurrent high-grade tumors, these options are less likely to result in meaningful survival. Patients and families have to be guided through a very difficult decision-making process. For some, palliative or supportive care alone is sufficient. For others, additional tumor-directed therapy is sought. Regardless, families often seek out multiple providers to discuss options.

Palliative Care

Many children diagnosed with a brain tumor will die from their disease. In some cases, the prospect of death from cancer is a sorrowful certainty from the time of diagnosis. For other patients, it becomes clear only after multiple failed attempts at therapy. The supportive care of a patient with a brain tumor patient does differ from care for children dying from other diseases. Maintenance of comfort, pain control, hydration, and nutrition are common issues, but seizure control, neurologic disabilities, and alterations in consciousness present distinct challenges to caregivers and the health care team. Ultimately, the continuing, compassionate involvement of the treating team together with the skills of trained pediatric hospice staff can ameliorate the suffering of the patient and prepare the grieving family for life without their loved one.

Summary

Tumors of the CNS in childhood comprise a wide variety of neoplasms with different presentations and outcomes. Early recognition is not always possible, but prompt referral to a pediatric center with appropriate neuro-oncology expertise is critical. Access to clinical trials is an important consideration in referral not only from the standpoint of the advancement of knowledge but also from the standpoint of patient care, routine aspects of which may be enhanced indirectly by the rigor required for its investigational aspects. Effective communication between the primary physician and the neuro-oncologist allow some elements of follow-up, surveillance for late effects, and palliative care to revert to the less threatening environment of the medical home.

Web Sites

Clinical Trials

NIH Clinical Trials: www.clinicaltrials.gov

Children's Oncology Group: www.curesearch.org

Pediatric Brain Tumor Consortium: www.pbtc.org

Brain Tumor Associations

American Brain Tumor Association: www.abta.org

Children's Brian Tumor Foundation: www.cbtf.org

The Brain Tumor Society: www.tbts.org

Childhood Brain Tumor Foundation: www.childhoodbraintumor.org

Pediatric Brain Tumor Foundation: www.pbtf.org

Brain Tumor Foundation of Canada: www.braintumour.ca

Information for Families

American Cancer Society: www.cancer.org

Candlelighters Childhood Cancer Foundation: www.candlelighters.org

Bibliography

General Considerations

Carpentieri SC, Waber DP, Pomeroy SL, et al. Neuropsychological functioning after surgery in children treated for brain tumor. *Neurosurgery.* 2003;52:1348–1356

The Childhood Brain Tumor Consortium. The epidemiology of headache among children with brain tumor. Headache in children with brain tumors. *J Neurooncol.* 1991;10:31–46

Cochrane DD, Gustavsson B, Poskitt KP, Steinbok P, Kestle JR. The surgical and natural morbidity of aggressive resection for posterior fossa tumors in childhood. *Pediatr Neurosurg.* 1994;20:19–29

Lew SM, Morgan JN, Psaty E, Lefton DR, Allen JC, Abbott R. Cumulative incidence of radiation-induced cavernomas in long-term survivors of medulloblastoma. *J Neurosurg.* 2006;104:103–107

Mehta V, Chapman A, McNeely PD, Walling S, Howes WJ. Latency between symptom onset and diagnosis of pediatric brain tumors: an Eastern Canadian geographic study. *Neurosurgery.* 2002;51:365–372

Ostergaard L, Hochberg FH, Rabinov JD, et al. Early changes measured by magnetic resonance imaging in cerebral blood flow, blood volume, and blood-brain barrier permeability following dexamethasone treatment in patients with brain tumors. *J Neurosurg.* 1999;90:300–305

Poussaint TY, Rodriguez D. Advanced neuro-imaging of pediatric brain tumors: MR diffusion, MR perfusion, and MR spectroscopy. *Neuroimaging Clin N Am.* 2006;16:169–192, ix

Gliomas

Bucci MK, Maity A, Janss AJ, et al. Near complete surgical resection predicts a favorable outcome in pediatric patients with nonbrainstem, malignant gliomas: results from a single center in the magnetic resonance imaging era. *Cancer.* 2004;101:817–824

Donaldson SS, Laningham F, Fisher PG. Advances towards and understanding of brainstem gliomas. *J Clin Oncol.* 2006;24:1266–1272

Goumnerova L, Drzymalski D, Kieran M, Pomeroy S, Scott RM, Tarbell N. Long-term neurological and neurosurgical outcomes after surgery only in children with low-grade brain tumors. *J Neurosurg Pediatrics.* 2008;1:A354–A355

Gropman AL, Packer RJ, Nicholson HS, et al. Treatment of diencephalic syndrome with chemotherapy: growth, tumor response, and long term control. *Cancer.* 1998;83:166–172

Healey EA, Barnes PD, Kupsky WJ, et al. The prognostic significance of postoperative residual tumor in ependymoma. *Neurosurgery.* 1991;28:666–671

Marcus KJ, Goumnerova L, Billett AL, et al. Stereotactic radiotherapy for localized low-grade gliomas in children: final results of a prospective trial. *Int J Radiat Oncol Biol Phys.* 2005;61: 374–379

Pollack IF, Pang D, Albright AL. The long-term outcome in children with late-onset aqueductal stenosis resulting from benign intrinsic tectal tumors. *J Neurosurg.* 1994;80:681–688

Poussaint TY, Barnes PD, Nichols K, et al. Diencephalic syndrome: clinical features and imaging findings. *AJNR Am J Neuroradiol.* 1997;18:1499–1505

Poussaint TY, Kowal JR, Barnes PD, et al. Tectal tumors of childhood: clinical and imaging follow-up. *AJNR Am J Neuroradiol.* 1998;19:977–983

Raffel C, Hudgins R, Edwards MS. Symptomatic hydrocephalus: initial findings in brainstem gliomas not detected on computed tomographic scans. *Pediatrics.* 1988;82:733–737

Robertson PL, Zeltzer PM, Boyett JM, et al. Survival and prognostic factors following radiation therapy and chemotherapy for ependymomas in children: a report of the Children's Cancer Group. *J Neurosurg.* 1998;88:695–703

Smoots DW, Geyer JR, Lieberman DM, Berger MS. Predicting disease progression in childhood cerebellar astrocytoma. *Childs Nerv Syst.* 1998;14:636–648

Sposto R, Ertel IJ, Jenkin RD, et al. The effectiveness of chemotherapy for treatment of high grade astrocytoma in children: results of a randomized trial. A report from the Children's Cancer Study Group. *J Neurooncol.* 1989;7:165–177

Wisoff JH, Boyett JM, Berger MS, et al. Current neurosurgical management and the impact of the extent of resection in the treatment of malignant gliomas of childhood: a report of the children's cancer group trial no. CCG-945. *J Neurosurg.* 1998;89:52–59

Medulloblastoma and Primitive Neuroectodermal Tumors

Albright AL, Wisoff JH, Zeltzer PM, Deutsch M, Finlay J, Hammond D. Current neurosurgical treatment of medulloblastomas in children. A report from the Children's Cancer Study Group. *Pediatr Neurosci.* 1989;15:276–282

Evans AE, Jenkin RD, Sposto R, et al. The treatment of medulloblastoma. Results of a prospective randomized trial of radiation therapy with and without CCNU, vincristine, and prednisone. *J Neurosurg.* 1990;72:572–582

Gajjar A, Chintagumpala M, Ashley D, et al. Risk-adapted craniospinal radiotherapy followed by high-dose chemotherapy and stem-cell rescue in children with newly diagnosed medulloblastoma (St Jude Medulloblastoma-96): long-term results from a prospective, multicentre trial. *Lancet Oncol.* 2006;7:813–820

Krischer JP, Ragab AH, Kun L, et al. Nitrogen mustard, vincristine, procarbazine, and prednisone as adjuvant chemotherapy in the treatment of medulloblastoma. A Pediatric Oncology Group study. *J Neurosurg.* 1991;74:905–909

Ladanyi M, Heinemann FS, Huvos AG, Rao PH, Chen QG, Jhanwar SC. Neural differentiation in small round cell tumors of bone and soft tissue with the translocation t(11;22)(q24;q12): an immunohistochemical study of 11 cases. *Hum Pathol.* 1990;21:1245–1251

Packer RJ, Gajjar A, Vezina G, et al. Phase III study of craniospinal radiation therapy followed by adjuvant chemotherapy for newly diagnosed average-risk medulloblastoma. *J Clin Oncol.* 2006;24:4202–4208

Tait DM, Thornton-Jones H, Bloom HJ, Lemerle J, Morris-Jones P. Adjuvant chemotherapy for medulloblastoma: the first multi-centre control trial of the International Society of Paediatric Oncology (SIOP I). *Eur J Cancer.* 1990;26:464–469

Zeltzer PM, Boyett JM, Finlay JL, et al. Metastasis stage, adjuvant treatment, and residual tumor are prognostic factors for medulloblastoma in children: conclusions from the Children's Cancer Group 921 randomized phase III study. *J Clin Oncol.* 1999;17:832–845

Atypical Teratoid/Rhabdoid Tumor

Packer RJ, Biegel JA, Blaney S, et al. Atypical teratoid/rhabdoid tumor of the central nervous system: report on workshop. *J Pediatr Hematol Oncol.* 2002;24:337–342

Germ Cell Tumor

Calaminus G, Bamberg M, Jürgens H, et al. Impact of surgery, chemotherapy and irradiation on long term outcome of intracranial malignant non-germinomatous germ cell tumors: results of the German Cooperative Trial MAKEI 89. *Klin Padiatr.* 2004;216:141–149

Diez B, Balmaceda C, Matsutani M, Weiner HL. Germ cell tumors of the CNS in children: recent advances in therapy. *Childs Nerv Syst.* 1999;15:578–585

Hardenbergh PH, Golden J, Billet A, et al. Intracranial germinoma: the case for lower dose radiation therapy. *Int J Radiat Oncol Biol Phys.* 1997;39:419–426

Hoffman HJ, Otsubo H, Hendrick EB, et al. Intracranial germ-cell tumors in children. *J Neurosurg.* 1991;74:545–551

Kellie SJ, Boyce H, Dunkel IJ, et al. Primary chemotherapy for intracranial nongerminomatous germ cell tumors: results of the second international CNS Germ Cell Study Group protocol. *J Clin Oncol.* 2004;22:846–853

Kochi M, Itoyama Y, Shiraishi S, Kitamura I, Marubayashi T, Ushio Y. Successful treatment of intracranial nongerminomatous malignant germ cell tumors by administering neoadjuvant chemotherapy and radiotherapy before excision of residual tumors. *J Neurosurg.* 2003;99:106–114

Kretschmar C, Kleinberg L, Greenberg M, Burger P, Holmes E, Wharam M. Pre-radiation chemotherapy with response-based radiation therapy in children with central nervous system germ cell tumors: a report from the Children's Oncology Group. *Pediatr Blood Cancer.* 2007;48:285–291

Choroid Plexus Papilloma and Carcinoma

Ellenbogen RG, Winston KR, Kupsky WJ. Tumors of the choroid plexus in children. *Neurosurgery.* 1989;25:327–335

Craniopharyngioma

Albright AL, Hadjipanayis CG, Lunsford LD, Kondziolka D, Pollack IF, Adelson PD. Individualized treatment of pediatric craniopharyngiomas. *Childs Nerv Syst.* 2005;21:649–654

Carpentieri SC, Waber DP, Scott RM, et al. Memory deficits among children with craniopharyngiomas. *Neurosurgery.* 2001;49:1053–1057

Cavazzuti V, Fischer EG, Welch K, Belli JA, Winston KR. Neurological and psychophysiological sequelae following different treatments of craniopharyngioma in children. *J Neurosurg.* 1983;59:409–417

Fischer EG, Welch K, Shillito J, Jr., Winston KR, Tarbell NJ. Late effects associated with treatment of craniopharyngiomas in childhood. *J Neurosurg.* 1990;73:534-540

Kalapurakal JA, Goldman S, Hsieh YC, Tomita T, Marymont MH, Lustig RH. Clinical outcome in children with craniopharyngioma treated with primary surgery and radiotherapy deferred until relapse: risk factors for the development of obesity in children surviving brain tumors. *Med Pediatr Oncol.* 2003;40:214–218

Merchant TE, Kiehna EN, Kun LE, et al. Phase II trial of conformal radiation therapy for pediatric patients with craniopharyngioma and correlation of surgical factors and radiation dosimetry with change in cognitive function. *J Neurosurg.* 2006;104:94–102

Merchant TE, Kiehna EN, Sanford RA, et al. Craniopharyngioma: the St. Jude Children's Research Hospital experience 1984–2001. *Int J Radiat Oncol Biol Phys.* 2002;53:533–542

Sanford RA. Craniopharyngioma: results of survey of the American Society of Pediatric Neurosurgery. *Pediatr Neurosurg.* 1994;21:39–43

Weiss M, Sutton L, Marcial V, et al. The role of radiation therapy in the management of childhood craniopharyngioma. *Int J Radiat Oncol Biol Phys.* 1989;17:1313–1321

Yasargil MG, Curcic M, Kis M, Siegenthaler G, Teddy PJ, Roth P. Total removal of craniopharyngiomas. Approaches and long-term results in 144 patients. *J Neurosurg.* 1990;73:3–11

Hematologic Neoplasia

Grois N, Flucher-Wolfram B, Heitger A, Mostbeck GH, Hofmann J, Gadner H. Diabetes insipidus in Langerhans cell histiocytosis: results from the DAL-HX 83 study. *Med Pediatr Oncol.* 1995;24:248–256

Hund E, Steiner H, Jansen O, Sieverts H, Sohl G, Essig M. Treatment of cerebral Langerhans cell histiocytosis. *J Neurol Sci.* 1999;171:145–152

Minkov M, Grois N, Heitger A, Pötschger U, Westermeier T, Gadner H. Treatment of multisystem Langerhans cell histiocytosis. Results of the DAL-HX 83 and DAL-HX 90 studies. DAL-HX study group. *Klin Padiatr.* 2000;212:139–144

Titgemeyer C, Grois N, Minkov M, Flucher-Wolfram B, Gatterer-Menz I, Gadner H. Pattern and course of single-system disease in Langerhans cell histiocytosis data from the DAL-HX 83- and 90-study. *Med Pediatr Oncol.* 2001;37:108–114

Womer RB, Raney RB Jr, D'Angio GJ. Healing rates of treated and untreated bone lesions in histiocytosis X. *Pediatrics.* 1985;76:286–288

Neurofibromatosis

Es VS, North KN, McHugh K, De Silva M. MRI findings in children with neurofibromatosis type 1: a prospective study. *Pediatr Radiol.* 1996;26:478–487

Farmer JP, Khan S, Khan A, et al. Neurofibromatosis type 1 and the pediatric neurosurgeon: a 20-year institutional review. *Pediatr Neurosurg.* 2002;37:122–136

Hersh JH, American Academy of Pediatrics Committee on Genetics. Health supervision for children with neurofibromatosis. *Pediatrics.* 2008;121:633–642

Listernick R, Charrow J, Greenwald M, Mets M. Natural history of optic pathway tumors in children with neurofibromatosis type 1: a longitudinal study. *J Pediatr.* 1994;125:63–66

Listernick R, Charrow J, Tomita T, Goldman S. Carboplatin therapy for optic pathway tumors in children with neurofibromatosis type-1. *J Neurooncol.* 1999;45:185–190

Listernick R, Ferner RE, Liu GT, Gutmann DH. Optic pathway gliomas in neurofibromatosis-1: controversies and recommendations. *Ann Neurol.* 2007;61:189–198

Listernick R, Louis DN, Packer RJ, Gutmann DH. Optic pathway gliomas in children with neurofibromatosis 1: consensus statement from the NF1 optic pathway glioma task force. *Ann Neurol.* 1997;41:143–149

Molloy PT, Bilaniuk LT, Vaughan SN, et al. Brainstem tumors in patients with neurofibromatosis type 1: a distinct clinical entity. *Neurology.* 1995;45:1897–1902

Pollack IF, Shultz B, Mulvihill JJ. The management of brainstem gliomas in patients with neurofibromatosis 1. *Neurology.* 1996;46:1652–1660

Chapter 16

Hydrocephalus

Andrew Jea, MD
Abhaya V. Kulkarni, MD, PhD

Introduction

Hydrocephalus is the excess accumulation of cerebrospinal fluid (CSF), usually as the result of obstruction in CSF absorption, resulting in raised intracranial pressure (ICP). In children, hydrocephalus can result from many different underlying conditions, with a spectrum that is very different from adult hydrocephalus. Most children with hydrocephalus need surgical treatment and face the possibility of need for repeat surgical interventions throughout their lives.

Cerebrospinal fluid is produced by the choroid plexus, which is located within all 4 ventricles in the brain. Under normal conditions, the CSF flows from the lateral ventricles to the third ventricle, through the foramen of Monro, and from the third ventricle to the fourth ventricle, through the aqueduct of Sylvius. Then it exits the fourth ventricle to circulate in the subarachnoid space. Cerebrospinal fluid is generally thought to be absorbed back into the venous system largely through arachnoid villi, which are protrusions of the subarachnoid space into the superior sagittal sinus and the other dural venous sinuses, although there is mounting laboratory animal evidence that a good deal of CSF absorption occurs through the nasal lymphatics, especially in infants in whom there appear to be very few arachnoid villi. Hydrocephalus has traditionally been categorized as *obstructive,* meaning that mechanical obstruction of bulk flow does not allow the CSF to leave the ventricular system, and *non-obstructive* or *communicating,* meaning that the obstruction to CSF absorption occurs outside the ventricular system in the subarachnoid space or at the arachnoid villi.

Common causes of obstructive hydrocephalus include stenosis of the aqueduct by congenital malformations, midbrain tumors, posterior fossa tumors, hemorrhage, or infection. Common causes of communicating hydrocephalus include fibrosis of the subarachnoid space and arachnoid villi following intraventricular hemorrhage (IVH) in premature infants or meningitis. In congenital conditions such myelomeningocele, the cause of hydrocephalus is likely multifactorial and may involve both communicating and obstructive elements.

Epidemiology

True congenital hydrocephalus has an estimated incidence of 0.2 to 0.8 per 1,000 live births in the United States; however, most cases of pediatric hydrocephalus, even cases of congenital origin, are not diagnosed until later in infancy rather than right at birth. There is evidence to suggest that the incidence of pediatric hydrocephalus may be decreasing, based on a trend of reduced CSF shunt surgery across Canada. The reasons for this decline are not clear, but it may reflect changes in practice patterns, such as rising clinical thresholds for treatment, or it may be the consequence of the falling incidence of myelomeningocele. This decreasing incidence, therefore, may be only a regional phenomenon not reflective of other areas of North America.

Infections are a common cause of hydrocephalus in infants and children. In a minority of cases, meningitis may lead to permanent obliteration of the CSF absorptive surfaces and pathways. An estimated 1% of pediatric patients who survive bacterial meningitis develop progressive hydrocephalus. Other less common infectious causes of hydrocephalus in children include tuberculosis meningitis, whose worldwide prevalence is rising; toxoplasmosis or other members of the TORCH (toxoplasmosis, other agents, rubella, cytomegalovirus, herpes simplex) group; and viral meningitis and encephalitis.

Head trauma has been recognized as a common cause of hydrocephalus. As management schemes for traumatic brain injury have improved over recent years, more patients are surviving to develop hydrocephalus as a delayed complication. About 4% of patients develop posttraumatic hydrocephalus requiring surgical CSF diversion.

Tumors related to the ventricular system can cause hydrocephalus by obstruction of the CSF pathways, most often in the vicinity of the fourth ventricle. Tumors may also cause hydrocephalus by spilling blood or protein into the CSF, making the CSF more viscous, overloading the absorptive capacity of the arachnoid villi, and resulting in a communicating hydrocephalus.

Some of the common underlying causes of pediatric hydrocephalus are summarized in Table 16-1.

Table 16-1. Some Common Causes of Pediatric Hydrocephalus	
Etiology (Relative Frequency)	**Examples**
Myelomeningocele (20%)	
Intraventricular hemorrhage of prematurity (15%)	
Congenital aqueductal stenosis (12%)	
Communicating hydrocephalus of unknown origin (10%)	
Neoplasm (8%)	• Posterior fossa tumor • Third ventricular tumor • Pineal region tumor • Choroid plexus papilloma
Postinfectious (7%)	• Bacterial, viral, fungal, or tuberculous meningitis • TORCH encephalitis
Posttraumatic (3%)	
Arachnoid cyst (5%)	• Suprasellar arachnoid cyst
Syndrome-related	• Dandy-Walker malformation • X-linked recessive hydrocephalus • Achondroplasia • Mucopolysaccharidosis, type VI • Neurofibromatosis, type I • Pfeiffer syndrome • Apert syndrome • Crouzon syndrome

Abbreviation: TORCH, toxoplasmosis, other agents, rubella, cytomegalovirus, herpes simplex.

Other than cases of congenital X-linked hydrocephalus, which constitutes less than 4% of all cases of hydrocephalus, there is no gender predilection for hydrocephalus. X-linked hydrocephalus accounts for about 8% to 15% of primary idiopathic hydrocephalus in boys. The abnormal gene is located on Xq28. This congenital abnormality occurs with a deficiency of the L1 cell adhesion molecule and is associated with partial or complete agenesis of the corpus callosum, a peculiar block deformity of the midbrain tectum, and hypoplasia of the anterior cerebellum. The clinical picture features mental retardation, adducted thumbs, and lower limb spasticity. Aside from this distinctive and rare syndrome, genetic factors contributing to hydrocephalus remain obscure.

Symptoms

Pediatric hydrocephalus most commonly presents in infancy. The presenting symptoms usually relate to raised ICP and include excessive irritability, lethargy, or vomiting.

In older children, the more common presenting symptoms include headache, nausea, or vomiting. These symptoms tend to be more common in the mornings, when ICP is higher after hours of nighttime recumbency. Rarely, older children may present with visual deficits, which may be either the result of severe papilledema or a consequence of the underlying cause of hydrocephalus (eg, a large suprasellar tumor causing obstructive hydrocephalus and compression of the optic chiasm). Diplopia may be described as well, usually from unilateral or bilateral abducens nerve palsy—a classic, nonspecific, false-localizing sign of raised ICP. Some of the common signs and symptoms of hydrocephalus are presented in Box 16-1.

Signs

Macrocephaly, bulging of the anterior fontanel, and separation of the calvarial sutures are common signs of active hydrocephalus in infancy. The fontanel should be assessed with the baby calm and in an upright position. Scalp veins may appear dilated. Among eye findings, forced downgaze (so-called sun-setting) is a well-described sign. It usually occurs later in the clinical course and may be associated with other components of Parinaud syndrome, including downward eye deviation, lid retraction, and convergence-retraction nystagmus. As ICP rises acutely, infants may develop bradycardia and apneic episodes. In severe and chronic cases, the skull may be so grossly enlarged with CSF that it can be transilluminated. In older children, papilledema or abducens palsy may be present. Focal neurologic deficits attributable to the underlying cause of the hydrocephalus, such as ataxia from a posterior fossa tumor or bitemporal hemianopsia from a suprasellar tumor, may be present as well.

> ## Box 16-1. Some Common Signs and Symptoms of Pediatric Hydrocephalus
>
> **Symptoms**
> - Headache
> - Nausea/vomiting
> - Lethargy
> - Developmental delay or regression
> - Cognitive decline
> - Increased seizure frequency
>
> **Signs**
> - Accelerated head growth
> - Bulging fontanel, separated sutures
> - Forced downgaze (sun-setting) or paresis of upgaze
> - Papilledema
> - Abducens nerve palsy

Differential Diagnosis

In an infant presenting with macrocephaly, the most common differential diagnosis—and one that is much more common than true hydrocephalus—is simple benign macrocephaly. The typical infant, more commonly male, has a head circumference at or above the 98th percentile but without a bulging fontanel and with no clinical signs or symptoms of truly raised ICP. Frequently parental head circumference will also be large. Brain imaging shows deep subarachnoid spaces over the convexities of the cerebral hemispheres, in the interhemispheric fissure, and sometimes in the cisterns at the base (Figure 16-1). There may be mild dilation of the ventricular system, but not in proportion to the prominence of the subarachnoid spaces. This condition has sometimes been misunderstood as *extraventricular obstructive hydrocephalus*,

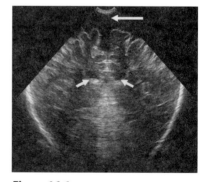

Figure 16-1.

Coronal transfontanel ultrasound showing typical findings of benign macrocephaly, or so-called external hydrocephalus. There is prominence of the subarachnoid spaces (long arrow) and normal-size ventricles (short arrows).

although there is no evidence for obstruction of CSF flow. It has sometimes been mislabeled *subdural effusions of infancy,* even though the excess fluid is not in the subdural space. Another widely used term is *external hydrocephalus,* which carries the incorrect connotation of a progressive course. The accelerated head growth invariably stabilizes without treatment, and brain imaging generally normalizes in early childhood. The etiology of this common condition is not clear, but the benign clinical course suggests an exaggerated responsiveness of the developing membranous bones of the calvarium to the push of the growing brain. Chronic subdural hematoma may also present with macrocephaly (Figure 16-2). In such cases, the possibility of abusive injury must be considered. Chronic subdural hematoma of infancy can generally be distinguished from benign macrocephaly on clinical grounds because affected infants are ill. Typical presentations include developmental delay, failure to thrive, irritability, bulging fontanel, and seizures. Other intracranial space-occupying lesions in infants can also present with macrocephaly even in the absence of hydrocephalus, including brain tumors and large arachnoid cysts. Differential diagnoses for macrocephaly and ventriculomegaly are presented in Box 16-2.

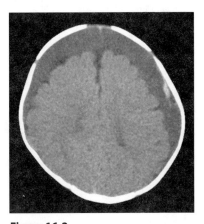

Figure 16-2.
An axial computed tomography scan showing acute-on-chronic subdural hematoma in an infant with progressive macrocephaly. The imaging density of the extensive subdural fluid is slightly higher than that of cerebrospinal fluid.

Diagnostic Imaging

The diagnosis of hydrocephalus is confirmed by brain imaging. Computed tomographic (CT) scanning provides sufficient detail to make the diagnosis, it is readily available, and it can be performed very quickly. It does, however, expose the child to some radiation. Axial CT scanning shows enlarged ventricles. Acute, severe hydrocephalus usually demonstrates periventricular, interstitial edema manifest as low-density in the white matter surrounding the ventricles (Figure 16-3). The cause for the hydrocephalus must always be sought. Magnetic resonance imaging (MRI) provides greater anatomical

---

Box 16-2. Differential Diagnoses for Macrocephaly

- Benign familial macrocephaly
- Chronic subdural hematoma (abusive traumatic brain injury)
- Megalencephaly
- Tumor
- Arachnoid cyst
- Metabolic diseases (leukodystrophies, lipidoses, mucopolysaccharidoses)
- Primary diseases of bone (achondroplasia, osteogenesis imperfecta, osteopetrosis, rickets)

---

detail of the brain and ventricles. It can provide vital information about congenital anomalies affecting the CSF pathways, such as aqueductal stenosis, and it can demonstrate tumors, such as gliomas of the tectum, that are undetectable by CT scan. Its various sequences and its multiplanar imaging capacities are indispensable for preoperative planning for patients who might be candidates for endoscopic third ventriculostomy. The FLAIR (fluid-attenuated inversion recovery) sequence shows ventriculomegaly and the periventricular edema to best advantage (Figure 16-4).

For the infant who presents with

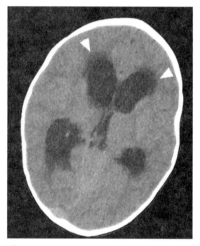

Figure 16-3.
An axial computed tomography scan in the setting of acute hydrocephalus, showing evidence of periventricular edema, represented by the hypodensities in the region of the frontal horns (white arrowheads).

only gradual macrocephaly and who fits the clinical picture of a benign, familial macrocephaly, brain imaging can be done electively with ultrasound. Computed tomography is the modality of choice for urgent assessment of the acutely ill patient. Magnetic resonance imaging, which necessitates sedation or even general anesthesia to yield technically adequate images in infants and young children, may be obtained at the discretion of the treating neurosurgeon.

Although the term *brain atrophy* sometimes appears in radiologic interpretations of childhood imaging studies, in the pediatric setting atrophy cannot be assessed on an imaging basis alone without reference to clinical context. Infants with benign macrocephaly who have deep subarachnoid spaces, wide sulci, and mild ventriculomegaly are often mistakenly said to exhibit atrophy when in fact they simply have cranial cavities that are too big for their normal-sized brains, a state sometimes called *craniocerebral disproportion*. Children with microcephaly children who have suffered some early, catastrophic brain insult often show sulcal prominence and ventricular dilation on brain imaging, but even in this context, the term *atrophy* is not necessarily appropriate, because such brains often have suffered developmental arrest rather than true tissue loss. True diffuse brain atrophy can be seen among children, as among adults, in the setting of hypoxic-ischemic injury, infection, and metabolic or degenerative conditions. Identification of hydrocephalus complicating such conditions can be a genuine clinical challenge, in which imaging features such as ventricular morphology or degrees of sulcal enlargement are seldom conclusive.

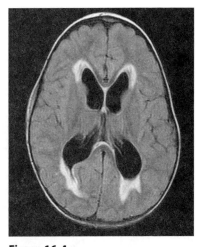

Figure 16-4.
Axial FLAIR (fluid-attenuated inversion recovery) magnetic resonance imaging vividly showing periventricular edema associated with acute hydrocephalus.

A list of differential diagnoses for macrocephaly and ventriculomegaly is shown in Box 16-2.

Treatment

Management of the child with a new diagnosis of hydrocephalus depends on the acuity of the child's clinical condition. Extreme irritability, lethargy, obtundation, and bradycardia are the immediate predecessors of ventilatory arrest and indicate urgent airway control and neurosurgical assessment. On the other hand, the asymptomatic child with accelerated head growth can be evaluated as an outpatient and treated on an elective basis. Most new cases fall somewhere between these extremes, but as a general rule, patients who are symptomatic in any way must be admitted to a neurosurgical service for investigation and treatment.

Treatment is always surgical. In some cases, there may be a discrete tumor mass, typically in the suprasellar region or the fourth ventricle, causing obstruction of ventricular CSF drainage, and the goal of surgery will be tumor resection, which will in many cases relieve the hydrocephalus. More commonly there is no mass lesion to resect, and treatment will require diversion of the CSF itself, either by a CSF shunt or by endoscopic third ventriculostomy (ETV).

Cerebrospinal Fluid Shunts

Cerebrospinal fluid shunting is by far the most common treatment for pediatric hydrocephalus and has been practiced for more than 50 years with, unfortunately, little technical refinement during that time. The shunt system consists of silastic tubing about 2.5 mm in outer diameter that is placed, via a burr hole in the skull, through the cortical mantle of the brain into the lateral ventricle. Cerebrospinal fluid drainage is regulated by a mechanical valve system through which CSF passes into distal silastic tubing. This subcutaneous tubing conveys the CSF to a remote site in the body where it can be reabsorbed into the vascular tree at low pressure, most commonly the peritoneal cavity. In children in whom the peritoneal cavity is not accessible because of previous infection or postsurgical adhesions, the distal end of the tubing may be placed into the right atrium of the heart via the jugular vein, into the pleural cavity, or occasionally into the gall bladder.

Endoscopic Third Ventriculostomy

Endoscopic third ventriculostomy is an alternative to CSF shunting suitable for selected children with mechanical obstruction of CSF drainage at the level of the aqueduct or downstream. An endoscope is introduced into the lateral ventricle through a burr hole and then is navigated through the foramen of Monro into the third ventricle. Under visual control through the optical system of the endoscope, by means of specially designed instruments introduced through the working channel of the endoscope, a small hole can be created in the floor of the third ventricle, just anterior to the mammillary bodies, which are actually visible through the attenuated floor, and posterior to the infundibular recess (Figure 16-5). This hole allows CSF to exit the ventricles directly into the subarachnoid space of the basal cisterns, thereby bypassing obstruction downstream from the third ventricle. Endoscopic third ventriculostomy is a technically more demanding operation than CSF shunt insertion and carries the possibility, although small, of catastrophic complications, because major vascular and neural structures are within millimeters of the operative site. Nevertheless, a successful ETV can have many advantages over a CSF shunt, the most compelling of which is avoidance of the burden of multiple reoperations for the virtually inevitable mechanical and infectious complications of shunts. Selection of patients for recommendation of ETV remains a matter of neurosurgical judgment. Endoscopic third ventriculostomy is a popular treatment for older children with discrete obstructive lesions (Figure 16-6), but there is wide variation in its employment among infants and among children with posthemorrhagic and postinfectious etiologies.

Natural History and Prognosis

Shunt Complications

The child with shunt-treated hydrocephalus remains forever susceptible

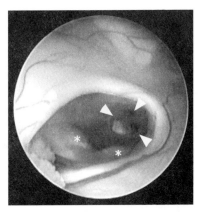

Figure 16-5.

A view from the lateral ventricle through the foramen of Monro after completion of a third ventriculostomy. In the lower left is the choroid plexus of the lateral ventricle passing through the foramen to become continuous with the choroid plexus in the roof of the third ventricle. The mammillary bodies are visible in the floor of the third ventricle (white asterisks). A large ventriculostomy has been created (bordered by white arrowheads), through which the light of the endoscope can be seen reflected off the dura of the diaphragm of the sella.

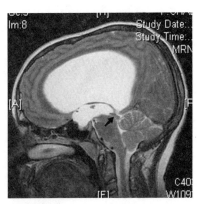

Figure 16-6.

A sagittal T2-weighted magnetic resonance image showing hydrocephalus and stenosis of the aqueduct of Sylvius (arrow). This older child is an ideal candidate for endoscopic third ventriculostomy.

to the development of complications that require surgical management. The parents of an infant with a new diagnosis of hydrocephalus can expect 4 operations to insert or to revise the shunt in the first 10 years. Roughly 40% of all new shunts fail and require reoperation for some reason within the first year. The most common reason for reoperation is obstruction of the CSF shunt. Mechanical obstruction happens in more than 50% of children within 2 years, and the lifetime risk is at least 80%. The symptoms and signs of CSF shunt obstruction are the same as the symptoms and signs of untreated hydrocephalus, except that they often progress more precipitously. Irritability, vomiting, bulging of the fontanel, separation of the sutures, sunsetting, and tense collections of CSF under the skin along the course of the shunt are common among infants. Headaches, vomiting, lethargy, paresis of upgaze, and papilledema are common among older children. Examination of the shunt itself can disclose fractures of the catheter with separation of the broken ends. Tenderness along the course of a shunt is very common in younger adolescents, but it is not a reflection of shunt failure. The cause is presumed to be tension in the fibrotic sleeve around the distal catheter occasioned by growth spurts. Most shunt valves have a depressible reservoir that can be pumped to move fluid anterograde through the tubing. Refill of the valve reservoir is an unreliable indicator of CSF shunt function. The clinical picture of shunt failure is generally progressive, although young school-aged children sometimes experience brief remissions lasting from days to a few weeks due to separation of the calvarial sutures, a phenomenon demonstrated readily on skull radiographs (Figure 16-7) or on the scout view of a CT scan.

Confirmation of suspected CSF shunt failure requires diagnostic imaging. Radiographs of the shunt system, the so-called shunt series, are readily available in most emergency departments, but they are difficult to interpret correctly, they have very low yield, and they often delay definitive investigations and neurosurgical

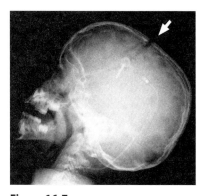

Figure 16-7.
This lateral radiograph of the skull of a child with cerebrospinal fluid shunt failure and elevated intracranial pressure shows separation of the coronal sutures (white arrow).

consultation. The decision to order radiographs of the shunt is best left to the discretion of the responsible neurosurgeon. The mainstay of the investigation of suspected shunt obstruction is imaging of the ventricular system— in the acute setting most commonly by CT scan. In general, ventricular volume will decrease after successful CSF shunt treatment and, in general, CSF shunt obstruction will be manifest by some increase in ventricular volume in comparison to the previous postoperative baseline. The increase may be quite subtle, and in a fraction of cases, even experienced interpreters may agree that ventricular volume is unchanged—a genuinely false-negative test result (Figure 16-8). In the face of suspicious clinical circumstances, a negative radiologic interpretation of a CT scan must never be a stopping point in the assessment of the child with a CSF shunt. Neurosurgical consultation is required.

The treatment for a shunt obstruction is surgery to remove and replace the failed shunt component. The ventricular catheter is the component most susceptible to obstruction due to adherence of choroid plexus and ependymoglial tissue of the ventricular wall. The distal silastic catheter can become brittle with age and fracture. Adhesions can loculate the peritoneal cavity and interfere with CSF reabsorption. Infrequently the valve itself can become obstructed by particulate or proteinaceous debris. Unfortunately, the survival expectations for revised shunt are no better than for new shunts; in many clinical circumstances they are worse.

Infection is perhaps the most serious complication after CSF shunting. It occurs in roughly 8% of cases and typically presents within the first 6 months following surgery. Cerebrospinal fluid shunt infection is exceedingly rare after this period. An infection can present as bacterial meningitis, peritonitis, shunt obstruction, wound infection, or some combination of these phenomena. The diagnosis of shunt infection must be made by aspiration of CSF from the shunt for culture, a procedure best performed by a neurosurgeon familiar with the design of the shunt system. Among patients with ventriculoatrial shunt systems, blood cultures are equally sensitive. Unfortunately, management of CSF shunt infection generally requires removal of the infected system and replacement of a new system after parenteral antibiotics have sterilized the CSF.

Shunts cannot restore normal CSF physiology. Although mechanical obstruction with insufficient CSF drainage is by far the most common mode

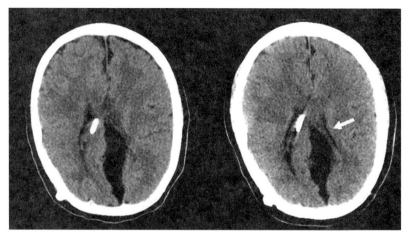

Figure 16-8.
The computed tomography (CT) on the left shows the ventricular system of a child in a stable, asymptomatic state with a functioning cerebrospinal fluid shunt. The CT on the right shows the ventricular system during an episode of shunt obstruction. Note that there is scarcely any change in ventricular volume—the left lateral ventricle is just visible in the symptomatic scan (arrow).

of failure, shunts can fail by excessive drainage of CSF as well. In the early postoperative period, excessive drainage can cause collapse of the cerebral hemispheres with collection of blood or CSF in the subdural spaces. This complication most commonly occurs following initial treatment of infants with large heads and markedly dilated ventricles, and if it is symptomatic, it may require revision of the shunt, drainage of the subdural collection, or both. In the long term, excessive CSF drainage can have adverse effects on the growth of the calvarium and the mechanical properties of the brain, leading to a constellation of troublesome complications that have in common very small ventricular volumes, the so-called slit ventricle syndrome. Subsumed under this term are shunt-related migraine headaches, chronic postural headaches, neurocognitive disturbances, and frequent episodes of ventricular catheter obstruction, often with minimal or absent interval change on CT scan. A number of clever valve designs have been introduced to reduce the frequency of complications related to excessive CSF drainage without any impact on short-term rates of shunt failure. Whether such modifications of valve design or any other technical surgical refinement can prevent the chronic complications of excessive CSF drainage is unknown.

The adverse effects of non-physiological CSF drainage arguably constitute the greatest unsolved problem in contemporary pediatric neurosurgery.

Complications of Endoscopic Third Ventriculostomy

The risks of ETV are greater than the risks of insertion of a CSF shunt, but they are probably much less than the risks of a lifetime of CSF shunt revisions. Acute perioperative complications include infection and subdural hygroma or hematoma. Creation of the opening in the floor of the third ventricle can disturb hypothalamic function, and endocrine deficiency states, particularly diabetes insipidus, have been reported in up to 5% of cases. Immediately below the floor of the third ventricle is the head of the basilar artery. Injury to the basilar artery is exceedingly infrequent, but it can cause catastrophic subarachnoid and intraventricular hemorrhage and pseudoaneurysm formation. As noted previously, failure rates for ETV depend heavily on patient selection, but like CSF shunts, most failures of ETV occur within the first year. Long-term control of hydrocephalus by ETV must not be mistaken for cure, as late failure can occur. Neurosurgical follow-up is required indefinitely.

Long-term Outcome

Quality of Life

The long-term outcome for children with hydrocephalus is highly variable. There are some children who lead seemingly normal or near-normal lives, while others are devastated. Figure 16-9 shows the wide distribution of quality-of-life (QOL) scores (0=worse QOL, 1= best QOL) for a large, typical sample of children with hydrocephalus at long-term follow-up. The factors that determine outcome are still not definitively known, but certainly the underlying etiology of the hydrocephalus seems to be important. For example, children with myelomeningocele tend to have greater difficulty, owing to their other neurologic, urological, and orthopedic issues. As well, children with severe congenital brain malformations or those with severe IVH of prematurity tend to do worse. Casey et al reported on a cohort of 155 children over a 10-year period. For children surviving until school age, 59% were able to attend a regular school. There was an 11% mortality rate during the 10-year follow-up for those with non-tumor–related hydrocephalus.

Kokkonen et al followed 42 patients shunted as children and found that social maturation lagged behind physical abilities. One-third of patients in this study had received some sort of vocational training but few had jobs. One-fourth of patients were at home without meaningful vocation. Sgouros et al reported on a series of 33 patients shunted as children. Most of the children (63%) graduated from a regular school or a school for physically handicapped children (21%). Sixty-seven percent of the patients were socially independent but lived at home with their parents; 16% left their parents' home and lived either on their own or with their partners.

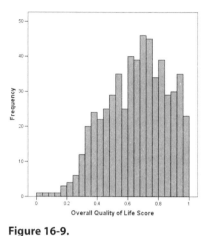

Figure 16-9.

A histogram showing the range in quality-of-life (QOL) outcomes from a typical, large sample of 569 children seen at the follow-up clinics of The Hospital for Sick Children, Toronto. Higher scores indicate better QOL. (Adapted from Kulkarni AV, Drake JM, Rabin D, Dirks PB, Humphreys RP, Rutka JT. Measuring the health status of children with hydrocephalus by using a new outcome measure. *J Neurosurg.* 2004;101:141–146.)

Neurocognitive Outcomes

Many aspects of cognitive functioning are detrimentally affected by hydrocephalus. Academic progress is significantly affected by the demonstrated difficulties that children with hydrocephalus have with reading comprehension and with inferencing skills. Further, these difficulties are not due to deficits in word recognition or vocabulary, and they occur regardless of the child's cognitive level. As a group, children with hydrocephalus have poor math skills. Suggestions for possible causes for difficulties in math include their relatively slow information processing skills and visuospatial deficits. Children with hydrocephalus have demonstrated lower scores on measures of fine motor, visual-motor, and spatial skills compared with controls. The evidence concerning memory performance in children with hydrocephalus is less clear. There have been few studies concerning memory function in children with hydrocephalus, and these studies have shown inconsistent results.

Children with hydrocephalus encounter social and emotional challenges common to many children with chronic illnesses, including maintenance of peer friendships, developing self-confidence, and worrying about their future. Such issues are particularly exacerbated in the case of hydrocephalus by prolonged or repeated hospital admissions, usually for shunt complications, which interrupt the child's usual routines and disrupt their participation in peer-related and academic activities.

Transition Into Adulthood

Unfortunately, significant clinical problems continue to arise during adulthood for patients shunted in infancy. Problems can happen unpredictably, even after long periods of stability. Continuing neurosurgical follow-up is therefore essential. The transition into the adult medical care system, however, is usually a challenge for most children with hydrocephalus. Frequently they must leave the familiar confines of the pediatric hospital in which they have been treated for many years. Comprehensive management strategies are frequently lacking for these children once they enter into adulthood. Local initiatives to improve this area of care use different models. For example, a multidisciplinary group might be set up to serve these children and might include internists, social workers, neurologists, and neurosurgeons with a special interest in hydrocephalus. In an alternate model, pediatric neurosurgeons might follow their shunt-treated patients right into adulthood.

The obstacles to successful transition to adult care settings are encountered at every step of the process from the training and practice patterns of medical specialists, to the organizations of pediatric and general adult hospitals, to the policies of social service agencies, to the benefit packages of public and private insurance carriers. Many of these obstacles are not at all unique to hydrocephalus but affect the care of patients with other chronic illnesses of childhood onset, such as congenital heart disease, diabetes, cystic fibrosis, and sickle cell disease.

Clinical Pearls

- Transfontanel ultrasound is an excellent initial screen for serious intracranial pathology in infants with macrocephaly of all causes, including hydrocephalus.
- Computed tomography scanning is the appropriate imaging modality for the acutely ill child with suspected hydrocephalus or CSF shunt failure.

- Magnetic resonance imaging is the gold standard imaging modality for diagnosis of the various forms and causes of hydrocephalus.
- The most common treatment for hydrocephalus is ventriculoperitoneal CSF shunting, but selected patients with macroscopic obstruction to CSF flow at the level of the aqueduct of Sylvius or downstream can be treated by ETV.
- While brain imaging for most children with CSF shunt failure exhibits an increase in the volume of the ventricles, false-negative brain imaging is not rare. The evaluation of the child with suspected shunt failure must be undertaken in close cooperation with the responsible neurosurgeon.
- Continued follow-up by a neurosurgeon and a medical team with a particular interest in and knowledge of hydrocephalus-related medical, cognitive, and social issues is essential, regardless of the age of the patient.

Bibliography

Epidemiology

Bondurant CP, Jimenez DF. Epidemiology of cerebrospinal fluid shunting. *Pediatr Neurosurg.* 1995;23:254–258

Chi JH, Fullerton HJ, Gupta N. Time trends and demographics of deaths from congenital hydrocephalus in children in the United States: National Center for Health Statistics data, 1979 to 1998. *J Neurosurg.* 2005;103:113–118

Cochrane DD, Kestle J. Ventricular shunting for hydrocephalus in children: patients, procedures, surgeons and institutions in English Canada, 1989–2001. *Eur J Pediatr Surg.* 2002;12(1):S6–S11

Cochrane DD, Kestle JR. The influence of surgical operative experience on the duration of first ventriculoperitoneal shunt function and infection. *Pediatr Neurosurg.* 2003;38:295–301

Fransen E, Schrander-Stumpel C, Vits L, Coucke P, Van Camp G, Willems PJ. X-linked hydrocephalus and MASA syndrome present in one family are due to a single missense mutation in exon 28 of the l1cam gene. *Hum Mol Genet.* 1994;3:2255–2256

Kanemura Y, Okamoto N, Sakamoto H, et al. Molecular mechanisms and neuroimaging criteria for severe l1 syndrome with x-linked hydrocephalus. *J Neurosurg.* 2006;105(5S):403–412

Patwardhan RV, Nanda A. Implanted ventricular shunts in the United States: the billion-dollar-a-year cost of hydrocephalus treatment. *Neurosurgery.* 2005;56:139–144

Symptoms, Signs, and Differential Diagnosis

Alvarez LA, Maytal J, Shinnar S. Idiopathic external hydrocephalus: natural history and relationship to benign familial macrocephaly. *Pediatrics.* 1986;77:901–907

Barkovich AJ, Edwards MS. Applications of neuroimaging in hydrocephalus. *Pediatr Neurosurg.* 1992;18:65–83

Garton HJ, Kestle JR, Drake JM. Predicting shunt failure on the basis of clinical symptoms and signs in children. *J Neurosurg.* 2001;94:202–210

Hamza M, Bodensteiner JB, Noorani PA, Barnes PD. Benign extracerebral fluid collections: a cause of macrocrania in infancy. *Pediatr Neurol.* 1987;3:218–221

Kim TY, Stewart G, Voth M, Moynihan JA, Brown L. Signs and symptoms of cerebrospinal fluid shunt malfunction in the pediatric emergency department. *Pediatr Emerg Care.* 2006;22:28–34

Maytal J, Alvarez LA, Elkin CM, Shinnar S. External hydrocephalus: radiologic spectrum and differentiation from cerebral atrophy. *AJR Am J Roentgenol.* 1987;148:1223–1230

Medina LS, Frawley K, Zurakowski D, Buttros D, DeGrauw AJ, Crone KR. Children with macrocrania: clinical and imaging predictors of disorders requiring surgery. *AJNR Am J Neuroradiol.* 2001;22:564–570

Piatt JH. Physical examination of patients with cerebrospinal fluid shunts: is there useful information in pumping the shunt? *Pediatrics.* 1992;89:470–473

Piatt JH Jr, Garton HJ. Clinical diagnosis of ventriculoperitoneal shunt failure among children with hydrocephalus. *Pediatr Emerg Care.* 2008;24:201–210

Complications

Brockmeyer D, Abtin K, Carey L, Walker ML. Endoscopic third ventriculostomy: an outcome analysis. *Pediatr Neurosurg.* 1998;28:236–240

Casey AT, Kimmings EJ, Kleinlugtebeld AD, Taylor WA, Harkness WF, Hayward RD. The long-term outlook for hydrocephalus in childhood. A ten-year cohort study of 155 patients. *Pediatr Neurosurg.* 1997;27:63–70

Drake JM, Kestle JR, Milner R Steinbok P. Randomized trial of cerebrospinal fluid shunt valve design in pediatric hydrocephalus. *Neurosurgery.* 1998;43:294–303

Feng H, Huang G, Liao X, et al. Endoscopic third ventriculostomy in the management of obstructive hydrocephalus: an outcome analysis. *J Neurosurg.* 2004;100:626–633

Garton HJ, Kestle JR, Cochrane DD, et al. A cost-effectiveness analysis of endoscopic third ventriculostomy. *Neurosurgery.* 2002;51:69–77

Iskandar BJ, McLaughlin C, Mapstone TB, Grabb PA, Oakes WJ. Pitfalls in the diagnosis of ventricular shunt dysfunction: radiology reports and ventricular size. *Pediatrics.* 1998;101:1031–1036

Kulkarni AV, Drake JM, Lamberti-Pasculli M. Cerebrospinal fluid shunt infection: a prospective study of risk factors. *J Neurosurg.* 2001;94:195–201

Piatt JH, Carlson CV. A search for determinants of cerebrospinal fluid shunt survival: retrospective analysis of a 14-year institutional experience. *Pediatr Neurosurg.* 1993;19:233–241

Piatt JH, Cosgriff MP. Monte Carlo simulation of cerebrospinal fluid shunt failure and definition of instability among shunt-treated patients with hydrocephalus. *J Neurosurg.* 2007;107(6 suppl):474–478

Sgouros S, Malluci C, Walsh AR, Hockley AD. Long-term complications of hydrocephalus. *Pediatr Neurosurg.* 1995;23:127–132

Smith R, Leonidas JC, Maytal J. The value of head ultrasound in infants with macrocephaly. *Pediatr Radiol.* 1998;28:143–146

Tuli S, Alshail E, Drake J. Third ventriculostomy versus cerebrospinal fluid shunt as a first procedure in pediatric hydrocephalus. *Pediatr Neurosurg.* 1999;30:11–15

Tuli S, Drake J, Lawless J, Wigg M, Lamberti-Pasculli M. Risk factors for repeated cerebrospinal shunt failures in pediatric patients with hydrocephalus. *J Neurosurg.* 2000;92:31–38

Long-term Outcome

Barnes MA, Dennis M. Discourse after early-onset hydrocephalus: core deficits in children of average intelligence. *Brain Lang.* 1998;61:309–334

Barnes MA, Dennis M. Reading in children and adolescents after early onset hydrocephalus and in normally developing age peers: phonological analysis, word recognition, word comprehension, and passage comprehension skill. *J Pediatr Psychol.* 1992;17:445–465

Dennis M, Barnes MA. Oral discourse after early-onset hydrocephalus: linguistic ambiguity, figurative language, speech acts, and script-based inferences. *J Pediatr Psychol.* 1993;18:639–652

Dennis M, Barnes MA, Hetherington CR. Congenital hydrocephalus as a model of neurodevelopmental disorder. In: Tager-Flusberg H, ed. *Neurodevelopmental Disorders: Contribution to a New Perspective From the Cognitive Neurosciences.* Cambridge, MA: MIT Press; 1999:505–532

Dennis M, Jacennik B, Barnes MA. The content of narrative discourse in children and adolescents after early-onset hydrocephalus and in normally developing age peers. *Brain Lang.* 1994;46:129–165

Fletcher JM, Brookshire BL, Bohan TP, Brandt ME, Davidson KC. Syndrome of nonverbal learning disabilities: neurodevelopmental manifestations. In: Rourke BP, ed. *Early Hydrocephalus.* New York, NY: Guilford Press; 1995:206–238

Fletcher JM, Dennis M, Northrup H. Hydrocephalus. In: Yeates KO, Ris MD, Taylor HG, eds. *Pediatric Neuropsychology: Research, Theory, and Practice.* New York, NY: Guilford Press; 2000:25–46

Fletcher JM, Landry SH, Bohan TP, et al. Effects of intraventricular hemorrhage and hydrocephalus on the long-term neurobehavioral development of preterm very-low-birthweight infants. *Dev Med Child Neurol.* 1997;39:596–606

Heinsbergen I, Rotteveel J, Roeleveld N, Grotenhuis A. Outcome in shunted hydrocephalic children. *Eur J Paediatr Neurol.* 2002;6:99–107

Kokkonen J, Serlo W, Saukkonen AL, Juolasmaa A. Long-term prognosis for children with shunted hydrocephalus. *Childs Nerv Syst.* 1994;10:384–387

Kulkarni AV, Drake JM, Rabin D, Dirks PB, Humphreys RP, Rutka JT. Measuring the health status of children with hydrocephalus by using a new outcome measure. *J Neurosurg.* 2004;101:141–146

Kulkarni AV, Rabin D, Drake JM. An instrument to measure the health status in children with hydrocephalus: the Hydrocephalus Outcome Questionnaire. *J Neurosurg.* 2004;101:134–140

Thompson NM, Fletcher JM, Chapieski L, Landry SH, Miner ME, Bixby J. Cognitive and motor abilities in preschool hydrocephalics. *J Clin Exp Neuropsychol.* 1991;13:245–258

Chapter 17

Skull Deformities: Plagiocephaly and Craniosynostosis

Robert Owen, MD
Thomas Pittman, MD

Introduction

Pediatricians frequently see children with skull deformities. Most have minor problems that are self-limited or respond to relatively innocuous intervention. A few, though, have either craniosynostosis or some other condition that requires more extensive evaluation or involved therapy; these patients require referral to a pediatric neurosurgeon.

A well-trained clinician can diagnose most infant skull deformities on the basis of physical examination. The patterns of deformity are specific and are described in the following text. Other variations in the development of the infant skull besides its shape can sometimes cause confusion and raise unnecessary concerns. Early closure or late persistence of the anterior fontanel, for instance, is unrelated to the presence or absence of craniosynostosis, although the latter phenomenon is rarely associated with metabolic bone disease or skeletal dysostoses. Neither positional plagiocephaly nor craniosynostosis causes deceleration of head growth. Nor, in the absence of a visible deformity of the skull, does a ridge along a calvarial suture have any diagnostic significance. The experienced clinician pauses at the doorway of the examination room to take in the shape of the infant's head. If there is no deformity, there is no craniosynostosis.

Plagiocephaly

Most infants with skull deformity have positional plagiocephaly. Plagiocephaly means skull asymmetry, and it encompasses a wide variety of abnormal head shapes. The deformity associated with unilateral coronal synostosis is sometimes called *anterior plagiocephaly*. Without specific qualifications, however, the term *plagiocephaly* is most often used to describe the cranial contour—flat on one side in the back with compensatory fullness of the forehead on the same side—that is associated with persistently positioning a child supine on a favored side. The prevalence of this deformity has increased substantially over the last 15 years. This change is thought to be due at least in part to the American Academy of Pediatrics Back to Sleep campaign to prevent sudden infant death syndrome and the subsequent, seemingly universal, use of the supine position for sleep in infants. Nevertheless, most infants who sleep supine do not develop a skull deformity. Another necessary factor is diminished mobility of the head and neck. Most infants with posterior plagiocephaly have some degree of congenital torticollis. In affected children, neck rotation is limited and the head is turned toward the involved side. Consequently, when placed on their backs, the children rest asymmetrically on the occiput. This leads to flattening and, ultimately, compensatory change in other parts of the skull.

Some children are born with skull asymmetry. This may reflect some facet of the intrauterine environment: persistent crowding or early engagement of the head in the pelvis. This type of asymmetry should be distinguished from cranial molding, which is not asymmetrical. After a vaginal delivery of a newborn with an occipital presentation, the molded skull is elongated in the direction of the vertex, and the parietal bones overly the frontal and occipital bones. Cranial molding is self-limited and generally resolves over a period of several days. Children born prematurely often have abnormal head shapes. Most have scaphocephaly, an elongated boat-shaped head, but many, in addition, have some occipital flattening and frontal asymmetry. Presumably, this type of asymmetry develops because premature babies are less active than full-term babies, and it may be exacerbated by the premature baby's greater osseous pliability.

Finally, many babies with significant neurologic abnormalities have plagiocephaly. These children are usually less active and may spend prolonged periods in one position. Although some have relatively typical plagiocephaly, others have unusual, but not characteristic, skull contours. It is important to recognize that the plagiocephaly is the effect, not the cause, of the neurologic disability. There is no convincing evidence that plagiocephaly causes any problems with cognitive development.

The diagnosis of positional plagiocephaly is made by physical examination. The head shape is characteristic and easily recognized. The occiput on the affected side is flat, and the ear is pushed forward. There is compensatory prominence of the contralateral parieto-occipital region. There is compensatory fullness of the forehead on the same side, and the forehead on the opposite side may be flattened. When viewed from above, the cranium has the shape of a parallelogram (Figure 17-1). The facial skeleton may be asymmetrical as well, sometimes out of proportion to the degree of calvarial asymmetry. There may be inequality of the palpebral fissures. There may be prominence of the malar eminence on the same side as the posterior flattening, and the anterior displacement of the ear on the flattened side can take the temporomandibular joint with it to cause an asymmetry of the mandible.

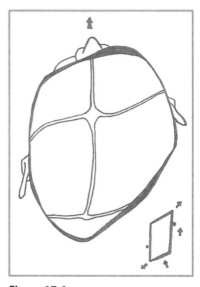

Figure 17-1.
Posterior positional plagiocephaly. The head assumes a parallelogram shape. The occiput is flattened. There is bossing of the ipsilateral forehead and anterior advancement of the ipsilateral ear.

Asymmetry of the posterior aspect of the head can raise the question of unilateral lambdoid synostosis. In unilateral lambdoid synostosis, as in positional plagiocephaly, the affected parieto-occipital region is flat. In lambdoid synostosis, however, the ear on the involved side is more frequently, but not always, displaced posteriorly. An even more distinctive feature of lambdoid synostosis is the situation of the affected ear in the vertical dimension: It is displaced inferiorly. Because the distinction between lambdoid synostosis and positional plagiocephaly can occasionally be difficult, it is important to remember 2 points: (1) positional plagiocephaly is much, much more common than lambdoid synostosis and (2) if the ears are set at the same altitude (ie, if they lie in the same axial plane), the question of lambdoid synostosis can be dismissed.

Children with obvious positional plagiocephaly do not require any radiographic examination. Treatment can be based solely on the physical examination. If there is some concern that the head shape is atypical for positional plagiocephaly, plain radiographs of the head can be obtained. Even with a radiograph, however, it can be difficult to eliminate the possibility that a patient has lambdoid synostosis. Irregular calcification and marginal sclerosis, generally signs of synostosis, can be seen in patent lambdoid sutures. Some authors assert that normal-appearing sutures can be sticky and functionally synostotic. Unless the suture has been replaced by dense bone, the physician can still be left unsure of the diagnosis. Primary physicians should not order computed tomographic (CT) scans for children who are suspected of having positional plagiocephaly. If there is uncertainty about the diagnosis, the patient should be referred to a pediatric neurosurgeon. Pediatric neurosurgical consultation entails no radiation exposure, is more reliable than interpretation of imaging, and is less expensive.

The natural history of positional plagiocephaly is poorly defined. In part, this lack of definition reflects a huge variation in the severity of the deformity. In most cases, the head shape will improve somewhat as the child ages and spends less time on his or her back; however, the degree of improvement is often less than might be anticipated. Physicians must never promise parents that the deformity will go away. Most children who have significant cranial asymmetry are likely to require some form of therapy.

The first step in treating plagiocephaly is to position the infant off the flat part of the head. This treatment, like all of the others available, is most effective when initiated at the earliest point in time. When the child is lying down, a foam wedge or a blanket roll can be placed under the torso to encourage the child to lie on the unaffected side. Unfortunately, only the youngest infants stay where they are put. Normal infant development usually defeats passive positioning tactics by 3 or 4 months of age. Active tactics can be helpful as well. Parents can move any mobiles or other playthings in the crib so that the child must lie on the opposite side to play with them or to see them. Finally, the crib can be positioned so that the child must lie opposite the preferred side to see out the door. Periods of supervised tummy time can also be very helpful.

Most infants with plagiocephaly have some degree of torticollis. Passive neck range of motion exercises can be demonstrated in the physician's office, but additional instruction, supervision, and encouragement by a physical therapist are helpful. Parents are encouraged to perform several repetitions of the passive stretching exercises with every diaper change.

Infants with severe asymmetry and infants who have not responded to positioning are treated with a molding helmet. Helmets are of 2 types: active and passive. Active helmets incorporate some mechanism to deliver a mild compressive force to the areas of the skull that are full. Passive helmets are padded and fit closely in the areas of fullness but leave room for growth in the areas that are flat. There is no clear indication that one type of helmet is preferable to the other; however, there is a difference in cost and provider availability.

There is no consensus as to when helmet therapy should be started or how long it should be continued. In general, the earlier a helmet is used the more likely it is to be effective. Treatment is frequently initiated by 6 months, and there is little reason to expect any benefit from treatment initiated after 12 months. Helmets generally are worn for 3 or 4 months, although some authors recommend continuing therapy for much longer periods. To be effective, a helmet must be worn essentially all of the time. It can be removed to bathe the child and check for pressure points.

In view of the substantial prevalence of plagiocephaly in infancy and in view of the expense of helmet therapy, the dearth of clinical research into the outcomes of treatment is disappointing. Although uncontrolled observations support the impression of most clinicians that helmets effect beneficial changes in the first 6 to 12 weeks after initiating therapy, Moss found no benefit from the orthotic treatment of "mild to moderate" deformities compared with a historical control group. No other controlled observations have appeared. Almost all reports have limited the period of observation to the duration of the course of treatment, but physicians and parents naturally want to know whether the deformity will be an obstacle to acceptance when the patient enters society later in childhood. The only description of outcomes among school-aged children is the work of Steinbok et al, who reported that 63 of 65 patients 5 years of age or older were judged by their parents to have normal or mildly abnormal head shapes. Parents perceived residual deformity in 58% of cases, but in only 21% were they concerned about it. There was no difference between children managed with cranial orthosis and children managed by other means, although no meaningful comparative analysis was possible. For many reasons in addition to its actual resolution, the deformity becomes less conspicuous as time passes. The growth of hair conceals the deformity. The development of neck musculature later in childhood and the increasing dominance of the face both tend to minimize the visual impact of the asymmetry of the calvarium. The asymmetry of the position of the ears persists, but it is of little concern except to the oculist. Reassurance of parents is a major component of the management of positional plagiocephaly.

Single-Suture Craniosynostosis

Sagittal

About 40% of patients with craniosynostosis have isolated involvement of the sagittal suture. The disease, which occurs in approximately 1 in 5,000 live births, is more frequent in boys. Premature closure of the sagittal suture causes an elongated cranium with a coincident reduction in the biparietal diameter. This head shape has been variously described as scaphocephaly, dolichocephaly or, less decorously, a boat-shaped head. Sagittal synostosis is usually sporadic but there have been instances of familial transmission.

The diagnosis is usually based on physical examination. There is often a prominent palpable ridge along the sagittal suture. The condition may involve the entire suture, but isolated posterior or anterior sagittal synostosis may also occur. Secondary calvarial changes become more obvious as the process advances: frontal bossing may be prominent, the occiput may be pointed, and bitemporal narrowing or "pinching" may be present (Figure 17-2).

Imaging studies usually reveal an absent suture replaced by a sclerotic ridge. While imaging studies may aid in diagnosis, many surgeons argue that they are not mandatory. One should note that premature infants often have a scaphocephalic head shape. True synostosis is rare among premature babies.

Surgical correction of sagittal synostosis is recommended by most, if not all, pediatric neurosurgeons. Although the primary goal of surgery is to improve appearance, this concern should not be taken lightly. Uncorrected sagittal synostosis usually causes significant deformity that does not improve as the patient ages, and the social implications of conservative management may be substantial.

The timing of surgical intervention depends on the technique preferred by the surgeon. Options range from a simple sagittal strip craniectomy, during which the involved suture is excised, to more elaborate, global calvarial reconstructions. In general, strip craniectomies are performed 4 weeks to 4 months after birth. Cranial vault remodeling is performed at 4 to 8 months of age. Older children are better able to tolerate the blood loss that occurs during more extensive procedures and the bone is stronger and easier to work with.

A strip craniectomy can usually be performed within an hour, blood loss is minimal, and transfusion is not often needed. With less extensive exposure and shortened operative time, the likelihood of an anesthetic, hemodynamic, or anatomical

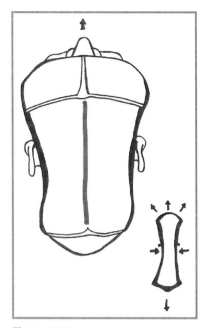

Figure 17-2.
Sagittal synostosis. Head shape is oblong and thin. Frontal bossing is usually more prominent than that in the posterior/parietal region. The bitemporal diameter is narrow.

complication is decreased. More extensive operations have greater risk but can completely correct the primary and secondary calvarial abnormalities associated with sagittal synostosis. There is no evidence that any technique is clearly superior. Surgical decisions should be based on the surgeon's preference, the parents' expectations and desires, and the age of the patient. Because the calvarium is less plastic, simple synostectomy is less successful in children older than 6 months.

Metopic

About 20% of patients with craniosynostosis have metopic synostosis. The metopic suture, the first calvarial suture to close, usually closes by the second year. Premature closure results in trigonocephaly—a triangular head as viewed from above with a pointed forehead (Figure 17-3). The appearance of children with metopic synostosis can vary widely: defects range from a palpable but not visible midline forehead keel, which causes no cosmetic problem, to a prominent frontal ridge with significant secondary flattening of the supraorbital ridges and hypotelorism causing noticeable craniofacial dysmorphism. The severity of the defect may be related to the degree of involvement of the sutures along the anterior fossa skull base.

The natural history of trigonocephaly associated with metopic synostosis is less clear-cut than the natural history of the deformities associated with other forms of single-suture synostosis. The elaboration of the frontal sinuses and the development of the brow in adolescence

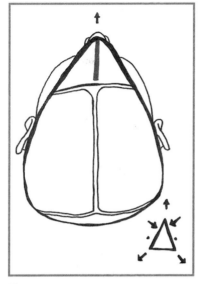

Figure 17-3.

Metopic synostosis. Trigonocephaly is present. The forehead is pointed. Biparietal bossing may be present, and the head assumes a triangular configuration.

tend to mitigate the deformity of the forehead, and the expansion of the ethmoid sinuses may have a similar effect on the associated hypotelorism. Although adults with scaphocephaly adults with never treated or poorly treated sagittal synostosis are not so uncommon, recognizably adults with trigonocephaly adults are exceptionally rare. Nevertheless, documentation of the natural history of metopic synostosis is very limited, and most authorities recommend surgical correction in infancy.

Unlike sagittal synostosis, metopic synostosis is associated with intracranial developmental anomalies. Associated abnormalities, such as holoprosencephaly and dysgenesis of the corpus callosum, usually involve midline structures. Metopic synostosis is also more frequently part of a syndrome than are other single suture synostoses. Because of this relation to intracranial abnormalities and some craniofacial syndromes, patients with metopic synostosis are more likely to have neurocognitive and intellectual deficits. In such cases, the problem is caused by the associated neurodevelopmental problems and not by the synostosis. Preoperative counseling should make clear that surgical intervention is aimed at correcting the head shape rather than improving neurologic or cognitive performance.

Surgical correction is usually undertaken when the child is a few months old. The surgical procedure involves a bifrontal craniotomy with remodeling of the forehead. The orbital rim is advanced and widened to correct flattening and hypotelorism. In an older child with a less severe case, a prominent forehead keel may be drilled down through a bicoronal exposure. More aggressive approaches afford a more complete cosmetic correction. Less aggressive approaches should be reserved for older children with milder defects and less severe secondary changes.

Unicoronal

The incidence of unicoronal synostosis is similar to that of metopic synostosis. Whereas patients with bicoronal involvement are likely to have one of a number of craniofacial syndromes, unicoronal synostosis is associated only rarely with other systemic abnormalities. The ipsilateral forehead and orbital rim are flat, resulting in forehead asymmetry often exaggerated by compensatory contralateral frontal prominence (Figure 17-4). A palpable coronal ridge is usually present. The eyebrow is elevated on the affected side, and the palpebral fissure is widened. Infants often have facial scoliosis with deviation of the nasion toward the affected side and with consequent rotation of the nose in the plane of the face. Skull radiographs show that the superior margin of the orbit on the involved side is elevated resulting in a "harlequin eye" deformity. Secondary to the orbital changes, strabismus is often present.

Surgical correction is pursued when the child is a few months of age. Techniques range from a unilateral frontal craniotomy and

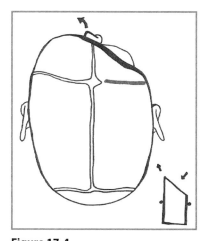

Figure 17-4.
Unicoronal synostosis. The forehead ipsilateral to the synostotic suture is flattened. The nose deviates away from the fused coronal suture. Secondary changes involving the ears and posterior region are usually not as pronounced as posterior plagiocephaly.

unilateral orbital bar advancement to bilateral craniotomies and orbital bar reconstructions.

Lambdoid

Lambdoid synostosis is rare. Probably fewer than 5% of patients with craniosynostosis have isolated lambdoid involvement. As previously discussed, it can be confused with deformational posterior plagiocephaly (Figure 17-5).

If true lambdoid synostosis is present, surgical correction may not be recommended unless the cosmetic defect is profound.

Facial dysmorphism is often less pronounced than in other types of craniosynostosis, and the primary area of abnormality is covered by hair. The risks of surgical correction may be higher than with other types of craniosynostosis because posterior calvarial reconstruction is performed in the vicinity of the superior sagittal sinus, transverse sinus, and torcular.

Imaging

Skull radiographs may be helpful in cases of suspected craniosynostosis. Radiographic findings vary, but in general a synostotic suture will be sclerotic, absent, or enostotic. Occasionally an involved suture

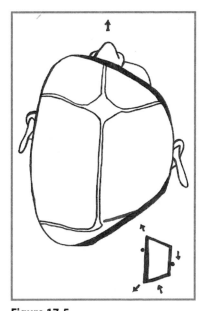

Figure 17-5.
Lambdoid synostosis. Head shape is rhomboidal. Ipsilateral occipital and frontal regions are flattened. The ipsilateral ear is usually posteriorly displaced toward the synostotic lambdoid suture.

may appear normal but be functionally tight. In such cases, secondary skull changes may still suggest the diagnosis. Plain films have specificity greater than 90% and sensitivity of approximately 80% for the diagnosis of synostosis.

When plain films are equivocal, a CT scan can be performed. Three-dimensional reconstructed scans are generally most helpful. The sensitivity and specificity of 3-dimensional CT scans approaches 100%, and the studies are also useful for presurgical evaluation and planning. Computed tomography better delineates the extent of suture involvement, involvement at the skull base, bony architecture near the dural venous sinuses, associated facial abnormalities, and the relationship of sutures involved in the calvarium and skull base than do plain radiographs. Computed tomography also allows evaluation of the brain, extra-axial cerebrospinal fluid spaces, and the ventricular system so that gross brain malformations and hydrocephalus can be detected.

Although imaging studies are useful adjuncts to the diagnosis of craniosynostosis, they are not mandatory. Diagnosis is generally on the basis of physical examination. Experienced surgeons may not perform any imaging study before undertaking surgical correction in straightforward cases.

The same reservations apply to the radiologic investigation of craniosynostosis as to the investigation of plagiocephaly. If the primary physician cannot make a confident clinical diagnosis, or if craniosynostosis is suspected, direct referral to a pediatric neurosurgeon is expeditious. The consulting surgeon can determine whether and what type of secondary imaging studies are required.

Syndromic Craniosynostosis

Although management of single-suture craniosynostosis is a challenging problem, syndromic cases are significantly more complicated. Syndromic craniosynostosis often involves multiple sutures and serious associated abnormalities of the face and airway. Surgical correction is more complicated and often requires multiple cranial and facial procedures. Hydrocephalus, which is rarely an associated finding in nonsyndromic cases but relatively common in syndromic synostosis, makes correction of the deformity more difficult. Children with syndromic synostosis frequently have psychosocial and neurocognitive abnormalities. Although cosmetic results of surgical intervention can be good, the severity of the deformities results in less satisfactory correction than straightforward single suture cases.

Crouzon Syndrome (Craniofacial Dysostosis)

Crouzon syndrome, initially described in 1912, is an autosomal dominant disorder with variable expression. It occurs in approximately 1 in 25,000 births. Bilateral coronal involvement is the most frequent pattern of synostosis, but sagittal and metopic synostosis can occur. Affected children have a characteristic facial morphology: midface hypoplasia and retrusion with prominent exophthalmos and a beaked nose. Airway problems and obstructive apnea are common, and a tracheostomy may be required. Pulmonary abnormalities occur occasionally, and hydrocephalus is seen in 30% to 70% of cases. Neurocognitive function and intellect are not usually affected, although psychological and social problems are common.

Apert Syndrome (Acrocephalosyndactyly)

Apert syndrome, first reported in 1894, affects approximately 1 in 55,000 children. Inheritance is autosomal dominant, but a large number of cases are sporadic. Its hallmark is craniosynostosis in conjunction with fusion of the digits of the hands and feet. The coronal sutures are most frequently involved. Typical craniofacial morphology includes brachycephaly, midface hypoplasia and retrusion with associated underbite, hypertelorism, exophthalmos, downwardly slanted palpebral fissures, and a beaked nose. Brain, cardiac, genitourinary, and pulmonary abnormalities occur occasionally. Hearing loss and neurocognitive and intellectual deficiencies are prevalent. True hydrocephalus is much less common than in Crouzon syndrome.

Pfeiffer Syndrome

Pfeiffer syndrome, initially described in 1964, is a rare but very severe craniofacial disorder. Its hallmark is craniosynostosis with broad thumbs and great toes. Partial digit fusion may also be present. The syndrome occurs in 1 in 210,000 births, and inheritance is autosomal dominant. Sporadic cases are common and often severe. Bicoronal synostosis, sometimes with sagittal involvement, is common but cloverleaf deformity (pan-sutural synostosis) can occur. Like Apert syndrome, there is associated midface hypoplasia and retrusion, exophthalmos, downward slanted palpebral fissures, hypertelorism, prominent jaw and chin, and malocclusion of the teeth. Hearing loss can be caused by external canal abnormalities, and severe neurocognitive deficits are not uncommon. The severity of neurodevelopmental deficits may be lessened if early surgery is performed to release multiple synostotic sutures.

Carpenter Syndrome

Carpenter syndrome, first described in 1901, is a rare disorder that typically follows an autosomal recessive inheritance pattern. Sagittal, coronal, and lambdoid sutures can be affected and cloverleaf deformities have been reported. Malformations of the extremities are common, especially polydactyly. Cardiac abnormalities are very common and may be severe. Neurocognitive and intellectual deficits are usually present and may be significant.

Saethre-Chotzen Syndrome

Saethre-Chotzen syndrome, initially described in the 1930s, is a rare autosomal dominant disorder. Phenotypic expression is very variable. In the past, many patients were probably misclassified as having Crouzon syndrome. Synostosis usually affects coronal sutures, although the metopic and lambdoid can be affected. A low hairline, flat face, maxillary hypoplasia, ptosis, beaked nose, hypertelorism, facial asymmetry, and prominent ear crus are present. Syndactyly may be present. Skeletal anomalies occur occasionally. Intellectual function may be diminished.

Others

Other primary craniosynostosis syndromes not mentioned above include Antley-Bixler syndrome, Greig cephalopolysyndactyly syndrome, craniofrontonasal dysplasia, Muenke craniosynostosis, and Baller-Gerold syndrome. Craniosynostosis is an associated feature in approximately 60 identified syndromes.

Multiple Suture Synostosis and Kleeblattschädel

Multiple suture synostosis is relatively uncommon and is usually seen in the context of a syndromic disorder. If more than one suture is involved, the incidence of significantly elevated intracranial pressure is high and much more likely to be clinically significant. In these cases, reduction in intracranial pressure is a goal of surgery.

The kleeblattschädel or cloverleaf deformity results from synostosis of most or all calvarial sutures. As a result, the head assumes a trilobular configuration that resembles a cloverleaf as viewed *en face*. It is seen most often in Pfeiffer syndrome but can occur in any of the syndromic craniosynostoses. There is marked temporal and frontal bossing, proptosis may be severe, and airway problems are frequent. Surgical intervention should be undertaken within the first few weeks of life because of the severe brain constriction.

Craniosynostosis, Intracranial Pressure, and Neurocognitive Outcomes

As noted in the previous section, craniosynostosis involving more than one calvarial suture generally places an infant at high risk for abnormally elevated intracranial pressure. Potential functional complications include neurocognitive disability and papilledema, optic atrophy, and blindness. These complications may be exacerbated by the hydrocephalus that is associated with the syndromic forms of craniosynostosis.

The question of functional outcomes among children with single-suture craniosynostosis is much more difficult to address. Mild elevations of intracranial pressure can be recorded in a minority of infants and young children with not yet treated sagittal, metopic, and unicoronal synostosis, but the clinical significance of such elevations is uncertain. Some authorities have asserted a correlation with developmental delay, but contrary observations have been reported as well. Children with single-suture synostosis have a higher prevalence of abnormalities on formal developmental testing than their siblings. Some craniofacial centers have reported that earlier surgical treatment is associated with a lower prevalence of developmental problems than later treatment, but as treatment time has never been randomized for experimental purposes, later treatment generally reflects social circumstances that limit access to medical care and that are therefore likely to have a confounding effect on developmental outcomes. Starr et al recently reported interim results of a large, prospective, multicenter, controlled study of neurodevelopmental outcomes among young children with single-suture craniosynostosis. Patients were slightly but significantly more likely than controls to score in the delayed range on a variety of developmental tests, but no effect of suture location or timing of surgery was demonstrable. The current understanding can be summarized by noting that no beneficial effect of surgery on neurocognitive outcome has been demonstrated for infants with single-suture synostosis, but the possibility of a quantitatively small benefit has not been excluded conclusively. The principal indication for treatment of single-suture synostosis is cosmetic.

Multidisciplinary Care

The management of the deformity associated with craniosynostosis is intrinsically surgical, but many patients have functional complications of deformity that require the services of a great variety of medical specialists and therapists in addition to the craniofacial plastic surgeon and the neurosurgeon. A team approach is appropriate. Patients with orbital deformity, as in unicoronal, metopic, and syndromic craniosynostosis, require assessment and follow-up by an ophthalmologist for strabismus and for detection of papilledema. Patients with midface hypoplasia related to a craniofacial syndrome require the services of an otolaryngologist for management of hearing loss related to eustachian tube dysfunction and often for management of airway insufficiency. Many syndromic patients have tracheostomies. Underbite requires the attention of the pediatric dentist and the oral/maxillofacial surgeon. The medical geneticist/dysmorphologist serves a critical diagnostic function that facilitates anticipation of complications and future therapy needs. The psychologist, speech and language pathologist, audiologist, and nutritionist all provide important services. The American Cleft Palate–Craniofacial Association has published guidelines for the composition and operation of the model team (www.acpa-cpf.org/teamcare/ccteam.htm).

Conclusion

Most children with skull deformities have positional plagiocephaly, a problem a pediatrician can recognize and often treat. It is important to identify those few children who may have craniosynostosis; they require early referral to allow them the best opportunity for good cosmetic correction with potentially less extensive operations.

Bibliography

Plagiocephaly

American Academy of Pediatrics Task Force on Infant Positioning and SIDS. Positioning and SIDS. *Pediatrics.* 1992;89:1120–1126

Kelly KM, Littlefield TR, Pomatto JK, Manwaring KH, Beals SP. Cranial growth unrestricted during treatment of deformational plagiocephaly. *Pediatr Neurosurg.* 1999;30:193–199

Moss SD. Nonsurgical, nonorthotic treatment of occipital plagiocephaly: what is the natural history of the misshapen neonatal head? *J Neurosurg.* 1997;87:667–670

Peitsch WK, Keefer CH, LaBrie RA, Mulliken JB. Incidence of cranial asymmetry in healthy newborns. *Pediatrics.* 2002;110:e72

Persing J, James H, Swanson J, Kattwinkel J. Prevention and management of positional skull deformities in infants. *Pediatrics.* 2003;112:199–202

Ripley CE, Pomatto J, Beals SP, Joganic EF, Manwaring KH, Moss SD. Treatment of positional plagiocephaly with dynamic orthotic cranioplasty. *J Craniofac Surg.* 1994;5:150–159

Steinbok P, Lam D, Singh S, Mortenson PA, Singhal A. Long-term outcome of infants with positional occipital plagiocephaly. *Childs Nerv Syst.* 2007;23:1275–1283

Craniosynostosis

Dominguez R, Oh KS, Bender T, Girdany BR. Uncomplicated trigonocephaly. A radiographic affirmation of conservative therapy. *Radiology.* 1981;140:681–688

Mathijssen I, Arnaud E, Lajeunie E, Marchac D, Renier D. Postoperative cognitive outcome for synostotic frontal plagiocephaly. *J Neurosurg.* 2006;105:16–20

Pollack IF, Losken HW, Biglan AW. Incidence of increased intracranial pressure after early surgical treatment of syndromic craniosynostosis. *Pediatr Neurosurg.* 1996;24:202–209

Renier D. Intracranial pressure in craniosynostosis: pre- and postoperative recordings—correlation with functional results. In: Persing JA, Edgerton MT, Jane JA, eds. *Scientific Foundations and Surgical Treatment of Craniosynostosis.* Baltimore, MD: Williams & Wilkins; 1989:263–269

Ruiz-Correa S, Starr JR, Lin HJ, Kapp-Simon KA, Cunningham ML, Speltz ML. Severity of skull malformation is unrelated to presurgery neurobehavioral status of infants with sagittal synostosis. *Cleft Palate Craniofac J.* 2007;44:548–554

Starr JR, Kapp-Simon KA, Cloonan YK, Collett BR, Cradock MM, et al. Presurgical and postsurgical assessment of the neurodevelopment of infants with single-suture craniosynostosis: comparison with controls. *J Neurosurg (2 suppl Pediatrics).* 2007;107:103–110

Chapter 18

The Chiari Malformation and Syringomyelia

Joseph H. Piatt Jr, MD

Introduction

In 1890 Hans Chiari first described the 4 malformations that have come subsequently to bear his name. This nomenclature is unfortunate. Aside from attachment of his name and involvement of the cerebellum, the Chiari malformations have very little in common. The most prevalent, Chiari malformation type 1 (CM1), is defined as displacement of normally developed cerebellar tonsils more than 5 mm below the plane of the foramen magnum (Figure 18-1). To refer to this entity as a malformation is misleading in so much as the term implies an anatomically fixed consequence of an error in development, when in fact CM1 is now recognized to reflect a variety of dynamic pathophysiological processes. A more descriptive and less connotative designation might be chronic tonsillar herniation, but this chapter will conform to the standard terminology of the substantial and rapidly expanding literature on this topic.

What accounts for the explosion of clinical and investigative interest in CM1 is proliferation of magnetic resonance imaging (MRI) units. Prior to the appearance of MRI, the diagnosis of CM1 required myelography with air, oil-based iodinated contrast, or most recently with water-soluble iodinated contrast. The requisite diagnostic investigations were unpleasant for patients and challenging for radiologists. They entailed substantial radiation exposure and complications such as post-lumbar

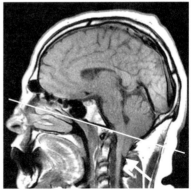

Figure 18-1.
This sagittal, T1-weighted magnetic resonance image of the head shows a severe Chiari malformation type 1. The white line marks the plane of the foramen magnum. The white arrow marks the tips of the tonsils of the cerebellum, which are displaced and deformed.

puncture headache and encephalopathy from contrast toxicity. Only patients with serious clinical problems specifically localized to the craniocervical junction ever received a diagnosis. Magnetic resonance imaging, on the other hand, yields detailed pictures of any part of the body without risk or discomfort in sessions that generally last less than an hour. The enormous diagnostic power of MRI has blossomed, in this country at least, in a very fertile economic environment for medical imaging services, and MRI units are now everywhere. The clinical threshold for ordering MRI has fallen to a very low level, and patients with mild symptoms and with no neurologic impairment are routinely subjected to studies of the brain and spine.

Magnetic resonance imaging has demonstrated that Chiari malformations are rather common among patients who have undergone diagnostic imaging for unrelated reasons. Meadows et al reviewed 22,591 consecutive MRI studies of the head and cervical spine. There were 175 instances of CM1, as defined by tonsillar displacement greater than 5 mm. Twenty-five cases had no symptoms that could be associated with CM1, for a prevalence of asymptomatic CM1 in the general population of 1.1 per 1,000. Not surprisingly, since Chiari malformation seems to be present in so many people who are otherwise perfectly well, MRI has also opened the possibility of associations between Chiari malformation and a long list of nonspecific and non-disabling neurologic symptoms. In the modern era the challenge is not the diagnosis of Chiari malformation, but the selection of patients who really require treatment from among the many who carry the diagnosis.

Anatomy and Physiology

Chiari malformation type 1 was originally conceptualized as an error of brain development, but recent investigation has shifted blame to maldevelopment of the surrounding skull and has directed attention to disturbances of cerebrospinal fluid (CSF) and cerebrovascular physiology. Logically, displacement of the tonsils of the cerebellum through the foramen magnum admits a limited number of explanations: The room available for normal brain structures within the osseous confines of the posterior fossa may be insufficient. The tonsils may be pushed down from above. Or they may be pulled down from below. Each of these considerations seems to play a role to varying degrees in particular patients. Volumetric studies employing both computed tomography scanning and MRI have shown that many cases of

CM1 are associated with relatively small posterior fossa volumes. Patients who respond favorably to surgical decompression have smaller volumes than patients who do not. A very recent report by Sgouros et al noted that posterior fossa volumes are smaller in children with CM1 complicated by syringomyelia but are no different from controls among children with uncomplicated CM1. Among cases with normal posterior fossa volume, CSF pressure gradients or decreased cerebral compliance due to cerebral venous hypertension or other causes may generate forces that push the tonsils downward. Alternatively, low spinal CSF pressures may pull or suck the tonsils inferiorly. To emphasize further the dynamic nature of the CM1, there are case reports of spontaneous resolution and de novo development of these lesions.

Probably the most important complication of CM1 is syringomyelia (Figure 18-2). *Syringomyelia* means "cavitation of the spinal cord." Syrinx is the term for an individual cavity. The development of a syrinx cavity necessarily reflects destruction of spinal cord tissue. A related concept is *hydromyelia,* or dilation of the central canal of the spinal cord. Syringomyelia and hydromyelia cannot be distinguished reliably on MRI, and autopsy specimens often demonstrate the concurrence of the 2 processes. For these reasons, *hydromyelia* and the elided term *hydrosyringomyelia* are falling into disuse.

Syringomyelia is an acquired condition that reflects a regional disturbance of CSF physiology in the spine. Syringomyelia may be seen in

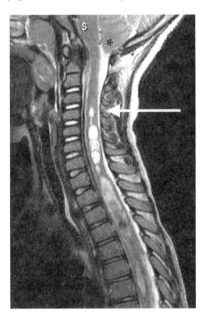

Figure 18-2.
This sagittal, T2-weighted magnetic resonance image of the cervical spine shows a septated syrinx cavity beginning at the C4 level (white arrow) and extending inferiorly. The signal intensity of the cerebrospinal fluid (CSF) within the syrinx is not homogeneous because it varies with the amplitude and the phase of CSF pulsation. In this case the inferior displacement of the tonsils of the cerebellum (black asterisk) is not very severe, but it fills the foramen magnum and suffices to establish a dissociation of CSF pulse pressures between the cranial and the spinal compartments. This syrinx collapsed after craniocervical decompression.

the setting of a variety of conditions, including myelomeningocele, trauma, intrinsic spinal cord tumor, and arachnoiditis, but the most common association is with CM1. Elucidation of the pathophysiology of syringomyelia in association with CM1 has been a long process, but it has been accelerated recently by data from MRI. The contemporary understanding derives from the work of Williams, who first hypothesized that CSF flow back and forth across the foramen magnum might be obstructed by the displaced tonsils of Chiari malformations. He actually measured the resulting pressure differentials in humans by means of simultaneous lumbar and ventricular recordings. This concept was elaborated and refined by Oldfield et al, who imagined the displaced tonsils of the cerebellum, snug in the dural sleeve of the cervical spinal canal, to be like a piston driven downward by the systolic expansion of the brain. The downward stroke of the tonsillar piston is easily demonstrated by ultrasound in the operating room, and it is believed to cause sharply enhanced CSF pulsatility within the spinal compartment. Cerebrospinal fluid is driven into the substance of the spinal cord along perivascular extensions of the subarachnoid space, the so-called Virchow-Robin spaces, and it collects there as interstitial edema, microcysts, and eventually gross syrinx cavities.

Clinical Contexts and Associations

Most cases of CM1 seem to arise spontaneously without any explanation and without association with any other recognized condition, but occasionally, CM1 is a complication of another disease process that provides a context for the pathophysiological processes described in the preceding section. Such disease processes can have complex interrelationships with CM1 and with each other (Figure 18-3).

Craniofacial dysostoses, such as Crouzon and Pfeiffer syndromes, and skeletal dysplasias, such as achondroplasia, feature not only small posterior fossa volumes on the basis of craniosynostosis or other disturbance of skull growth but also decreased intracranial compliance related to venous hypertension. Venous hypertension appears in these syndromes as a consequence of maldevelopment of the skull base with jugular foraminal stenosis. Another vivid association is with rickets, which causes thickening of the skull that encroaches on the volume available to the neural contents of the posterior fossa. Rickets in infancy can also cause global impairment

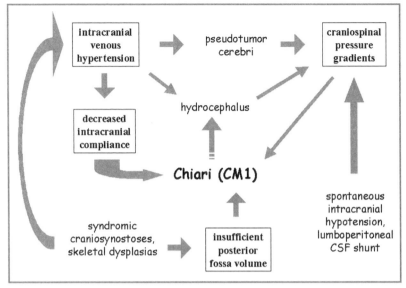

Figure 18-3.
Clinical conditions associated with Chiari malformation type 1 and intermediary pathophysiological mechanisms.

of skull growth and craniosynostosis affecting multiple calvarial sutures. This impairment of skull growth is the basis for the classical observation of the bulging anterior fontanel in the rachitic infant. Over time the growing brain expands in the direction of least resistance—out the open anterior fontanel—causing a distinctive "towering" deformity of the skull, so-called turribrachycephaly. Simultaneous expansion of the brain in the opposite direction—out the foramen magnum—leads to an association with CM1 as well. This syndrome is seldom seen any longer among children born in developed countries, but it is particularly well recognized among North African immigrants.

The arrow of causality points in many different directions in the association of CM1 with hydrocephalus. The 2 conditions seem to share an underlying congenital or developmental cause in some instances, as roughly 10% of patients with CM1 also have hydrocephalus at presentation. Successful treatment of the hydrocephalus can lead occasionally to resolution of CM1. In the setting of syndromic craniosynostosis and skeletal dysplasia, the common cause of both hydrocephalus and CM1 may be impaired intracranial venous drainage. Hydrocephalus is a well-recognized complication of the surgical treatment of CM1 as a consequence of infection, sterile meningitis, or posterior fossa subdural hygroma. Conversely, CM1 can be acquired as a complication of treatment of hydrocephalus in infancy. Excessive decompression of the infant head by a CSF shunt causes overriding of the bones of the calvarium, abnormal ossification of the apposed sutures, and possible skull deformity and craniocerebral disproportion. Although the bones that delimit the posterior fossa cannot override, decompression of the posterior fossa by CSF shunting during a sensitive stage in early infancy seems to alter the developmental program for the skull base and lead to impaired growth and eventual appearance of CM1.

Chiari malformation type 1 also has important and illustrative associations with 2 less common disturbances of CSF circulation, pseudotumor cerebri, and spontaneous intracranial hypotension. Pseudotumor cerebri is a clinical syndrome characterized by elevated intracranial pressure (ICP) without any explanatory structural finding on brain imaging. Typical presenting symptoms are headache, transient visual obscurations, and diplopia. Typical physical findings are papilledema with enlargement of the blind spots and variable degrees of visual impairment ranging all the way to complete blindness. Unilateral or bilateral sixth cranial nerve palsies can be present as well, as nonspecific signs of elevated ICP. A complete review of the clinical events that have been known to precipitate the development of pseudotumor cerebri is beyond the scope of this chapter, but what all these events seem to have in common is elevation of dural venous sinus pressures. Among obese young women, who are particularly subject to pseudotumor cerebri, the elevated venous pressures can be tracked to the right atrium. In other clinical contexts, such as in the setting of mastoiditis, there is obstruction to venous drainage within a major dural sinus by thrombus or by fibrotic stenosis. From whatever cause, the elevated dural venous sinus pressures not only raise the pressure gradient required for CSF reabsorption but also impair intracranial compliance. As noted previously, impaired compliance is observed in a large fraction of patients with CM1 and presumably plays a role in displacement of the tonsils. This association of elevated venous pressures with CM1 accounts for the occasional patient who exhibits papilledema at the time of original presentation. It is believed also to account for the persistence of symptoms and the development of tense CSF wound collections in some patients after surgical treatment. Pseudotumor cerebri can be treated by correcting the underlying cause, such as over-weight, by acetazolamide, a diuretic that both lowers right atrial pressures and inhibits CSF secretion, or by lumboperitoneal CSF shunt.

Spontaneous intracranial hypotension is a rare syndrome characterized by disabling postural headaches, that is, headaches that are exacerbated by upright posture and relieved by recumbency much like post-lumbar puncture headaches. The precipitating event seems to be development of an intraspinal CSF fistula from rupture a previously unsuspected meningeal diverticulum or perineural cyst or from erosion of the dura by a degenerative spinal osteophyte. Drainage of CSF into the spinal epidural space lowers intrathecal CSF pressure and can create a pressure gradient between the cranial cavity and the spine that essentially sucks the contents of the posterior fossa down into the cervical spinal canal to establish an acquired CM1. From a hydrodynamic standpoint, spontaneous intracranial hypotension is very similar to the physiological state of the patient with a valveless lumboperitoneal shunt, another clinical setting in which acquisition of CM1 has been described. The diagnosis of spontaneous intracranial hypotension is confirmed by myelography or by radionuclide CSF cisternography, and it is treated by surgical obliteration of the dural CSF fistula.

Symptoms and Signs

Chiari malformation type 1 can cause symptoms either by compression of neural structures by the displaced cerebellar tonsils or by damage to spinal cord tissue by syringomyelia. The possibilities are legion. Box 18-1 lists symptoms that can be caused by, or have been attributed to, tonsillar compression of the cervicomedullary junction. Box 18-2 lists symptoms that can be caused by syringomyelia. A moment's reflection will show that many of the symptoms on these lists are nonspecific in the sense that they have other, more common explanations. Hence the primary clinical challenge in the management of CM1: to determine whether the imaging findings are really responsible for the presenting symptoms.

The question of headache deserves special attention, because headache is by far the most frequent indication for the MRI that discloses previously unsuspected CM1. Typical is a headache at the nape of the neck occurring in brief paroxysms precipitated by coughing, laughter, vigorous physical exercise, or straining to defecate. The patient's description is not often as

---

Box 18-1. Symptoms of Cerebellar Tonsillar Compression of the Cervicomedullary Junction

Headache

Neck pain

Inconsolable crying

Torticollis

Dysphagia, feeding difficulties; failure to thrive

Dysphonia

Sleep-disordered breathing

Abnormalities of ocular motility, especially downbeat nystagmus

Scoliosis

Gait disturbance

Impairment of limb, especially hand, movements

---

crisp as the textbook's, but location over the posterior aspect of the head and neck and exacerbation by Valsalva—especially by cough—are salient features that are useful to distinguish pain related to CM1 from other much more common headache patterns. The spectrum of symptoms among children old enough to give a history is not dissimilar from adults. The addition of dizziness or syncope to posterior headache enhances the specificity of the association with CM1. The mechanism for the production of pain is hypothesized to be abnormally large and abnormally sustained pressure differences between the cranial cavity and the spinal canal caused by the obstruction of the craniospinal junction by the displaced cerebellar tonsils. Of course patients with CM1 can be expected to have ordinary migraine and tension headaches at the same prevalence as the general population. McGirt and associates have found prognostic value in measurements of CSF flow at the craniocervical junction by cine MRI. In these studies, patients with typical headache patterns commonly had abnormal CSF flow, and patients with abnormal flow were much more likely to obtain symptom relief from craniocervical decompression than patients with normal flow. These authors mentioned occasional, exceptional patients with abnormal CSF flow but atypical frontal headaches who nevertheless benefited from surgery.

There is growing awareness of the possibility of symptomatic CM1 among preverbal children. The first descriptions of this phenomenon

---

Box 18-2. Symptoms of Syringomyelia

Neck or back pain

Paresthesia in limbs or trunk

Pain in limbs or trunk

Loss of sensation in limbs or trunk

Impairment of limb, especially hand, movements

Muscle wasting, especially the intrinsic muscles of the hands

Gait disturbance

Scoliosis

Incontinence or other disturbance of bladder function

Disturbance of sexual function

---

featured reports of infants with otherwise unexplained paroxysms of extreme irritability, crying, and other pain behavior who were eventually determined to have CM1 and were treated surgically with success. Greenlee and associates reported 16 patients younger than 3 years who came to medical attention predominantly with oropharyngeal dysfunction, by which was meant feeding disorders, failure to thrive, aspiration, dysphonia, and sleep-disturbed breathing. Several patients had undergone gastrostomy and fundoplication prior to recognition of CM1. Nearly all of these patients were treated surgically, with relief of presenting complaints in more than 90% of cases and with no permanent surgical morbidity. As is true for so many facets of current understanding of CM1, there is limited documentation of the natural history of Chiari-associated, early childhood oropharyngeal dysfunction. The author of this chapter has seen several young children with sufficiently troublesome symptoms to have been subjected to MRI by their primary physicians whose syndromes nevertheless resolved without treatment before additional diagnostic investigations could be completed and before surgery could be scheduled. Current published data do not provide useful guidance about which children with oropharyngeal dysfunction should be evaluated.

The classical clinical syndrome attributed to syringomyelia relates closely to the basic neuroanatomy of the spinal cord. A syrinx in the lower cervical region, for instance, might be expected to cause lower motor neuron signs in the upper limbs, such as weakness and atrophy of the intrinsic muscles of the hands, and upper motor neuron signs in the lower limbs, such as spasticity and a so-called dissociated sensory deficit in a cape-like distribution over the shoulders and upper limbs corresponding to the involved cervical segments. The dissociation is among sensory modalities—crossing fibers mediating pain and temperature sensation being destroyed by central spinal cord cavitation with sparing of uncrossed fibers mediating proprioceptive sensation that ascend in the posterior columns. The classical concept is virtually never realized among children. By far the most common presentation of syringomyelia in childhood is scoliosis, which presumably relates to disturbed axial muscle tone corresponding to cavitation in the central gray matter of the thoracic and lumbar segments. Careful neurologic examination sometimes discloses focal, most often lateralized or asymmetrical neurologic signs, such as foot deformity or asymmetry, ankle instability, leg muscle atrophy, reflex asymmetry, an abnormal plantar response, or missing superficial abdominal reflexes, but focal neurologic deficits are very seldom symptomatic. These lateralized neurologic signs can sometimes be correlated with high-quality MRI of the spinal cord, which may show asymmetrical cavitation of the central gray matter on the side of greater involvement.

Natural History

Although CM1 and syringomyelia have been known as autopsy findings since the 19th century, they both remained very obscure from a clinical standpoint well into the last decade of the 20th century. As noted in the introduction, MRI has essentially overwritten all previous knowledge of both conditions, but even with access to the most detailed and effortless imaging technology, passage of time is necessary for acquisition of an understanding of natural history. Our notions of the natural history of CM1 and syringomyelia are still preliminary.

Before MRI, only patients with the most troublesome symptoms were subjected to radiologic investigation, but since MRI has become so widely available, a substantial prevalence of patients with asymptomatic CM1 has been recognized in the general population, as high as 1.1 per 1,000 in the study of Meadows et al. Although there is a case report literature describing both spontaneous progression and spontaneous regression, the degree of displacement of the cerebellar tonsils seems to remain relatively stable in most instances. Whether—or at what rate—asymptomatic patients become symptomatic later in life is entirely unknown.

Another small set of case reports has raised the disturbing possibility that patients with CM1 may be at risk for sudden death or quadriplegia after minor trauma. Such cases must be very infrequent, but because they are so sensational, they are very likely to stimulate the writing of manuscripts. The risk may be small but real, or the apparent risk may be an artifact of publication bias. The experiences reported are so few that there has been no meaningful analysis of predisposing factors, although the tightness of the impaction of the tonsils in the upper cervical spinal canal, deformity of the odontoid process and other associated skeletal anomalies, and latent cranio-cervical instability are all likely possibilities. Concern for the potential for catastrophic disability after minor trauma to the head or neck weighs heavily on recommendations about the safety of activities such as football and soccer. In the absence of guidance from the literature, a cautious judgment based on careful analysis of the patient's clinical presentation and imaging findings qualified by a frank explanation of the risk and the uncertainty is the best that a physician can offer.

Many questions about the natural history of syringomyelia remain unanswered as well. The prevalence of asymptomatic syringomyelia in the general population is unknown. In the work of Meadows et al, among 22,591 MRIs of the head and neck and among 25 cases of asymptomatic CM1, there was only one example of asymptomatic syringomyelia. The fraction of the imaging study set that included the entire cervical spine was not stated, and images of the thoracic spine were not reviewed. The burden of consultations for incidentally discovered, asymptomatic syringomyelia in a pediatric neurosurgical practice is certainly greater than reflected in the report by Meadows et al.

For purposes of prognostication and management, distinctions are made among syringes based on axial dimensions (ie, width, breadth, and the degree to which they expand the profile of the spinal cord). Intuitively, a 2-mm cavity in the center of an otherwise normal appearing spinal cord seems less threatening than a distended 10-mm cavity surrounded by an attenuated rim of stretched spinal cord tissue. Indeed, among adult patients who come to surgical treatment at least, the presence of a large, distended syrinx cavity is associated with brief duration of rapidly progressive symptoms. Thin, slit-like syringes deserve special mention because they are believed to represent persistence of the central canal of the spinal cord. They are infrequently seen in association with CM1 or any other recognized cause of syringomyelia, and they are static over years of follow-up. Holly and Batzdorf warn that the discovery of a slit-like syrinx must not be accepted as the end point of an investigation, because 16 of their 32 patients were later determined to have other, specific medical diagnoses responsible for the symptoms that served as the indications for MRI. In confirmation of the benign nature of slit-like syrinx cavities, there is evidence that symptomatic, distended syringes do not develop from slits; rather, the pre-syrinx state is characterized by expansion of the spinal cord and diffuse, intrinsic magnetic resonance signal intensity changes that precede the coalescence of actual cavities. In the pediatric setting, the slit-like syrinx most often presents in the course of imaging evaluation of scoliosis. It must not be considered the cause of the scoliosis. It may represent a minor, inconsequential anomaly that shares an underlying developmental etiology with the scoliosis, or it may be genuinely incidental.

Because the diagnosis is easy and the surgical treatment is straightforward, the natural history of symptomatic but untreated syringomyelia is never witnessed in contemporary practice, but the classical descriptions indicate that it is slowly but relentlessly disabling, often in a stepwise pattern resembling demyelinating disease. In some instances sudden deterioration seems to be precipitated by straining, as though abdominal pressure is transmitted to the spinal canal and squeezing of the syrinx cavity causes it to rupture into previously uninvolved segments of the spinal cord. For this reason, patients with significant syrinx cavities are often counseled not to lift weights or wrestle. There is, however, uncertainty whether asymptomatic, incidentally discovered syringomyelia associated with CM1 pursues a similar course. Evidence is scant. Nishizawa et al described 9 such patients, all adults, who were followed with periodic clinical assessments and surveillance MRI. Only one patient developed neurologic symptoms and required surgical intervention, at 7 years. The remaining 8 patients were stable from clinical and imaging standpoints for more than 10 years. No similar experience with long-term observation of children has been reported. Many surgeons view distended syrinx cavities as reflecting a potentially irreversible destructive process, and the threshold for recommending surgical intervention is low.

Management

As the preceding discussion makes plain, there are important gaps in our understanding of CM1, but decisions about management of this condition must be made nevertheless. When knowledge is incomplete, physicians must feel their way based on reasoning and experience, and variation of practice from physician to physician is great. What follows is a description of this writer's perspective on the most important management questions. The reader must understand that at almost every point a contradictory opinion might be found either in the published medical literature or at the offices of other neurosurgical practitioners. Hopefully, as medical knowledge advances, this document will require revision soon to reflect growing consensus about the most critical matters.

Because of the association of CM1 with both hydrocephalus and syringomyelia, every patient deserves complete imaging of the brain and spine before treatment decisions can be addressed. About 10% of patients with CM1 have associated hydrocephalus, and treatment of CM1 must not be undertaken without preceding or simultaneous treatment of the hydrocephalus.

When the relationship of symptoms to CM1 is clear, and when symptoms are intolerable, the indication for treatment is indisputable. If symptoms are mild, and, in this writer's view, if there is no syringomyelia, a decision about treatment may be deferred safely in favor of clinical and imaging observation. If the relationship of symptoms to CM1 is not certain, judgment is required. Most often the symptom that creates such a degree of uncertainty is headache. Qualities that distinguish headaches caused by CM1—and therefore likely to be relieved by surgery—from other more common headaches have been discussed. A vigorous attempt at pharmacologic control of symptoms under the supervision of a pediatric neurologist is appropriate in most cases. For medically intractable and disabling headaches, surgical treatment may be considered.

The child with CM1 and syringomyelia at the time of diagnosis deserves special consideration. There is little disagreement that surgical treatment is indicated for the child with scoliosis, neurologic disabilities, or neuropathic pain. The question of asymptomatic syringomyelia is more problematic. The markedly distinct implications of prominence of the central canal and distention of an asymptomatic syrinx cavity have been discussed. Some surgeons withhold treatment unless symptoms develop or unless there is imaging evidence of expansion of the syrinx cavity. Other authorities view syringomyelia as a destructive and progressive process. Although long periods of clinical stability are common, eventual neurologic losses are the expectation, and such losses are not necessarily reversible by subsequent treatment.

If treatment is deferred, the patient deserves surveillance for the development of new symptoms and disabilities and for the development or progression of syringomyelia. As the long-term natural history of syringomyelia has been documented so poorly, the schedule for follow-up must be a matter of judgment based on the severity of the CM1 and the age of the patient. Magnetic resonance imaging of the cervical spine is the appropriate surveillance study for the development of syringomyelia. Surveillance imaging of the head is not necessary. Imaging surveillance does not need to be as frequent as office assessment, and the interval between encounters can be lengthened gradually if the patient remains stable.

A vexing question is whether the child with untreated CM1 should be subjected to restrictions of activity. The concern about sudden death or catastrophic paralysis after minor injury has been discussed previously. Judgment must be based on the severity of the CM1 on MRI and on the presence or absence of associated skeletal anomalies at the craniocervical junction. The nature of the activity must be weighed as well. The inclination of most pediatric neurosurgeons is to encourage vigorous physical activity, including participation in athletics, but collision sports may be unwise for the child with a severe malformation. If particular clinical circumstances do not indicate a firm proscription of activities, the physician must transfer responsibility to the patient and the family by a thorough and well-documented sharing of the current state of knowledge. Directors of high school and college athletic programs may sometimes request written assurance that the child with CM1 is at no greater risk of injury than any other child. Effectively, what they are asking is that the physician's malpractice carrier indemnify their athletic program against claims arising from Chiari-related injuries. Compliance with such requests is impossible. Chiari malformation type 1 complicated by syringomyelia is a special case. Patients should refrain from weight lifting and wrestling because of theoretical concerns, reinforced by anecdotal reports, about rupture and extension of the syrinx cavity precipitated by straining.

Surgery

The goal of surgery is to relieve compression of the brain stem and the spinal cord by the displaced cerebellum and to restore CSF pulsation back and forth across the craniocervical junction. Many variations of surgical technique have been described, and no 2 techniques have ever been compared in a credibly controlled fashion. The common first step is to remove the posterior rim of the foramen magnum together with variable portions of the squamous occipital bone and the posterior arch of the atlas. Beyond this point, surgical practices diverge with regard to whether to open the dura; whether to resect or coagulate the tips of the cerebellar tonsils; whether to inspect, open, or stent the foramen of Magendie; and whether or how to close the dura. The cerebellum, the medulla, and the spinal cord can be examined by ultrasound through the dura after removal of the overlying bone, and some surgeons base decisions about subsequent surgical maneuvers on the appearance of the subarachnoid spaces and the pulsatile motion of the tonsils.

The risk of neurologic complications of the surgical treatment of CM1 is extremely low, but wound complications can be troublesome. The disturbances of CSF circulation that accompany CM1 can lead to development of a tense, painful pseudomeningocele at the surgical site that may threaten the integrity of the closure. Reexploration of the wound or insertion of a CSF shunt may be necessary. The risk of deep infection is less than 1%, but more frequently observed is a syndrome of headache, fever, nausea, and nuchal rigidity with sterile CSF cultures—so-called chemical meningitis. This syndrome must be managed with non-narcotic analgesics, steroids, and reassurance, because it may persist for days to weeks. Bacterial meningitis, chemical meningitis, and postoperative, posterior fossa subdural hygromas can precipitate hydrocephalus. Except in cases of skeletal dysostosis associated with anomalous cranial venous drainage, such as Crouzon or Pfeiffer syndrome, transfusion is almost never necessary.

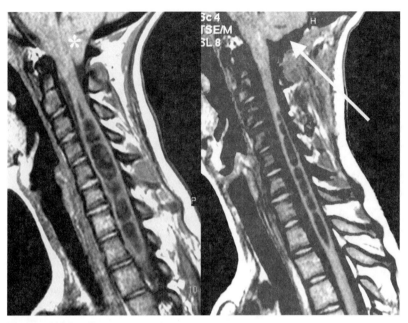

Figure 18-4.
Preoperative (left) and postoperative (right) sagittal, T1-weighted magnetic resonance images of the cervical spine show a typical syrinx regression after decompression of the craniocervical junction for Chiari malformation type 1. The syrinx is still visible, but it no longer distends the spinal cord. Before surgery the tonsils were tapered and protruded below the arch of the atlas (white asterisk). After surgery, which included bipolar coagulation of the pia-arachnoid of the tonsils, they have retracted into the posterior fossa (white arrow).

The results of surgery for CM1 are directly related to the duration of symptoms and the objectivity of the indications for treatment. Perhaps the most objective indication for treatment is the association of a syrinx with CM1. Craniocervical decompression effects a decrease in syrinx volume (Figure 18-4) or complete disappearance in roughly 80% of cases. Neurologic symptoms and signs of acute or subacute onset respond at a similar rate, but long-standing disabilities can only be stabilized, not reversed. Mild and moderate degrees of scoliosis usually are stabilized and occasionally improve, but scoliosis that is severe at presentation often progresses to require instrumented fusion despite successful treatment of the underlying syringomyelia. The course of neuropathic pain—a very poorly understood phenomenon fortunately uncommon among pediatric patients—is impossible to predict. It can persist or even progress in the face of an excellent imaging result. Symptoms and signs that are clearly related to cervicomedullary compression, such as dysphonia, dysphagia, sleep-disordered breathing, and quadriparesis, tend to respond in relation to their preoperative duration. Although CM1 by itself can cause cervicomedullary compression, such syndromes are seen more commonly in the setting of craniovertebral junction anomalies, such as basilar invagination, which combine ventral osseous compressive lesions with the dorsal tonsilar compression of CM1. In distinction from such objective presentations, relief of headache is much more difficult to predict. As a generalization, the likelihood of relief from decompression depends on the degree to which the patient's headache resembles the sharp, brief, posterior craniocervical pain precipitated by cough, laughter, straining, or exertion that typifies CM1. Other headache patterns respond variably to surgery. As mentioned previously, cine MRI of CSF flow patterns at the craniocervical junction may be a useful guide to treatment.

Even if it successfully relieves all symptoms, surgical treatment for CM1 should not be considered a cure, especially if there is associated syringomyelia. The long-term outlook for treated patients is really not known. Periodic neurosurgical reassessment and, at the surgeon's discretion, periodic MRI are appropriate to monitor for complications.

Bibliography

Pathophysiology

Ball MJ, Dayan AD. Pathogenesis of syringomyelia. *Lancet.* 1972;2:799–801

Caldemeyer KS, Boaz JC, Wappner RS, Moran CC, Smith RR, Quets JP. Chiari I malformation: association with hypophosphatemic rickets and MR imaging appearance. *Radiology* 1995;195:733–738

Fagan LH, Ferguson S, Yassari R, Frim DM. The Chiari pseudotumor cerebri syndrome: symptom recurrence after decompressive surgery for Chiari malformation type I. *Pediatr Neurosurg.* 2006;42:14–19

Karahalios DG, Rekate HL, Khayata MH, Apostolides PJ. Elevated intracranial venous pressure as a universal mechanism in pseudotumor cerebri of varying etiologies. *Neurology.* 1996;46:198–202

Oldfield EH, Muraszko K, Shawker TH, Patronas NJ. Pathophysiology of syringomyelia associated with Chiari I malformation of the cerebellar tonsils. Implications for diagnosis and treatment. *J Neurosurg.* 1994;80:3–151

Pollack IF, Losken HW, Biglan AW. Incidence of increased intracranial pressure after early surgical treatment of syndromic craniosynostosis. *Pediatr Neurosurg.* 1996;24:202–209

Sgouros S, Kountouri M, Natarajan K. Posterior fossa volume in children with Chiari malformation type I. *J Neurosurg.* 2006;105:101–106

Tubbs RS, Webb D, Abdullatif H, Conklin M, Doyle S, Oakes WJ. Posterior cranial fossa volume in patients with rickets: insights into the increased occurrence of Chiari I malformation in metabolic bone disease. *Neurosurgery.* 2004;55:380–383

Williams B. Cerebrospinal fluid pressure-gradients in spina bifida cystica, with special reference to the Arnold-Chiari malformation and aqueductal stenosis. *Dev Med Child Neurol Suppl.* 1975:138–150

Williams B. Simultaneous cerebral and spinal fluid pressure recordings. 2. Cerebrospinal dissociation with lesions at the foramen magnum. *Acta Neurochir (Wien).* 1981;59:123–142

Headache and Other Presentations

Gagnadoux F, Meslier N, Svab I, Menei P, Racineux JL. Sleep-disordered breathing in patients with Chiari malformation: improvement after surgery. *Neurology.* 2006;66:136–138

Greenlee JD, Donovan KA, Hasan DM, Menezes AH. Chiari I malformation in the very young child: the spectrum of presentations and experience in 31 children under age 6 years. *Pediatrics.* 2002;110:1212–1219

Hudgins RJ. Paroxysmal rage as a presenting symptom of the Chiari I malformation. Report of two cases. *J Neurosurg.* 1999;91:328–329

McGirt MJ, Nimjee SM, Floyd J, Bulsara KR, George TM. Correlation of cerebrospinal fluid flow dynamics and headache in Chiari I malformation. *Neurosurgery.* 2005;56:716–721

McGirt MJ, Nimjee SM, Fuchs HE, George TM. Relationship of cine phase-contrast magnetic resonance imaging with outcome after decompression for Chiari I malformations. *Neurosurgery.* 2006;59:140–146

Nightingale S, Williams B. Hindbrain hernia headache. *Lancet.* 1987;1:731–734

Pascual J, Oterino A, Berciano J. Headache in type I Chiari malformation. *Neurology.* 1992;42:1519–1521

Sansur CA, Heiss JD, DeVroom HL, Eskioglu E, Ennis R, Oldfield EH. Pathophysiology of headache associated with cough in patients with Chiari I malformation. *J Neurosurg.* 2003;98:453–458

Stovner LJ. Headache associated with the Chiari type I malformation. *Headache.* 1993;33: 175–181

Acquired Chiari Malformation

Atkinson JL, Weinshenker BG, Miller GM, Piepgras DG, Mokri B. Acquired Chiari I malformation secondary to spontaneous spinal cerebrospinal fluid leakage and chronic intracranial hypotension syndrome in seven cases. *J Neurosurg.* 1998;88:237–242

Johnston I, Jacobson E, Besser M. The acquired Chiari malformation and syringomyelia following spinal CSF drainage: a study of incidence and management. *Acta Neurochir (Wien).* 1998;140:417–427

Mokri B, Piepgras DG, Miller GM. Syndrome of orthostatic headaches and diffuse pachymeningeal gadolinium enhancement. *Mayo Clin Proc.* 1997;72:400–413

Payner TD, Prenger E, Berger TS, Crone KR. Acquired Chiari malformations: incidence, diagnosis, and management. *Neurosurgery.* 1994;34:429–434

Susceptibility to Neurologic Catastrophe

Bondurant CP, Oro JJ. Spinal cord injury without radiographic abnormality and Chiari malformation. *J Neurosurg.* 1993;79:833–838

Bunc G, Vorsic M. Presentation of a previously asymptomatic Chiari I malformation by a flexion injury to the neck. *J Neurotrauma.* 2001;18:645–648

Callaway GH, O'Brien SJ, Tehrany AM. Chiari I malformation and spinal cord injury: cause for concern in contact athletes? *Med Sci Sports Exerc.* 1996;28:1218–1220

Couldwell WT, Zhang W, Allen R, Arce D, Stillerman CB. Cerebellar contusion associated with type I Chiari malformation following supratentorial head trauma: case report. *Neurol Res.* 1998;20:93–96

Erlich V, Snow R, Heier L. Confirmation by magnetic resonance imaging of bell's cruciate paralysis in a young child with Chiari type I malformation and minor head trauma. *Neurosurgery.* 1989;25:102–105

Martinot A, Hue V, Leclerc F, Vallee L, Closset M, Pruvo JP. Sudden death revealing Chiari type 1 malformation in two children. *Intensive Care Med.* 1993;19:73–74

Murano T, Rella J. Incidental finding of Chiari I malformation with progression of symptoms after head trauma: case report. *J Emerg Med.* 2006;30:295–298

Quebada PB, Duhaime AC. Chiari malformation type I and a dolichoodontoid process responsible for sudden cardiorespiratory arrest. Case report. *J Neurosurg.* 2005;103:567–570

Riviello JJ Jr, Marks HG, Faerber EN, Steg NL. Delayed cervical central cord syndrome after trivial trauma. *Pediatr Emerg Care.* 1990;6:113–117

Tomaszek DE, Tyson GW, Bouldin T, Hansen AR. Sudden death in a child with an occult hindbrain malformation. *Ann Emerg Med.* 1984;13:136–138

Vlcek BW, Ito B. Acute paraparesis secondary to Arnold-Chiari type I malformation and neck hyperflexion. *Ann Neurol.* 1987;21:100–101

Clinical Pediatric Neurosciences for Primary Care

Ziegler DK, Mallonee W. Chiari-1 malformation, migraine, and sudden death. *Headache.* 1999;39:38–41

Treatment

Alzate JC, Kothbauer KF, Jallo GI, Epstein FJ. Treatment of Chiari I malformation in patients with and without syringomyelia: a consecutive series of 66 cases. *Neurosurg Focus.* 2001;11:e3

Dyste GN, Menezes AH. Presentation and management of pediatric Chiari malformations without myelodysplasia. *Neurosurgery.* 1988;23:589–597

Navarro R, Olavarria G, Seshadri R, Gonzales-Portillo G, McLone DG, Tomita T. Surgical results of posterior fossa decompression for patients with Chiari I malformation. *Childs Nerv Syst.* 2004;20:349–356

Tubbs RS, McGirt MJ, Oakes WJ. Surgical experience in 130 pediatric patients with Chiari I malformations. *J Neurosurg.* 2003;99:291–296

Miscellaneous

Holly LT, Batzdorf U. Slitlike syrinx cavities: a persistent central canal. *J Neurosurg.* 2002;97:161–165

Koehler PJ. Chiari's description of cerebellar ectopy (1891): with a summary of Cleland's and Arnold's contributions and some early observations on neural tube defects. *J Neurosurg.* 1991;75:823–826

Meadows J, Kraut M, Guarnieri M, Haroun RI, Carson BS. Asymptomatic Chiari type I malformations identified on magnetic resonance imaging. *J Neurosurg.* 2000;92:920–926

Milhorat TH, Chou MW, Trinidad EM, et al. Chiari I malformation redefined: clinical and radiographic findings for 364 symptomatic patients. *Neurosurgery.* 1999;44:1005–1017

Nishizawa S, Yokoyama T, Yokota N, Tokuyama T, Ohta S. Incidentally identified syringomyelia associated with Chiari I malformations: is early interventional surgery necessary? *Neurosurgery.* 2001;49:637–640

Chapter 19

Spinal Dysraphism and Neurogenic Bladder Dysfunction

Nathan R. Selden, MD, PhD
R. Guy Hudson, MD
Steven R. Skoog, MD

Introduction

The topics of spinal dysraphism and voiding dysfunction lie at the interface of neurosurgery, urology, and pediatrics, and recent pressure to expand the concept of spinal cord tethering has made mutual understanding among these disciplines critical to the management of a wider spectrum of clinical problems. Virtually all patients with symptomatic spinal dysraphism have some degree of voiding dysfunction, and lately the question has arisen whether some substantial fraction of children with voiding dysfunction may have physiological spinal cord tethering even in the absence of gross anatomical evidence of dysraphism. Although practice patterns for the diagnosis and management of voiding dysfunction in patients with major spinal dysraphism, such as myelomeningocele and lipomyelomeningocele, are well established, evidence and practice guidelines are often lacking. Furthermore, the natural history of more minor forms of dysraphism is poorly understood, and indications for surgery are debated. A familiarity with the physiology and neurology of voiding is essential to contemporary management of the child with spinal dysraphism.

Voiding function is complex and depends on subtle interplay of anatomical, neurologic, psychological, and social factors. Voiding dysfunction may result in significant social and medical disability, including in the worst cases complete renal failure or death. The diagnosis and management of voiding dysfunction often requires specialty expertise. Pediatric urologists and neurosurgeons, as members of an interdisciplinary team, are often called on to diagnose and manage patients with neurogenic voiding dysfunction arising from central or peripheral nervous system abnormalities.

Development of Normal Continence

The neurophysiological mechanisms resulting in urinary continence are complex. These processes result in several observed developmental stages of urinary control. In newborns, micturition is a reflex that can occur 20 or more times per day. Bladder filling to an appropriate degree stimulates the efferent response of detrusor contraction preceded by sphincteric relaxation and bladder emptying. By 6 months of age a noticeable increase in voided volume and decrease of urinary frequency is seen. This is attributed to unconscious inhibition of the voiding reflex. Between 1 and 2 years of age, the child develops a conscious sensation of bladder fullness, which sets the stage for voluntary control of voiding. Volitional voiding and inhibition of voiding at any degree of bladder fullness develops in the second and third years of life. By the age of 4 or 5 years, most children have developed an adult pattern of urinary control. The usual sequence of attainment of bowel and bladder control is (1) nocturnal bowel control, (2) daytime bowel control, (3) daytime urinary control, and (4) nocturnal urinary control. Children between 3 and 12 years of age void 5 to 6 times per day and have a bowel movement each day.

Enuresis in children can be attributed to either non-neurogenic or neurogenic causes. Most non-neurogenic cases reflect a learned behavior that consists of contraction of the external urinary sphincter during voiding. This increase in intravesical pressure can lead to changes in detrusor compliance and function, compromise of the ureterovesical junction, vesicoureteral reflux, and upper urinary tract damage. Although, as the name implies, there is no central or peripheral nervous system etiology, the consequences of unrecognized and untreated dysfunction of the lower urinary tract can mimic the severity of neurologic disease.

Neuroanatomy/Physiology of Continence

The process of normal micturition is dependent on a coordinated interaction between various levels of the central and peripheral nervous systems. The coordinated control of the lower urinary tract results in a low-pressure storage of urine followed by effective bladder emptying.

In the central nervous system (CNS), the most significant area for detrusor control is the superior frontal gyrus. There is evidence that micturition is predominantly controlled by the right side of the brain. The pontine micturition center plays an important role in bladder storage and release by means of coordinated excitatory and inhibitory innervation that maintains bladder and sphincter synergy. Neurons in this center provide direct excitatory synaptic inputs to sacral preganglionic neurons and provide inhibitory innervation to the neurons controlling the external urethral sphincter.

Peripheral neural control of the lower urinary tract involves branches of the parasympathetic, sympathetic, and somatic nerves. The parasympathetic nerves originate in the sacral spinal cord (predominantly S2–S4) with preganglionic neurons located in the sacral parasympathetic nucleus in the intermediolateral column of the gray matter. Usually the innervation of the detrusor and urethra is predominantly S3 in origin; however, S2 and S4 may predominate in some cases. The parasympathetic neural control causes contraction of the detrusor and relaxation of the urethra. Sympathetic innervation originates at the T10–L2 levels of the spinal cord and passes to the sympathetic paraspinal ganglia. These inferior splanchnic nerves travel to the inferior mesenteric ganglia through the hypogastric nerves to the pelvic plexus. The sympathetic nerves cause relaxation of the detrusor and contraction of the bladder neck and urethra and thereby promote urine storage.

The somatic pathway involves activation and relaxation of the striated muscle fibers of the external urethral sphincter. The efferent pathway originates in the Onuf nucleus on the lateral border of the ventral horn of the spinal cord. The external urethral sphincter receives its motor neuron innervation by the pudendal nerve (S2–S4). Micturition involves precise coordination of the central and peripheral, autonomic, and somatic nervous system pathways to achieve normal continence.

Based on an understanding of the relevant neuroanatomy, patterns of bladder and sphincter disturbance can be predicted for various lesions of the nervous system. Lesions typically occur in 1 of 4 areas: peripheral sacral nerves, distal sacral spinal cord, suprasacral spinal cord, or a cerebral location. A lesion involving the peripheral sacral nerves can be expected to cause an underactive or acontractile detrusor, a flaccid sphincter, and impairment of sensation of bladder stimuli. Distal sacral spinal cord lesions cause an underactive or acontractile detrusor, a flaccid sphincter, lost or diminished bulbocavernosus reflexes, loss of perineal sensation, and impairment of sensation of bladder stimuli. Lesions of the brain stem or suprasacral spinal cord are associated initially with a period of spinal shock with suppression of all reflex activity. As spinal shock resolves, there is development of detrusor overactivity and loss of coordination of sphincter and detrusor action, so-called detrusor-sphincter dyssynergia (DSD). Detrusor-sphincter dyssynergia is characterized by involuntary contraction of the detrusor against a contracting external sphincter, and it therefore features sudden surges of intravesical pressure that can cause vesicoureteral reflux and renal damage. Cerebral lesions such as infarction or trauma result in an inability to suppress reflexive voiding with maintenance of normal coordination between detrusor and sphincter activity.

Patterns of Non-Neurogenic Dysfunction of the Lower Urinary Tract

A variety of patterns of dysfunction of the lower urinary tract are demonstrable in children without evidence of neurologic disease. These functional disorders can contribute to significant urologic sequelae including infection, incontinence, and renal compromise. These patterns vary in their clinical significance and include urge syndrome (overactive bladder), dysfunctional voiding, infrequent voiding syndrome, primary bladder neck dysfunction, giggle incontinence, and non-neurogenic neurogenic bladder (Hinman Syndrome) (Table 19-1).

Urge syndrome is characterized by frequent episodes of urgency to void caused by detrusor overactivity during filling. These contractions are involuntary and often countered by contraction of the pelvic floor muscles (guarding reflex) and holding maneuvers to maintain continence. Vincent's curtsy, squatting on the heel of one foot, obstructs the urethra to maintain continence during an involuntary detrusor contraction. Factors including constipation and encopresis can contribute to this syndrome and must be elucidated and treated if present. Urodynamic evaluation confirms bladder instability without evidence of urinary outlet obstruction. Contraction of the bladder against a closed external sphincter (DSD) is not present during the voiding phase of urodynamics.

Classic dysfunction of the lower urinary tract is characterized by an inability to fully relax the external urethral sphincter and/or pelvic muscles during voiding. This results in an abnormal flow pattern consisting of

Table 19-1. Patterns of Non-Neurogenic Dysfunction of the Lower Urinary Tract in Children

Type	Voiding Characteristics	Ultrasound Findings	Urodynamic Findings
Urge syndrome	Urgency, holding maneuvers	Normal	Bladder instability without outflow obstruction or DSD
Dysfunction of the lower tract	Interrupted urinary stream	Normal to thickened detrusor Increased post-void residual Hydronephrosis	Variation of bladder capacity Changes in bladder contractility DSD
Infrequent voiding syndrome (lazy bladder syndrome)	Infrequent voiding with variable pattern	Large, non-thickened bladder No hydronephrosis	Normal compliance Large capacity No outflow obstruction
Primary bladder neck dysfunction	Urgency, frequency Decreased force of stream Occasional dysuria, pelvic pain	Usually normal	Decreased flow rate Delayed bladder neck opening in voiding phase
Giggle incontinence	Incontinence with laughing	Normal	Normal
Non-neurogenic neurogenic bladder (Hinman syndrome)	Diurnal and nocturnal enuresis Recurrent UTIs Variable voiding pattern	Thickened bladder Possible bladder diverticula Hydronephrosis/ hydroureter	Decreased volume Decreased compliance Detrusor instability Increased PVR DSD Low/intermittent flow rate Increased voiding pressure Functional bladder outlet obstruction

Abbreviations: DSD, detrusor-sphincter dyssynergy; UTI, urinary tract infection; PVR, post-void residual.

staccato or interrupted voiding. These patients often present with recurrent urinary tract infections, incontinence, and constipation or encopresis. Ultrasound of the bladder can demonstrate a thickened detrusor and increased post-void residual along with potential upper tract changes, including hydronephrosis. These patients can show evidence of a small bladder capacity, decreased detrusor contractility, and impaired relaxation of the external urethral sphincter.

Infrequent voiding syndrome, also known as *lazy bladder syndrome* or *underactive detrusor,* is a spectrum of disorders ranging from infrequent voiding to bladder decompensation and may represent a latter stage of dysfunction of the lower urinary tract. Patients are usually dry at night, do not void on awakening, void infrequently during the day, and notably have issues with fecal retention. These patients have a large bladder capacity with normal compliance and lack normal detrusor contraction with micturition. Ultrasound demonstrates a large non-thickened bladder with no evidence of hydronephrosis. Often urodynamic evaluation is helpful to exclude an underlying neurologic or obstructive diagnosis. Behavioral training and bladder rehabilitation with a frequent voiding program and treatment of constipation are usually successful.

Primary bladder neck dysfunction is more often diagnosed in young adult males with lower urinary tract symptoms. Symptoms of urinary frequency, urgency, decreased force of urinary stream, incomplete emptying, dysuria or pelvic pain with voiding, and diurnal or nocturnal enuresis are the various manifestations of this disorder. Urodynamic evaluation demonstrates delayed or incomplete bladder neck opening during the voiding phase and a decreased urinary flow rate. Treatment with alpha-blockers has been shown to decrease outlet resistance and improve urinary flow rates.

Giggle incontinence was first described in 1964 by MacKeith and further by Williams in 1984. Giggle incontinence is more common in girls, and there is some evidence of inheritance. Although the exact etiology is unknown, several theories have been put forward. It is postulated that laughter may induce urethral relaxation by creating a generalized hypotonic state. It is also postulated that laughter may activate the micturition reflex by overriding central inhibitory mechanisms. History establishes the diagnosis, and radiographic imaging is not routinely used in the absence of urinary infection. Treatment initially consists of a voiding program designed to empty the bladder prior to an inciting event. Stimulants, such as methylphenidate, have been tried with some success.

Non-neurogenic neurogenic bladder, or Hinman syndrome, was first formally described by Hinman and Allen in 1971 and reviewed by Hinman in 1986. Initially thought related to an acquired personality disorder or stressful family environment, this syndrome may be the end stage of dysfunction of the lower urinary tract. Some authors believe it represents a voluntary dyssynergia between the striated muscle of the external urinary sphincter and detrusor during voiding. This creates high voiding pressures due to a functional outlet obstruction. These patients typically present with diurnal and nocturnal enuresis, recurrent urinary tract infections, variable voiding patterns, and fecal elimination issues. Physical and neurologic examinations are normal. Radiographic evaluation demonstrates evidence of a thickened, nonspherical bladder with evidence of diverticula formation with no evidence of an anatomical obstruction. Severe hydroureteronephrosis on renal ultrasound and renal insufficiency can be present in the latter stages of this syndrome. One-half will have vesicoureteral reflux. Urodynamic evaluation reveals a decrease in bladder volume and bladder compliance with evidence of detrusor instability, low or intermittent flow rate, an increase in voiding pressures, an increase in residual volume, and contraction of the pelvic floor muscles, which creates a functional outlet obstruction during voiding. Treatment is individualized to the patient but is often similar to those patients with true neurogenic bladder. Behavioral modification, biofeedback, restoration of normal bowel function, pharmacologic therapy, psychological counseling, and clean intermittent catheterization can be involved in the treatment regimen of these patients. These patients need to be followed closely given the increased risk of upper urinary tract compromise. The voiding issues often continue into adulthood requiring continued care.

Patterns of Neurogenic Voiding Dysfunction

Normal voiding is dependent on the functional coordination of the detrusor, bladder neck, and external sphincter mechanisms. A lesion at any level of the nervous system can lead to an abnormality of coordination among these mechanisms. The most common etiology of neuropathic bladder dysfunction in children is abnormal development of the spinal cord. Neurogenic bladder dysfunction in such children presents with various patterns of detrusor-sphincter dysfunction with a wide range of severity. Spinal dysraphism, including abnormalities of the filum terminale, lipomyelomeningocele, myelomeningocele, and various forms of caudal regression sequence, may cause tethered cord syndrome and be associated with neurogenic voiding dysfunction. Neurogenic bladder may also result from acquired conditions, including cerebral palsy, multiple sclerosis, tumors, spinal cord trauma or infection, vascular malformations of the spinal cord, or iatrogenic trauma to the pelvic plexus. Various other congenital malformations may also be associated with tethering or abnormal spinal cord function, including sacral agenesis, imperforate anus, cloacal malformations, and OEIS syndrome (omphalocele, bladder extrophy, imperforate anus, and sacral anomaly).

In children with spinal cord maldevelopment, such as myelomeningocele, bladder function cannot be reliably determined from the level of the malformation. After initial neurosurgical intervention to close the defect, a period of spinal shock is quite common, characterized by an areflexic detrusor requiring intermittent catheterization that may last for days to weeks. Baseline radiographic studies are obtained initially in all patients: a renal/bladder ultrasound and voiding cystourethrogram (VCUG). Hydronephrosis can be demonstrated in 7% to 30% with ultrasound, and up to 20% of newborns have vesicoureteral reflux on initial VCUG. Most patients have videourodynamic evaluation after the period of spinal shock has subsided to determine potential risk of upper tract deterioration and need for clean intermittent catheterization (usually 2–3 months). All radiographic procedures and clinical interventions should use latex-free products given the increased incidence of latex sensitivity or allergy, which is sometimes congenital.

Patients with neurogenic bladder dysfunction due to a spinal cord lesion can be categorized as high and low risk based on urodynamic assessment. High-risk patients demonstrate a detrusor leak point pressure greater than 40 cm H_2O on urodynamic testing. This high leak point pressure is believed to be related to fixed outlet resistance due to denervation of the external sphincter mechanism. The resultant functional bladder outlet obstruction causes increased intravesical pressure, decreased bladder compliance with subsequent decrease in bladder capacity, and upper tract changes.

Investigation of Bladder Function

All children who present with evidence of dysfunction of the lower urinary tract should undergo a comprehensive clinical history, physical examination, and review of a voiding diary. The goal is to distinguish functional enuresis from anatomical and neurogenic incontinence. The clinical history should include a thorough voiding history with attention to development of urinary and fecal continence, current voiding patterns, timing of incontinence, and any potential of neurologic disease. A voiding diary is used to document frequency of voids, timing and amount of incontinence episodes, and demonstration of dry periods. Appropriate accomplishment of developmental milestones should also be noted. Most parents have limited knowledge of their child's bowel and voiding habits. Hence a voiding diary is a critical component of a comprehensive evaluation.

Some patients with non-neurogenic bladder dysfunction and all patients with neurogenic bladder dysfunction require imaging of the urinary tract. The goals of imaging are to evaluate the morphology and function of the upper urinary tract and to evaluate the bladder.

Renal bladder ultrasound is a noninvasive imaging technique that provides anatomical information about the upper and lower urinary tract. It provides good visualization of the renal parenchyma, collecting system, and bladder in most cases. It offers the advantages of lack of radiation and portability, and it can be administered without sedation in children. Length and growth of the renal parenchyma can be determined and followed over time. Doppler evaluation of the vasculature of the kidneys can be performed without the use of intravenous contrast. Although this imaging technique does not provide functional information regarding the upper urinary tract, it is a first-line imaging technique for children with functional or neurologic causes of incontinence.

A VCUG is an integral part of evaluation of children with a suspected bladder or urethral abnormality. Although invasive, it provides anatomical information of the lower urinary tract and is the best test to evaluate for vesicoureteral reflux. The initial scout radiograph can also reveal evidence of a bony spinal abnormality, stone disease, or fecal elimination disorder. Examination of the physiological appearance of the bladder, bladder neck, and urethra can be demonstrated during bladder filling and voiding.

However, radiation exposure, risk of urinary infection, and potential contrast reactions do exist with this modality.

The most thorough test in the evaluation of incontinence with a suspected neurologic component is urodynamics. This procedure requires the use of a urinary catheter, rectal balloon catheter, and monitoring of the external urethral sphincter by patch or needle electrodes. Sensate children usually require either the use of topical anesthetic prior to catheter placement or sedation. Urodynamics can be performed in the office setting with or without the use of fluoroscopy. The urodynamic evaluation consists of several steps designed to give a complete picture of bladder and urethral function.

Filling cystometry measures the pressure/volume relationship of the bladder during filling. Intravesical pressure, abdominal pressure, and detrusor pressure are recorded. Electromyography is performed simultaneously. A physiological fill rate with warmed normal saline is used. Bladder sensation during the filling process is recorded. Simultaneous recording of these parameters allows a complete evaluation of bladder filling.

After bladder filling, the voiding phase is recorded. Patch or needle electrodes indicate proper relaxation of the external sphincter mechanism during this phase. Improper relaxation of this mechanism indicates DSD.

Voiding pressure monitoring can indicate a normal bell-shaped voiding pattern, a plateau pattern consistent with outlet obstruction, or an intermittent pattern usually in association with DSD. Bladder compliance is measured; a normal value is greater than or equal to 20 mL/cm H_2O. Urethral pressure profiles are measured in some cases.

Innervation of the external urethral sphincter can vary widely in children with neurogenic bladder and can evolve over time. Up to one-third of patients experience a change in innervation of the external sphincter in the first 3 years of life. Hence frequent monitoring of the upper tracts with ultrasound is critical in patients with neurogenic bladder. Hydronephrosis can indicate an early change in intravesical pressure and appropriate intervention can prevent upper tract compromise.

Abnormal urodynamic criteria suggestive of potential neurologic disease includes low total bladder volume (less than two-thirds of the expected bladder volume for age), abnormal bladder compliance, evidence of detrusor hyperreflexia or instability, and abnormal bladder sensation.

Behavioral and Pharmacologic Management of Voiding Dysfunction

The goal of urologic management in children with dysfunction of the lower urinary tract is preservation of renal function. Other goals include social continence, control of infection, and normal storage and passage of urine. The mainstay of treatment for most non-neurologic incontinence due to voiding dysfunction is behavioral modification. Motivational therapy, consisting of positive reinforcement and active patient involvement, is important for success. Initially, prior to the introduction of pharmacologic therapy, most patients are placed on a voiding schedule every 2 to 3 hours. Other changes in lifestyle, including dietary modification and good personal hygiene habits, are emphasized.

Biofeedback treatment is based on the recognition and correction of the poor coordination between the bladder and sphincter complex. The goal is to teach voluntary control of tone in the striated muscle of the pelvic floor. Electromyographic activity in the pelvic floor is transformed electronically into video images or sounds that the child can learn to manipulate. This method of therapy requires a motivated and cooperative child, and success rates range between 50% and 87%.

Pharmacologic treatment in patients with dysfunction of the lower urinary tract is based on the central and peripheral nervous system interactions that control bladder storage, bladder emptying, and sphincter function. In children with bladder overactivity (non-neurogenic etiology) or bladder hyperreflexia (neurogenic etiology), the pharmacologic treatment primarily involves the suppression of bladder contractility, the increase of bladder capacity, and/or the increase in outlet resistance. Bladder contraction is predominantly under the control of the parasympathetic nervous system, which acts through muscarinic cholinergic receptor sites on bladder smooth muscle. Muscarinic receptor subtypes M1–M3 have been identified. The M2 receptors are the most prevalent, but the M3 receptors are primarily responsible for the mediation of bladder contraction. Hence anticholinergic medications and, to a lesser degree, alpha-blockers are the most common medications used for children with dysfunction of the lower urinary tract (Table 19-2). The goals of anticholinergic therapy include an increase in functional bladder capacity and a decrease in bladder overactivity. These

Table 19-2. Medications for the Treatment of Dysfunction of the Lower Urinary Tract in Children

Medication (Trade Name) (Availability)	Mechanism of Action	Dose	Side Effects
Anticholinergic			
Oxybutynin (Ditropan) Immediate release (5 mg) Extended release (5, 10 mg) Suspension (1 mg/mL) Patch (3.9 mg)	Anticholinergic (M3, M1 receptors)	0.2 mg/kg/bid/tid	Dry mouth, constipation, headache, abdominal pain, blurred vision
Tolteridine (Detrol) Immediate release (1, 2, 4 mg) Extended release (4 mg)	Anticholinergic (M2, M3 receptors)	0.01 mg/kg/bid	Dry mouth, constipation, headache, abdominal pain,
Trospium chloride (Sanctura) (20 mg)	Anticholinergic (M2, M3 receptors)	10–25 mg/bid	Dry mouth, constipation, headache, palpitations, tachycardia
Alpha-Adrenergic Antagonists			
Phenoxybenzamine (Dibenzyline) (10 mg)	Nonselective alpha antagonist alpha-1, alpha-2 receptors	0.3–0.5 mg/kg/bid	Postural hypotension, dizziness, asthenia
Doxazosin (Cardura) (1, 2, 4, 8 mg)	Selective alpha receptor antagonist	0.5–2 mg/d	Hypotension, dizziness
Alfuzosin (Uroxatral) (10 mg)	Selective alpha-1 receptor antagonist	2.2–7.5 mg/d	Dizziness, sleepiness
Terazosin (Hytrin) (1, 2, 5, 10 mg)	Selective alpha receptor antagonist	2–5 mg/d	Postural hypotension, dizziness
Tamsulosin (Flomax) (0.4 mg)	Selective alpha-1 receptor antagonist	0.2–0.8 mg/d	Headache, somnolence, nasal congestion, nausea

Abbreviations: bid, twice a day; tid, 3 times a day, d, day.

pharmacologic actions lead to an increased dry interval between voids and an increase in voided volume. Although there are 6 anticholinergic medications on the market to treat overactive bladder, 3 are discussed regarding use in children.

Oxybutynin chloride (Ditropan) is a tertiary amine antimuscarinic medication with some selectivity for the M3 and M1 receptor subtypes and relative muscular relaxant activity. Oxybutynin is metabolized through a first pass mechanism through the liver to the active metabolite N-desethyl oxybutynin. This compound is also responsible for the numerous adverse effects of oxybutynin, including dry mouth, constipation, heat intolerance, headache, and abdominal pain. It crosses the blood-brain barrier and can lead to personality and psychological changes and blurred vision. The high incidence of side effects prohibits its use in some patients. Although this drug is available in oral tablet and liquid formulations, intravesical administration has been proven to lower detrusor pressure with fewer side effects compared with the immediate-release oral formulation. Other formulations have been developed to decrease the side effect profile of oxybutynin including a slow-release tablet, transdermal patch, and rectal suppository.

Tolterodine (Detrol) is a tertiary amine that acts as a muscarinic receptor antagonist without muscarinic receptor selectivity. It is available in an immediate- and extended-release formulation and does not cross the blood-brain barrier. Tolterodine was specifically formulated for the treatment of overactive bladder, because it exhibits functional selectivity for the muscarinic receptors in the urinary bladder over the salivary glands.

Trospium chloride (Sanctura) is a quaternary ammonium compound used for the treatment of overactive bladder. It has been available in Europe for more 20 years and was approved for use in the United States in 2004. Unlike other anticholinergic medications, it is not metabolized by the P450 system, and 60% of this drug is excreted unchanged in the urine.

The use of alpha-blockers in the management of voiding dysfunction has increased, although they are not currently approved by the US Food and Drug Administration for use in children. The rationale for the use of alpha-blockers stems from the presence of alpha-adrenergic receptors at the bladder outlet and proximal urethra. Stimulation of these receptors leads to smooth muscle contraction and increased outlet resistance. Receptor antagonism leads to smooth muscle relaxation at the bladder outlet and proximal urethra. In children with dysfunctional voiding, bladder emptying, post-void residuals, symptoms of overactive bladder, and symptoms related to DSD improved with the use of alpha-blockers. Doxazosin is the alpha-blocker that has been studied most thoroughly among children, but terazosin, alfuzosin, and tamsulosin have been used as well. Phenoxybenzamine is a nonselective agent of historical interest as the first alpha antagonist used in the treatment of patients with neuropathic bladder and voiding dysfunction. Side effects such as postural hypotension, dizziness, and asthenia limited its use in children.

Other options in the management of overactive bladder are available when pharmacologic therapy fails to improve symptoms. Botulinum toxin injection, neuromodulation, and bladder augmentation have been used in select patients. Botulinum A is a potent neurotoxin that blocks neuronal acetylcholine secretion at presynaptic nerve endings. Investigational use in children with neurogenic detrusor overactivity has yielded success in up to 86% of patients, but the results are usually only temporary. Periodic treatments are required. Neuromodulation may be performed by functional electrical stimulation or functional magnetic stimulation. Although the mechanism of action is not fully understood, the stimulation of afferent sacral nerves causes a change in the spinal reflex arc and the spino-ponto-spinal reflex arc with resultant inhibition in the efferent bladder innervation. Other potential actions include inhibition of C-fiber activity. Functional magnetic stimulation is less expensive and less invasive than functional electrical stimulation. Extracorporeal pelvic floor magnetic stimulation, transcutaneous neuromodulation, and percutaneous tibial nerve neuromodulation have been used in children to treat dysfunction of the lower urinary tract with some success. The limitation of such strategies is the requirement for long-term, continual treatments to prevent relapse. Bladder augmentation is a mainstay in the management of the end-stage neurogenic bladder, and when no less-aggressive options remain for the preservation of renal function in the child with non-neurogenic bladder overactivity, it may be considered in this class of patients as well.

Pathological Anatomy of Spinal Dysraphism

The term *spinal dysraphism* designates a large family of conditions that share some degree of developmental disturbance affecting the inferior terminus of the spinal cord, hence the clinical linkage to bladder dysfunction. Spinal dysraphism is divided traditionally into open (spina bifida aperta, Figure 19-1A) and closed (spina bifida occulta, Figure 19-1B) forms. Spina bifida aperta generally refers to myelomeningocele, which is defined by an open spinal dysraphic defect with exposed neural tissue. Myelomeningocele is also associated with hydrocephalus and with variable degrees of congenital brain and brain stem deformity (Chiari malformation type 2). Surgical closure of the dysraphic defect and often surgical cerebrospinal fluid (CSF) diversion to treat hydrocephalus are required within the first few days of life.

Myelomeningocele results from a failure of primary neurulation, the embryological process responsible for enfolding the central neuroectodermal plate into the primitive spinal cord. Up to 70% of open dysraphic defects may be prevented by periconceptional folate supplementation in women. Most patients with myelomeningocele have significant congenital neurologic

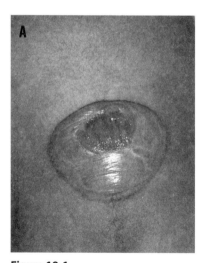
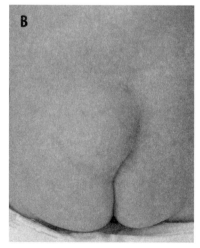

Figure 19-1.
Open and occult spina bifida. Myleomeningocele or spina bifida aperta (Figure 19-1A) features malformed spinal cord exposed by defective developmental closure of posterior vertebral elements, muscle, fascia, and skin. Lipomyelomeningocele, a type of major spina bifida occulta (Figure 19-1B), is manifest externally by only a subcutaneous lipoma covered with normal appearing skin. Notice how the gluteal fold is elongated and deflected to one side by the lipoma.

and urological deficits, including motor and sensory abnormalities, skeletal malformations of the feet and lower extremities, and neurogenic bowel and bladder dysfunction.

Spina bifida occulta refers broadly to skin-covered, and therefore hidden, dysraphic defects, which are not generally associated with hydrocephalus or other CNS anomalies. Occult dysraphic defects include lipomyelomeningocele, lipomas of the conus medullaris and filum terminale, dermal sinus tracts, and split cord malformations (SCM, also known as *diastematomyelia*), among others. The embryological mechanisms for these disorders may be mixed and remain to some degree less clearly understood than for myelomeningocele. These mechanisms include premature disjunction or failure of disjunction of the primitive spinal cord from the adjacent cutaneous ectoderm; failure of secondary neurulation, which is the embryological process responsible for the formation of the distal conus medullaris and filum terminale; and persistence of the neurenteric canal with incomplete separation of the primitive gut from the nervous system.

The conditions comprehended by the term *spina bifida occulta* exist on a spectrum of severity. The least severe abnormality is osseous spina bifida occulta which, in isolation, represents a normal variant that may be present in 8% to 20% of the general population. When simple osseous spina bifida occulta is identified incidentally, no further imaging, specialty referral, or follow-up is indicated. Next in the severity spectrum are simple deformities of the filum terminale, most commonly filum lipoma. A "fatty filum terminale" is sufficiently thickened to be visible on standard magnetic resonance imaging (MRI), and it may be associated with traction on the conus medullaris resulting in an abnormally low termination of the spinal cord within the spinal canal.

Other occult dysraphic defects are more complex. Conus medullaris lipomas involve not only the filum but also the tip of the spinal cord, itself, but they do not transgress the dura. By contrast, lipomyelomeningoceles extend from the spinal cord through dysraphic defects in the dura, ligament, bone, and fascia to connect directly to prominent deposits of subcutaneous fat. In addition to tethering the spinal cord, the intrinsic spinal cord portion of these lesions may produce mass effect on adjacent functional neural tissue.

Dermal sinus tracts may occur anywhere along the spine, but are most common in the lumbar region and at the lumbosacral junction. These epithelial lined pits and tracts typically extend via dysraphic defects all the way to the dorsal surface of the conus medullaris and may occasionally invade the substance of the spinal cord itself. They represent a breach in the normal epithelial barrier between the inside of the body and the outside, and CNS infection is a threat.

Diastematomyelia, by contrast, is characterized by a split or duplicated spinal cord. The split cord may be housed in separate dural sheaths separated by an osseous or cartilaginous spur extending from the vertebral body to the lamina (Type I SCM) or in a single dural sheath (Type II SCM). Concurrent terminal spinal cord tethering, often by a filum lipoma, is common.

Other rare forms of dysraphism include terminal myelocystocele, which consists of concentric, cystic CSF collections arising from the subarachnoid space and the central canal of the spinal cord, together with a fatty lesion tethering the distal spinal cord. Terminal myelocystocele is strongly associated with the OEIS syndrome, but may also occur independently. Other lipomatous spinal cord and filum lesions are also more common in patients with imperforate anus or congenital cloacal malformations.

Epidemiology

The incidence of myelomeningocele in the United States is approximately 0.05% of live births, representing a significant decrease in recent decades. This decrease is likely due to the adoption of periconceptional folic acid supplementation and improved maternal nutrition, as well as prenatal diagnosis and selective pregnancy termination in cases of major congenital anomaly. Myelomeningocele is more common in certain areas of the world, such as Ireland, and in first generation (but not subsequent) immigrants from such countries. The mechanisms of such variations in incidence are obscure.

The incidences of spina bifida occulta and of each of the individual entities covered by this umbrella designation are more difficult to determine. First, these lesions are by definition hidden, and therefore not all existing cases are diagnosed. Secondly, the diagnostic boundaries of some entities are controversial. For example, normal filum terminale anatomy may feature no more than "a streak" of fatty tissue, thickness less than 2 mm, and location of the conus-filum junction above the mid-L2 vertebral level in school-aged children. The first of these criteria, however, is subjective and the latter 2 are probably better represented by a normal distribution of anatomy in healthy individuals than a particular fixed cut-off point. Thus, without a clear definition of pathological anatomy, the incidence of the clinically most common form of occult dysraphism, fatty filum, is difficult to define.

Spinal Cord Tethering

Historically, untreated myelomeningocele resulted in death due to sepsis, renal failure, or other overwhelming complications early in life; however, many children with occult spinal dysraphism are neurologically and urologically normal at birth. What then is the imperative to diagnose occult dysraphic disorders early in life? Spina bifida occulta may cause neurologic complications and disabilities by 4 mechanisms, 3 of them progressive.

- First, major forms of dysraphism, lipomyelomeningocele in particular, may result in congenital functional lesions due to spinal cord maldevelopment.
- Mass effect from lipomatous tissue may also cause progressive injury to functional neural tissue over time.
- Dysraphic malformations share a strong tendency to tether the spinal cord to the spinal column and paraspinal structures, resulting in pathological traction on the neural elements. Experimental models suggest that traction on the spinal cord results in microvascular ischemia and impaired function. Surgical treatment of occult spinal dysraphism is predicated on the hypothesis that surgical separation of the spinal cord from structures to which it is not normally attached prevents or arrests progressive neurologic dysfunction from such traction.
- Finally, dermal sinus tracts may serve as conduits for the introduction of bacteria into the CNS, leading to meningitis or intraspinal suppuration.

Detecting Occult Spinal Dysraphism

History and Physical Examination
Tethered spinal cord is a clinical as well as an anatomical diagnosis. In addition to dysfunctional voiding, tethered cord syndrome consists of neurologic dysfunction, skeletal and gait abnormalities, and pain. The presence of

underlying spinal dysraphism may also be detected by the presence of typical cutaneous stigmata.

Neurologic abnormalities associated with tethered spinal cord include sensory loss, paresthesia, motor weakness and muscle wasting, and reflex abnormalities (both hyper- and hyporeflexia). Gait may be abnormal—toe walking is a common but very nonspecific sign. Asymmetrical neurological deficits are often manifest in gait asymmetry. Axial and radiating pain may be presenting complaints. Chronic muscle imbalance may result in musculoskeletal deformities: scoliosis, extremity asymmetry, pes cavus, etc. In severe cases, tethered cord syndrome may be associated with non-healing cutaneous ulcers in the legs and feet. The symptoms and signs of tethered spinal cord syndrome are typically limited to the lower extremities, but may also affect the trunk and arms in rarer cases of cervical or thoracic dysraphism.

There are a number of cutaneous stigmata of spinal dysraphism. The most common of these, dimples and vascular nevi, result in frequent referral for imaging or for pediatric neurosurgery consultation. However, there is some controversy about the exact implications of these clinical findings.

The common wisdom is that spinal dimples over the midline are benign if they occur within the gluteal fold; however, dimples near the top of the fold seem occasionally to be associated with abnormalities of the filum. Although evidentiary guidelines are lacking, dimples over the very tip of the coccyx itself seem to be uniformly benign. Fortunately, coccygeal dimples probably account for most incidentally noted spinal dimples. True coccygeal dimples in isolation do not indicate MRI or neurosurgical consultation.

Coccygeal dimples must be distinguished from the skin lesions associated with dermal sinus tracts. These lesions are often described as dimples or "pits" as well. They are located generally over the lumbar spine or at the lumbosacral junction. They may have small, coarse, or dysplastic hairs emanating from them (Figure 19-2). They may overlie a palpable dermoid cyst, and dermoid material, pus, or CSF may be expressible from them. The critical factor is location. Any dimple, pit, crease, or other topographic perturbation lying superior to the normal termination of the gluteal fold deserves spinal imaging and neurosurgical consultation. Any lesion draining pus or CSF deserves urgent consultation.

Vascular skin lesions over the spine are sometimes associated with dysraphism as well, but some lesions have more significance than others. Juvenile cutaneous hemangiomas are raised, bosselated, red to purple lesions that tend to involute in the latter part of infancy. They can occur at any site, and on a random basis they occur occasionally over the spine. They have no association with spinal dysraphism and are not indications for imaging. Flat vascular lesions, so-called strawberry nevi or stork bites, tend to be present at birth on the eyelids, at the glabella, over the nape of the neck, and in the midline of the lumbosacral region (Figure 19-3), and they tend to fade with age. The significance of the lumbosacral vascular nevus is uncertain. Recent reports have suggested that spinal

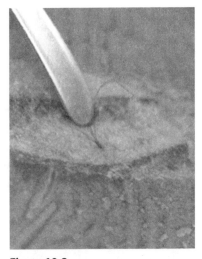

Figure 19-2.
A dissecting instrument points at a small bundle of long, thick, black hairs emerging from a cutaneous pit, which is the external orifice of a dermal sinus tract.

ultrasound evaluation of the newborn with a lumbosacral vascular nevus has a negligible yield, while MRI of similar skin lesions among school-aged children discloses spinal dysraphism is as many as 15% of cases. The discrepancy between these observations may be resolved by the hypothesis that stork bites fade while the vascular nevi associated with dysraphism persist into later childhood. In the absence of a valid rule for selection of patients for imaging, a low threshold for pediatric neurosurgical consultation is appropriate.

Other dysraphic markers, although less common, are more reliable indicators of underlying pathology. For example, discrete, dense patches of hair over the midline spine are highly associated with SCM (Figure 19-4). Midline subcutaneous lipomas (Figure 19-1B) and the exotic caudal appendage (or "tail," Figure 19-5) are highly suggestive of the presence of lipomyelomeningocele. Some markings may be seen in various conditions. Discrete round patches of atretic, waxy skin (sometimes referred to as *cigarette burns*) may be seen, with or without a ring of small dysplastic hairs, associated with SCMs or dermal sinus tracts. Multiple dysraphic markers in the same child are highly suggestive of an underlying dysraphic defect.

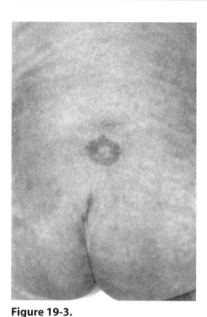

Figure 19-3.
A ring-shaped, flat, vascular nevus near the midline of the lumbar region signifies underling spinal dysraphism. In this case, a fibrovascular tract passed from the deep aspect of the dimple in the center of the ring (not visible at this magnification) through the subcutaneous adipose layer and through bifid posterior vertebral elements to penetrate the dura and to attach to the dorsal surface of the spinal cord.

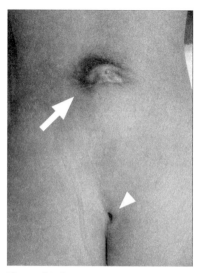

Figure 19-4.
This child with split cord malformation (SCM) exhibits a thick, sharply demarcated patch of black hair surrounding a dysplastic skin lesion (white arrow). SCM is often associated with a short, thick, lipomatous filum, which may, in this case, correlate with the deep, broad, cutaneous divot (white arrowhead) just above and to the right of the gluteal fold.

Of course, the presence of such markers in a child with neurologic or urological dysfunction, orthopedic deformity, gait abnormality, pain, or the presence of a coexisting cloacal malformation is highly suggestive of underlying dysraphism. Recognition of these patterns allows for appropriate detection and management of underlying dysraphic defects, imaging, and specialty referral.

Imaging

Radiographs of the spine may detect spinal dysraphism indirectly by disclosing associated osseous abnormalities: congenital intersegmental fusions, hemivertebrae, butterfly vertebrae, and defects of the posterior elements.

Ultrasound is often used to evaluate the spinal anatomy of infants. Ultrasound does not require sedation, and it entails no radiation exposure. Contemporary ultrasound units generate dynamic imaging sequences that allow analysis of spinal cord movement with respiratory and arterial pulsations, which can give indirect clues to the presence of spinal cord tethering. The quality of ultrasound images of the spine deteriorates rapidly beyond 3 months of age, but in the youngest infants spinal ultrasound yields anatomical detail comparable to—and sometimes complementary to—what can be obtained in this age group by MRI.

The imaging modality of choice for assessment of spinal dysraphism is MRI. An important datum easily determined from sagittal images

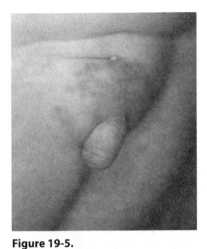

Figure 19-5.
A caudal appendage or "tail" emerges from the surface of a subcutaneous lipoma just to the left of the lumbosacral junction. Such appendages are not continuous with the end of the spinal column, and they do not contain any osseous or cartilaginous elements, so they are not real tails in any anatomical or developmental sense. Note the vascular nevus on the skin overlying the lipoma. This elaborate lesion overlies a lipomyelomeningocele.

is the level of termination of the spinal cord: In children older than 1 year, termination of the cord below the L2–L3 interspace is abnormal and is suggestive of dysraphism. Deposits of fat are particularly well seen on T1-weighted images. In autopsy studies the normal filum may contain some adipose tissue, but in only 5% of cases is it greater than 2 mm in thickness, which is roughly the threshold for detection of lipomatous infiltration of the filum on axial MRI. The significance of abnormalities of the filum will be discussed in greater detail below. T2-weighted images display intramedullary lesions, such as syringomyelia, to advantage. For evaluation of suspected lumbosacral dysraphism, imaging of the thoracic and lumbosacral spine is sufficient. In the exceptional instance of cervical dysraphism, the entire spine must be imaged. Brain imaging is not indicated in the assessment of occult spinal dysraphism.

Natural History and Efficacy of Surgical Intervention

Observational studies suggest that younger patients with major spinal dysraphism—that is, lipomyelomeningocele or SCM—tend to present for neurosurgical evaluation with relatively intact neurologic and urological function, while older children present with deficits. Although sudden major deterioration is rare, long-standing, static deficits are less likely to improve after surgery than recently apparent deficits. By contrast, 40% to 60% of patients with progressive deficits improve to some degree after surgery, while few, generally less than 5%, deteriorate due to complications of surgery. Urinary continence is more likely in children operated on for major dysraphism before 1 year of age (80% vs 50%). Up to 85% of patients with major dysraphism suffer functional deterioration by late childhood or adolescence. Together, these observations suggest that surgical correction of spinal cord tethering, at least for major forms of dysraphism, probably benefits both neurologic and urological function. Unfortunately, there is a significant rate of recurrent tethering in such patients due to postoperative scar formation, perhaps as high as 20% over the course of childhood.

The natural history of the minor forms of dysraphism, such as filum lipoma, is not clearly defined. Furthermore, as the prevalence of abnormal filum terminale is unknown, studies to answer questions about its natural history are inherently difficult to perform.

Minimal Tethered Cord Syndrome

Surgical correction of spinal cord tethering for major dysraphic spinal anomalies is accepted practice in North America despite limited availability of prospective evidence regarding the natural history and surgical treatment results. Making evidence-based treatment recommendations for children with minor forms of dysraphism is an even more daunting challenge.

Three clinical scenarios illustrate these difficulties.

1) A child with confirmed neurogenic voiding dysfunction, stiff gait, and back pain, but a normal neurologic examination is found on MRI to have a thickened or lipomatous filum, but the conus medullaris terminates at a normal level of the spine.

2) A child with no symptoms or signs of spinal cord tethering is imaged for unrelated reasons and is found to have minor dysraphic abnormalities, typically a filum lipoma.

3) A child with confirmed neurogenic voiding dysfunction, stiff gait, and back pain, but a normal neurologic examination has normal MRI of the spine, including a normal level of conus termination and a normal filum terminale. This entity has been referred to as *minimal tethered cord syndrome.*

In the first scenario of the symptomatic patient with a normal level conus but an abnormal filum, many North American pediatric neurosurgeons favor correction of spinal cord tethering by cutting of the filum terminale. Prospective evidence in favor of this practice is limited.

In the second scenario of the asymptomatic patient with an incidental filum lipoma, practice is variable. Some surgeons recommend cutting the filum if the associated lipoma is thick. Some surgeons intervene only if the conus is low, and some surgeons do not intervene at all. The relevant considerations seem to be that a small but unknown fraction of children with incidental filum lipomata become symptomatic later in childhood, that neurologic symptoms and signs may not be reversible by treatment once they have become established, and that complications of cutting the filum, including recurrent tethering, are very infrequent. The lack of a quantitative understanding of the natural history of filum lipoma hobbles rational deliberation about its management.

The third scenario, minimal tethered cord syndrome, is the most controversial and may also now account for the majority of surgical procedures to cut the filum among children in North America. At some centers, children with voiding dysfunction refractory to a year or more of medical and behavioral management are subjected to cutting of the filum in the absence of any structural abnormality on detailed MRI of the spine. What constitutes an adequate urological evaluation for the child with suspected minimal tethered cord syndrome varies greatly from center to center and probably bears an inverse relationship to surgical volume. The most judicious practice is to limit surgical intervention for minimal tethered cord syndrome to children with characteristic neurogenic findings on formal urodynamic testing performed and interpreted by a pediatric urologist experienced in the care of children with spinal dysraphism. The clinical data supporting even this conservative approach are nevertheless retrospective, uncontrolled, and collected by surgeons themselves without the benefit of validated outcome measures. A Canadian prospective trial employing rigorous criteria for diagnosis and outcome assessment and randomizing patients to best medical and behavioral management—without or with cutting of the filum—is slowly accruing subjects at the time of this writing.

Conclusion

Voiding dysfunction is a common disorder in children with multiple, sometimes interacting, causes. Both primary care physicians and specialists must consider behavioral, physiological, anatomical, and neurologic etiologies. Coexistence of neurologic complaints and/or cutaneous stigmata of dysraphism should increase suspicion of neurogenic voiding dysfunction. Pediatric urological management and evaluation of voiding dysfunction is necessary in complex and medically refractory cases. Pediatric neurosurgical evaluation with MRI of the spinal cord is required in cases of suspected dysraphism and tethered cord.

With appropriate intervention, the prognosis for children with voiding dysfunction is good. Some of the greatest current challenges in this area of patient care are posed by inadequate evidence regarding both diagnostic boundaries for neurogenic voiding dysfunction and the efficacy of surgical treatment for minor forms of spinal dysraphism.

Bibliography

Bladder Dysfunction

Allen TD, Bright TC III. Urodynamic patterns in children with dysfunctional voiding problems. *J Urol.* 1978;119:247–249

Austin PF, Homsy YL, Masel JL, Cain MP, Casale AJ, Rink RC. Alpha-adrenergic blockade in children with neuropathic and nonneuropathic voiding dysfunction. *J Urol.* 1999;162: 1064–1067

Chapple CR. Muscarinic receptor antagonists in the treatment of overactive bladder. *Urology.* 2000;55:33–46

Combs AJ, Glassberg AD, Gerdes D, Horowitz M. Biofeedback therapy for children with dysfunctional voiding. *Urology.* 1998;52:312–315

Greenfield SP, Fera M. The use of intravesical oxybutynin chloride in children with neurogenic bladder. *J Urol.* 1991;146:532–534

Herndon CD, Decambre M, McKenna PH. Interactive computer games for treatment of pelvic floor dysfunction. *J Urol.* 2001;166:1893–1898

Hinman F Jr. Nonneurogenic neurogenic bladder (the Hinman syndrome)—15 years later. *J Urol.* 1986;136:769-777

Hinman F, Baumann FW. Vesical and ureteral damage from voiding dysfunction in boys without neurologic or obstructive disease. *J Urol.* 1973;109:727–732

Koff SA. Estimating bladder capacity in children. *Urology.* 1983;21:248

Lopez Pereira P, Miguelez C, Caffarati J, Estornell F, Anguera A. Trospium chloride for the treatment of detrusor instability in children. *J Urol.* 2003;170:1978–1981

MacKeith R. Micturition induced by giggling. *Guys Hosp Rep.* 1964;113:250–260

Maizels M, King LR, Firlit CF. Urodynamic biofeedback: a new approach to treat vesical sphincter dyssynergia. *J Urol.* 1979;122:205–209

Massad CA, Kogan BA, Trigo-Rocha FE. The pharmacokinetics of intravesical and oral oxybutynin chloride. *J Urol.* 1992;148:595–597

Riccabona M, Koen M, Schindler M, et al. Botulinum-A toxin injection into the detrusor: a safe alternative in the treatment of children with myelomeningocele with detrusor hyperreflexia. *J Urol.* 2004;171:845–848

Williams DI. Giggle incontinence. *Acta Urol Belg.* 1984;52:151–153

Yoshimura N, Chancellor MB. Current and future pharmacological treatment for overactive bladder. *J Urol.* 2002;168:1897–1913

Spinal Dysraphism

Ackerman LL, Menezes AH. Spinal congenital dermal sinuses: a 30-year experience. *Pediatrics.* 2003;112:641–647

Allen RM, Sandquist MA, Piatt JH Jr, Selden NRW. Ultrasonographic screening in infants with isolated spinal strawberry nevi. *J Neurosurg.* 2003;98:247–250

Ben-Amitai D, Davidson S, Schwartz M, et al. Sacral nevus flammeus simplex: the role of imaging. *Pediatr Dermatol.* 2000;17:469–471

Bowman RM, McLone DG, Grant JA, Tomita T, Ito JA. Spina bifida outcome: a 25-year prospective. *Pediatr Neurosurg.* 2001;34:114–120

Bui CJ, Tubbs RS, Oakes WJ. Tethered cord syndrome in children: a review. *Neurosurg Focus.* 2007;23:1–9

Cabaret AS, Loget P, Loeuillet L, Odent S, Poulain P. Embryology of neural tube defects: information provided by associated malformations. *Prenat Diagn.* 2007;27:738–742

Cochrane DD. Cord untethering for lipomyelomeningocele: expectation after surgery. *Neurosurg Focus.* 2007;23:1–7

Finn MA, Walker ML. Spinal lipomas: clinical spectrum, embryology, and treatment. *Neurosurg Focus.* 2007;23:1–12

Gibson PJ, Britton J, Hall DM, Hill CR. Lumbosacral skin markers and identification of occult spinal dysraphism in neonates. *Acta Paediatr.* 1995;84:208–209

Guggisberg D, Hadj-Rabia S, Viney C, et al. Skin markers of occult spinal dysraphism in children: a review of 54 cases. *Arch Dermatol.* 2004;140:1109–1115

Herman JM, McLone DG, Storrs BB, Dauser RC. Analysis of 153 patients with myelomeningocele or spinal lipoma reoperated upon for a tethered cord. Presentation, management and outcome. *Pediatr Neurosurg.* 1993;19:243–249

Joo JG, Beke A, Papp Z, Csaba A, Rab A, Papp C. Risk of recurrence in major central nervous system malformations between 1976 and 2005. *Prenat Diagn.* 2007;27:1028–1032

Kanev PM, Park TS. Dermoids and dermal sinus tracts of the spine. *Neurosurg Clin North Am.* 1995;6:359–366

Liptak GS. Tethered spinal cord: update of an analysis of published articles. *Eur J Pediatr Surg.* 1995;5 (suppl) 1:21–23

McGuire EJ, Woodside JR, Borden TA, Weiss RM. Prognostic value of urodynamic testing in myelodysplastic patients. *J Urol.* 1981;126:205–209

McLone DG, La Marca F. The tethered spinal cord: diagnosis, significance, and management. *Semin Pediatr Neurol.* 1997;4:192–208

Pang D, Dias, MS, Ahab-Barmada M. Split cord malformation: part I: a unified theory of embryogenesis for double spinal cord malformations. *Neurosurgery.* 1992;31:451–480

Shaer CM, Chescheir N, Schulkin J. Myelomeningocele: a review of the epidemiology, genetics, risk factors for conception, prenatal diagnosis, and prognosis for affected individuals. *Obstet Gynecol Surv.* 2007;62:471–479

Tubbs RS, Wellons JC III, Iskandar BJ, Oakes WJ. Isolated flat capillary midline lumbosacral hemangiomas as indicators of occult spinal dysraphism. *J Neurosurg.* 2004;100:86–89

Yamada S, Won DJ, Pezeshkpour G, et al. Pathophysiology of tethered cord syndrome and similar complex disorders. *Neurosurg Focus.* 2007;23:1–10

Minimal Tethered Cord Syndrome

Drake J. Occult tethered cord syndrome: not an indication for surgery. *J Neurosurg.* 2006;104:305–308

Kesler H, Dias MS, Kalapos P. Termination of the normal conus medullaris in children: a whole-spine magnetic resonance imaging study. *Neurosurg Focus.* 2007;23:1–5

Selden NR, Nixon RR, Skoog SR, Lashley DB. Minimal tethered cord syndrome associated with thickening of the terminal filum. *J Neurosurg.* 2006;105:214–218

Selden NR. Minimal tethered cord syndrome: what's necessary to justify a new surgical indication? *Neurosurg Focus.* 2007;23:1–5

Selden NR. Occult tethered cord syndrome: the case for surgery. *J Neurosurg.* 2006;104:302–304

Steinbok P, Garton HJL, Gupta N. Occult tethered cord syndrome: a survey of practice patterns. *J Neurosurg.* 2006;104:309–313

Steinbok P, Kariyattil R, MacNeily AE. Comparison of section of filum terminale and non-neurosurgical management for urinary incontinence in patients with normal conus position and possible occult tethered cord syndrome. *Neurosurgery.* 2007;61:550–555

Steinbok P, MacNeily AE. Section of the terminal filum for occult tethered cord syndrome: toward a scientific answer. *Neurosurg Focus.* 2007;23:1–4

Warder DE, Oakes WJ. Tethered cord syndrome and the conus in a normal position. *Neurosurgery.* 1993;33:374–378

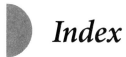

Index

DNA, *continued*
   mitochondrial disorders and, 93, 94,
      95–96
   myotonic dystrophy diagnosis, 386
   spinal muscular atrophy diagnosis, 370
   tissue biopsies and, 82
Dorsal rhizotomy, 69
Down syndrome
   congenital heart disease and, 192
   obstructive sleep apnea syndrome and, 420
Drop attacks, 297
Drugs. *See also* Antiepileptic drugs; *specific drug*
   accidental ingestion or abuse of, 123
   drug-induced tremor, 330, 331
Duchenne muscular dystrophy, 380
Dural laceration, 158
Dural venous thrombosis, 194
Dyschondrodysplasia, 247
Dyskinesias, 337–339
Dysplasia, of renal or carotid arteries, 220
Dystonia musculorum deformans, 336
Dystonias, 336–338
Dystrophinopathies, 380–383

E

Ehlers-Danlos syndrome, 180, 192
Electrical status epilepticus, 418
Electroencephalography
   encephalopathy and, 134
   for febrile seizures (deferred), 260
   for global developmental delay, 36
   headache evaluation and, 312
   in seizure diagnosis, 280–281
Embolism, 206
Emotional problems, Sturge-Weber syndrome and, 235
Encephalocutaneous lipomatosis, 247
Encephalomalacia, 22
Encephalopathy (acute), 119–142. *See also* Chronic static encephalopathies
   algorithm for management of children with, 133
   definitions, 120
   differential diagnosis, 134–139
      akinetic mutism, 138
      brain death, 138–139
      locked-in syndrome, 137–138
      minimally conscious state, 136–137
      vegetative state, 135–136

etiology, 120, 121
evaluation, 122–134
   blood pressure, 125–126
   breathing, 126
   diagnosis, 132
   electroencephalography, 134
   general examination, 126–127
   heart rate, 125
   history, 122–124
   laboratory evaluation, 132
   lumbar puncture, 134
   neuroimaging studies, 132–133
   neurologic examination, 127–131
   temperature, 124
Glasgow Coma Scale for Children, 128
pathophysiology, 120–122
prognosis, 140–142
treatment, 139–142
   of complications, 140
   etiological, 140
   vital support, 139–140
Endoscopic third ventriculostomy, 467–468
Endothelial cell-specific HIF activation, 233
Endovascular occlusion, 185
Endovascular stenting, 208
Energy metabolism disorders. *See* Mitochondrial disorders
Enzyme defects. *See* Inborn errors of metabolism (IEMs)
Enzyme replacement therapy, 105–106
Ependymomas, 432, 442
Ephedrine, 391
Epidermal nevus syndrome, 247
Epidural hematoma, 22, 24
Epidural hemorrhage, 159
Epigenetics, 41
Epilepsy, 267–298
   autism and, 49
   benign epilepsy of childhood with occipital spikes, 276
   benign rolandic epilepsy with centro-temporal spikes, 274, 275, 276
   childhood absence epilepsy, 272–273
   classification of, 267–268, 269, 270
   defined, 267
   diagnostic workup
      blood chemistries, 280
      electroencephalogram, 280–281
      lumbar puncture, 281
      neuroimaging studies, 281